CONTENTS

Acknowledgments ix

Introduction 1
The Ranch Kitchen Restaurant and Bakery ♦ Fruit Juice Concentrates ♦ My Own Story ♦ What's Wrong With Sugar?

1. The Fine Art of Baking 9
Love ♦ Technique ♦ Temperature ♦ Recipe ♦ Organization Tips ♦ Ingredients ♦ Recommended Equipment

2. Breads, Muffins, and Biscuits 25
Yeasted. . . ♦ . . . and Not: Quick Breads and Muffins

3. Cookies 62

4. Pies, Tarts, and Pastries 76
Pies and Tarts ♦ European Fruit Tarts and Tartlets ♦ Puff Pastry ♦ Cream Puff Pastry

5. Specialty Cakes for Every Occasion 132
The Basic Cakes . . . ♦ . . . Made into Masterpieces

6. Fillings, Frostings, Sauces, Glazes, and Garnishes 173

Index 195

Acknowledgments

I give my personal gratitude and acknowledgment to each of The Ranch Kitchen bakers, who have given of themselves with graciousness, dedication, and skill over the past ten years—without whom there would not be a Ranch Kitchen bakery or even this beautiful book in your hands;

to all of my teachers, beginning with my mother, who taught me to bake everything with joy—from my first snickerdoodle cookies to my first batch of puff pastry to today's three pumpkin pies and tomorrow's ten loaves of French bread;

and to my dear family, friends, and supporters, whose love and encouragement and willingness to be nutritional consultants, legal advisors, editors, typists, illustrators, photographers, stylists, tasters, peelers, hullers, kneaders, and choppers never flagged—and never ceased to touch my heart.

INTRODUCTION

THE RANCH KITCHEN RESTAURANT AND BAKERY

Just north of Yellowstone National Park on Montana's breathtaking Route 89 in the Paradise Valley is The Ranch Kitchen, a log-cabin-style restaurant offering the best of Montana home cooking.

The Ranch Kitchen is in Corwin Springs, just eight miles north of Gardiner, Montana, which is the northern entrance to Yellowstone Park. Actually, along with the Cinnabar General Store next door, The Ranch Kitchen *is* Corwin Springs. Built as a dude ranch lodge in the twenties and expanded to include a large dance hall during the thirties, the original building has been remodeled into a cozy country restaurant housing a professional dinner theater.

Since it became The Ranch Kitchen in the summer of 1982, its all-American breakfasts, hearty lunches, home-style dinners, and elaborate theater buffets have made the restaurant a favorite of local residents and park visitors.

The Ranch Kitchen's breads, muffins, and desserts have become a trademark of the restaurant. Many of the recipes developed that first summer have been grand-prize and blue-ribbon winners at the local county and state fairs. We still use those recipes today, along with many new ones, and have since switched to fruit sweeteners for all of our baked goods. No meal at The Ranch Kitchen is complete without something from the bakery.

Each of the recipes presented in this book has been developed and served at The Ranch Kitchen. Guests are always asking if, how, and when they can have the recipe for everything from the Very-Berry Syrup on their pancakes to the Apple Butter on their toast, to the French Bread with their spaghetti, to the Carrot Cake or Pumpkin Pie they had for dessert. People always want to know how we do it—how we get our desserts to taste and look so delicious without using refined white sugar.

Part of the answer stems from the standard of excellence held by everyone at the restaurant. Our goal is to offer the best—and to show that healthier food doesn't have to be heavy. We are always working to produce better, lighter, and tastier pastries, sweets, and breads, while lowering the content of sugar, fat, and cholesterol.

Through the years, as our techniques in the bakery improved and our palates were refined, our offerings evolved. As we studied more about healthier food and nutrition, we adapted our recipes accordingly. The first year we used a lot of white and brown sugars and dabbled with honey. Year two found us switching to fructose. Year three was our love affair with maple sugar and maple syrup. In year five we began experimenting with natural fruit sweeteners, and by year six we had found the mixed fruit sweetener we still prefer today.

We've also experimented with different flours—substituting brown rice flour and whole wheat pastry flour for unbleached white flour and using rolled oats and finely ground nuts where possible. We've also lowered the cholesterol in many items by eliminating eggs and dairy products and replacing them with oil, almond or soy milks, or unsweetened applesauce.

Working with alternative sweeteners and whole grains always puts one's skills to the test. Here I share with you the techniques and tips I've developed over the years, so that you can make your own quality baked goods at home.

Fruit Juice Concentrates

Natural fruit juice concentrates are an excellent alternative to refined white sugar in baked goods as they give excellent flavor and texture. They contain many micronutrients, the vitamins and minerals that are necessary for their assimilation and our metabolism. And their flavor is so rich and sweet that it is possible to reduce the total amount of sweetener by at least 50 percent in any recipe that uses them.

Fruit juice concentrates are fruit juices evaporated in a high vacuum using low temperatures (the mixtures boil at 110° F) until they reach a thicker consistency. Fruit concentrates come in a number of flavors and are readily available in the refrigerator section of most natural food stores in pints, quarts, or gallons.

If you can't find a commercially made fruit sweetener, you can substitute frozen fruit juice concentrates, such as unsweetened apple and orange juice, which are available in almost every grocery store, but you will have to cook them down to concentrate them. See page 16 for more information on purchasing and using these concentrates.

Here's my general rule for adapting a recipe that calls for sugar: Simply reduce the amount of sugar by half and replace that amount with a concentrated fruit sweetener. You will then have to adjust only your techniques and not the liquid or dry ingredients. If there is a slightly acidic aftertaste in the finished product, it is from too much sweetener and you can reduce it even more next time.

Another substitution we have made for refined white sugar is Coconut Powder (page 194) to replace powdered sugar. Once the coconut is finely powdered, it is mixed with a little dry milk powder and sifted over pastries to resemble the delicate look of powdered sugar. We also use raisin water (the liquid remaining from plumping raisins) and fruit-sweetened jams as other replacements for white sugar.

My Own Story

For myself, as I eat fewer sweet treats and a more balanced grain and vegetable diet, I can cut back the quantity of sweetener even more. I've discovered a whole range of new tastes as my taste buds begin to savor all flavors again, not just sweet.

Fruit sweeteners provide an excellent transition for those seeking to replace refined white sugar with whole foods. Since they can be used in smaller amounts than sugar with comparable results, they help you moderate your intake of sweets. For many people, fruit sweeteners do not produce the pronounced side effects often associated with excess sugar consumption—wide mood swings, uncontrolled emotions, crying spells, increased sleep requirements, headaches, out-of-control food binges, fidgeting, lack of appetite, and irritability.

I have had all of these symptoms myself. And because I had no idea of their cause, I thought I was going crazy.

In 1973, while working as the pastry chef at one of northern California's finest restaurants, I felt an incredible amount of mental, emotional, and physical stress. I thought I could no longer cope with life. I was concerned, but since I didn't know that there might be a physical cause for my problems, I chose to deal with the mental and emotional symptoms by spending the summer at a healing retreat on a small island in British Columbia. That it was an almost sugar-free summer was a bonus of which I took little notice. Our hosts served delicious vegetarian meals using the vegetables from their large organic garden. By the end of the summer, I had lost weight, grown tan and healthy, and was ready to deal with the world again.

Over the next few years, the symptoms returned. During those years, as I was not specializing exclusively in sweets, but cooking entrees also, the symptoms were not as severe. However, I would notice my head start to swim and my eyes begin to twitch on those mornings when I chose to sample a dessert left over from the evening before instead of eating a good breakfast.

In 1978, while living in a small town on the northern California coast, I heard a lecture on sugar, nicotine, alcohol, and drugs. I was overwhelmed and excited by what I heard, for I had never before realized the extent of sugar's effects. Here was the key to all that I had experienced during the previous six to seven years.

Changes were definitely in order. I did not work with sugar again until 1982, when I moved to Montana and began working as the pastry chef in The Ranch Kitchen restaurant. Since I then had a better understanding of what was wrong with sugar, I was able to begin to stop some of the excessive nibbling. However, just working with sugar eight hours a day (where it came in through the pores of my skin, and I breathed it in through my mouth and nose) was more than enough.

In 1985, wanting to improve my skills, I worked in a fine French hotel for almost a year under a very talented French pastry chef. It was a renewed struggle not to eat everything in sight! Everything was absolutely delicious and in such large quantities—60 quarts of magnificently light and fluffy cake batter and cheesecake and lemon mousse and 20 quarts of raspberry buttercream!

I often found it impossible to resist such overwhelming temptation. Even though I had a strong constitution, I became quite vulnerable to sugar, since products made with sugar had become the greater part of my diet. Many of the symptoms were returning, along with new ones, such as extreme sleepiness—I couldn't even drive the 45 minutes home without pulling off the freeway onto a side street to take a nap. My doctor was very concerned and had me take all the recommended supplements for hypoglycemia—large doses of vitamins B and C, chromium, calcium, magnesium, and protein—to try to stabilize and regulate my blood sugar levels.

Besides taking the supplements, I prayed a lot for strength to resist this addiction to sugar. Even though I knew the effects of sugar and knew what it was doing to me, I was unable to control my eating. I was addicted to sugar, plain and simple.

That winter, I attended another lecture on sugar and its connection with hypoglycemia. I knew it was an accurate lecture because I was experiencing almost every symptom.

It was after this lecture that The Ranch Kitchen bakery began working with fruit juice concentrates. When the mixed fruit concentrate was found, we knew we had discovered a realistic alternative. Its flavor was delicious, and we needed to use only half as much fruit concentrate as sugar to get comparable results. Best of all, its effects on the body and emotions were not as extreme.

Fruit concentrates are not the final answer to health. Moderation in your intake of sweets along with a well-balanced diet is the key. You should eat sweets only occasionally and make whole grains, legumes, and vegetables the focus of your diet, with fish or meat as needed. But for those special occasions when you want a sweet treat, you now have a delicious alternative. Isn't it nice to know that you can offer something beautiful and delicious to your friends and family without having to worry about the destructive effects of sugar?

What's Wrong with Sugar?

Over the past 25 to 30 years, more and more nutritionists, health care professionals, and people in all walks of life are finding out that, yes, indeed, there is a problem with sugar—refined white sugar, sucrose, with the chemical formula $C_{12}H_{22}O_{11}$.

Typical of the concern about the consumption of refined white sugar are the comments from the Center for Science in the Public Interest, a well-respected health advocacy organization in Washington, D.C. They have concluded, through their study of the available research, that sugar is not safe at all. They believe that there is substantial evidence that sugar contributes to tooth decay, obesity, and nutrient deficiencies, and may cause hypoglycemia and hyperactivity in children and in sensitive people. They also believe that it contributes to heart disease and diabetes. The Center adds that everybody has a different body chemistry and that sugar affects us all in different ways.

However, according to the United States Department of Agriculture's Dietary Guidelines, all Americans are advised to consume sugar only in moderation and to replace high-sugar foods with fruits, vegetables, whole grains, legumes, and other foods rich in complex carbohydrates. The guidelines also state that because sugars provide calories but few other nutrients, diets with large amounts of sugar should be avoided, especially by people with lower calorie needs.

It is very possible to eat too many calories and still not get enough nutrients. The main complaint that nutritionists have about sugar is that it gives the body empty, or naked, calories. Sugar is not only nothing, it is worse than nothing. In the refining process, sugar is stripped of all of its nutrients—vitamins, minerals, trace elements, enzymes, fatty acids, and amino acids. Yet our bodies have to use minerals to metabolize it. Thus sugar robs our bodies of essential elements, leaving us with nutritional deficiencies when we eat too much.

In order to digest refined sugar, the body must mobilize its stored vitamins and minerals, such as sodium, potassium, chromium, magnesium, and calcium, to deal with the rapid absorption of sugar into the bloodstream. If you eat sugar every day, your body must provide more and more minerals for digestion and assimilation, and then it must attempt to return your blood sugar level to normal.

When we eat white sugar, the rate at which it is absorbed into the blood as glucose is much too rapid. This rapid absorption causes the glucose level in the blood to increase drastically.

The pancreas can then overreact by rushing to produce enough insulin to allow the glucose to be absorbed by the individual body cells. This greatly reduces the blood glucose level and can even cause it to drop to a point lower than before the sugar was eaten. When this drop occurs, the adrenal glands have to work overtime to once again normalize the blood sugar level.

Now, of course, you may be among those people for whom sugar has no noticeable effects. But it is still wearing down your pancreas, your adrenals, and all of your organs.

Fruit sweeteners, on the other hand, still contain many vitamins, minerals, and even protein, along with their calories and sweetness. Fruit sweeteners are composed of monosaccharides in the form of fructose, which many health experts consider to be better than sucrose. Fructose is assimilated along a different metabolic pathway than sucrose, which places less stress on the pancreas.

The chart on page 7 compares the nutritional information on our favorite fruit sweetener (made from the combined juices of peaches, pears, and pineapples) with information on refined white sugar. The figures are for 100 grams of fruit sweetener (approximately 5 tablespoons) and 1 tablespoon. As *half the amount* of fruit sweetener is used in each recipe in comparison to the amount of sugar that would need to be used in the same recipe, the figures for sugar are for 200 grams (approximately 10 tablespoons of sugar) and for 2 tablespoons. As a point of reference, the Recommended Daily Allowances for adults of each of the nutrients are also included.

Americans have consumed one-fifth of the world's production of sugar every year but one since the Civil War. And consumption has risen at an amazing rate every year, so much so that white sugar is the third most frequently consumed food in the United States after coffee and white bread. For many Americans, sugar makes up 20 percent of their diet.

As sugar can increase the risk of nutritional deficiencies by diluting the total nutrient content of the diet, it is very likely to pose a threat to the nutritional status of many people—specifically those whose diets do include 15 to 20 percent added sugars (versus naturally occurring sugars from whole fruits). This means these people are getting too many calories with too few of the vitamins and minerals needed for the proper metabolism of the calories. These people would then need to fulfill 100 percent of their nutrient requirements from 80 to 85 percent of their diet. Yet it is highly unlikely that they would do so, because these classic junk food eaters are the very people who are least likely to be informed about nutrition.

The stressful lifestyle of modern society also takes its toll on our nutrient status. Psychological and environmental stresses increase our nutrient needs while decreasing the efficiency of intestinal absorption. Stress often leads to drug, tobacco, and alcohol use, which also increases nutrient needs. Therefore, it is more important than ever that every calorie we take in be worth the energy, vitamins, and minerals it needs to be metabolized.

The Sugar Association, an organization representing sugar manufacturers, has often stated in their advertising that there is a lack of "persuasive" or "conclusive" evidence regarding sugar's role in causing obesity, nutrient deficiencies, diabetes, adverse human behavior, or in contributing to heart disease and cancer. However, "conclusive" evidence is rarely available for diet–disease relationships. And this lack of evidence may indicate that too few studies

Comparison of Nutrients: Mixed Fruit Sweetener and White Sugar

	Mixed Fruit Sweetener		*White Sugar*		*RDA**
	5T	1T	10T	2T	
Calories	283	56	770	144	2400
Carbohydrates (grams)	70	14	192	36	300
Fats (grams)	0.5	0.1	0	0	66
Protein (grams)	2.3	0.46	0	0	46
Vitamin A (Int. Units)	738	148	0	0	4-5000
Vitamin C (milligrams)	43	86	0	0	60
Niacin (milligrams)	1.6	0.3	0	0	14-19
Riboflavin (milligrams)	0.12	0.2	0	0	1.2-1.6
Thiamine (milligrams)	0.23	0.05	0	0	1.0-1.4
Calcium (milligrams)	72	14.4	0	0	800
Iron (milligrams)	1.7	0.3	0.1	0.02	10-18
Phosphorus (milligrams)	41	8	0	0	800
Potassium (milligrams)	831	166	0	0	1525-4575
Sodium (milligrams)	6	1	1	0.2	900-2700

*RDA from the Food and Nutrition Board, National Academy of Sciences, National Research Council, 1980. Nutritional information for the mixed fruit sweetener, courtesy of American Fruit Processors, is based on estimated calculations derived from *Composition of Foods,* a Department of Agriculture Handbook.

have been conducted, rather than "proving" that sugar is not to blame. Even if sugar only plays a significant role, rather than being the sole cause of many twentieth-century problems, that is reason enough for sugar intake to be limited in a healthy diet.

The Food and Drug Administration has often considered sugar as a "food additive." As Dr. John Yudkin stated in his 1972 book *Sweet and Dangerous,* "If only a small fraction of what is already known about the effects of sugar were to be revealed in relation to any other material used as a food additive, that material would be promptly banned."

As sugar constitutes well over 10 percent of the average American's diet, it is considerably more than an additive; it is a substantial component of the diet. If you are interested in eating a nutritious diet and minimizing your risk of health problems, then cut down on sugar—or cut it out altogether!

From my own experiences with sugar and fruit sweeteners, I know that fruit sweeteners are a transitional solution toward the more moderate use of sweeteners. They are an excellent source of sweetness and they enable me (and you) to create delicious and beautiful pastries. They do not seem to cause the many side effects I had previously experienced with sugar.

People who cut down on sugar agree that their taste buds seem to come alive. They still get natural sweetness from foods but they discover a whole range of new tastes. And in the end, this may be the best reason to eat less sugar.

I hope you will try and enjoy these fruit-sweetened offerings from The Ranch Kitchen Restaurant and bakery. They are guaranteed to help you find new and delicious ways to satisfy your sweet cravings.

And the next time you are in Corwin Springs, Montana, do drop in and say hello.

1

The Fine Art of Baking

Baking and preparing all food is pleasurable both for yourself and for those whom you serve. As you develop the fine art of baking, master its techniques, and understand its philosophy, you will become freer to create and produce satisfying and nurturing works of beauty and flavor that can bring joy to all.

Allow me to share my own understanding of the fine art of baking and give you a few suggestions on how to make the whole process more efficient and enjoyable.

Over the years, I've come to understand that the four essential elements of fine baking are love, technique, temperature, and recipe—in that order.

Love

I learned about the element of love many years ago from the opening quote in one of my very first cookbooks, the *Tassajara Bread Book*:

> *Love is not only the most important ingredient, it is the only ingredient that really matters.*

Love is the ingredient that keeps your mistakes from being a problem; love is the ingredient that increases your patience and enables you to strive and do better next time; love fills you with joy, making every aspect of the baking process a new delight; love is the desire to work with each ingredient to bring forth its fullest potential; and love develops your senses, especially the sensitivity of your hands, nose, mouth, and eyes—the most important baking tools you possess.

Love is a somewhat intangible element. The other three elements are very tangible and can be learned easily.

TECHNIQUE

Technique is the reason why one person's cake is light and fluffy while another's is dense and heavy, even though both say they followed the recipe exactly. The difference can be that one person stopped beating the butter and sweetener too soon. Or she may have used a bowl too small for her hands and the volume of the ingredients, so that in folding the cake batter she deflated it before the cake even entered the oven. Such is the importance of technique.

Technique is the key to adapting recipes for use with liquid fruit sweeteners and whole grain flours. The introductory notes and baker's tips should give you the techniques you need for your own success in producing fine baked goods.

Organization is a very important aspect of technique. It is organization that enables The Ranch Kitchen bakery to daily produce its array of cakes, pies, custards, muffins, cookies, and breads. Everything that can be done in advance without compromising taste, texture, or appearance is done in advance: Nuts are sorted, toasted, chopped, and frozen; pie crusts and tart shells are formed and frozen unbaked; cake layers are baked and frozen; glazes and sauces are made and refrigerated; dry mixes for muffins or coffee cakes are precombined, etc. With so much done in advance, the preparation of everything from the simplest quick breads to the most elaborate cakes becomes simply a matter of skillfully assembling the parts.

These same principles of organization apply to the home baker. When you have extra time, stock your freezer and pantry. When you are well organized, you will be prepared for both the expected and the unexpected, making all of your baking more efficient and more enjoyable.

TEMPERATURE

The temperature of your ingredients, the room in which you work, and your oven or stove top are as important as your good techniques. Every aspect of baking requires its own temperature and technique. Pie crusts need quick handling under cool conditions; bread dough prefers thorough kneading and a warm room; feather-light cakes demand fast and gentle action with exact measurements and perfect oven conditions; and nondemanding apple butter requires long, slow cooking with a minimum of attention.

Knowing your ingredients and at which temperature they perform to their fullest saves time and avoids many frustrating mistakes. Knowing that your unusually hot hands would ruin pie crusts or biscuits by melting the butter while rubbing it into the flour, you instead use a food processor or an electric mixer. Knowing that your oven bakes 50 degrees too low, you adjust the temperature before you place your cakes or pie crusts or muffins into it. Knowing that egg yolks curdle if they get too hot, you remove your Lemon Curd from its hot water bath at just the right time to keep it creamy and smooth. And, knowing that cold cream cheese or cold butter won't blend with cold fruit sweetener, you save yourself much frustration by letting these ingredients come to room temperature before you start.

Recipe

Although most people think of the recipe as the most essential element, it is really the fourth element of importance in fine baking. Recipes don't stand on their own. They rely upon your good technique, your knowledge of your ingredients, and your understanding of the process for their success.

Here's how to get the most out of your recipes:

Read the recipe completely through before beginning—even if it's an old favorite. Try to visualize each step of the preparation and what equipment and ingredients you will need to complete it. I like to read everything I can about a specific cake or pie or bread, in a number of sources, before I attempt a new recipe. This way I become familiar with the many techniques and ideas for preparing, cooking, decorating, and serving it. Then I combine the information until I feel comfortable with what I am about to do and in what order.

I suggest that as you begin baking and cooking with fruit sweeteners you start with the simpler recipes, such as those for cookies, sauces, and muffins, and follow the recipes exactly. Then, as you refine your skills, progress to the more elaborate pies, cakes, and breads, developing your own ideas and variations and enjoyment in the process.

Organization Tips

Here are a few other suggestions that will help you better organize yourself for all of your cooking and baking.

• Know the specific requirements of the item or items you are to prepare. Are there special ingredients needed? Is the butter to be cold, room temperature, or melted? Are the nuts blanched, sliced, slivered, or chopped? Should the oven be preheated? To what temperature? Is extra time required for chilling or heating the ingredients? Is it necessary to wait before serving?

• Pay close attention to what you are doing while you work, giving special consideration to every detail, especially with new recipes or unfamiliar techniques. Allow yourself plenty of time to finish a recipe, including the final decoration.

• Always begin by preparing the baking pans, adjusting the oven shelves, and preheating the oven to the required temperature. Then, when the mixture is ready for the oven there will be no delay before baking. This is especially important with cakes, which may deflate and lose their lightness, with pie crusts, which may collapse, and with puff pastry, which will not rise if the oven temperature is not hot enough.

• Avoid opening the oven door during the early baking stage. Other than with small cookies which you can peek at after 5 minutes, generally you should wait at least 15 to 20 minutes, or until approximately half of the baking time has elapsed, before opening the door.

• Don't work against yourself by being a pot-saver in order to save clean-up time. Use all of the pots, pans, bowls, spoons, spatulas, equipment, and towels that you need to get the job done. But clean up after yourself frequently to avoid confusion.

And, most of all, enjoy yourself. Put your heart into everything you make, infuse it with love, and you will be transformed in the process, as will be everyone who works by your side or eats the food you prepare.

Ingredients

Choose the finest and freshest ingredients you can find. The quality of your ingredients and how you work with them will affect the quality, flavor, texture, and appearance of your finished products. Some of the items in this introduction may be new to you, or they may be used in unfamiliar ways. This information will assist you with all of your baking and most especially with the recipes in this book.

Almond Milk

Almond milk is a delicious, protein-rich alternative to cow's milk. It can be used in any recipe without alterations in amounts or techniques.

To make almond milk, blend blanched almonds and water on high speed for 5 minutes. Strain this mixture through a double thickness of dampened cheesecloth. The almond pulp remaining in the strainer will have almost no flavor and should be discarded.

The usual proportion of almond milk is 4 parts water to 1 part almonds (written as 4:1). However, this proportion of water to almonds can be varied depending on how rich a milk is desired. The lower the ratio of water to almonds, the richer the milk. A rich almond milk would be 3:1; i.e., 3 parts water to 1 part blanched almonds.

Keep almond milk under refrigeration and use it within 4 days.

Amazake

Amazake, or rice milk, is a whole-grain product made by adding cultured brown rice (koji) to sweet brown rice and water. The mixture is then fermented into a thick liquid that is used both as a sweetener and a beverage.

Amazake is about 21 percent sugar, mainly glucose and maltose, and it is high in carbohydrates and other nutrients, including vitamin B and iron.

Amazake comes in many flavors; however, plain or vanilla is preferred for baking. Amazake can be purchased in natural food stores in the freezer or the refrigerator section in half pint, pint, and quart bottles. Once opened, it will keep for a week under refrigeration.

Apples

Many varieties of apples are available all year long, but do experiment with some of the shorter-lived fall and winter varieties. For most recipes, tart, crisp apples are recommended, such as Granny Smiths, Pippins, and Gravensteins. Golden Delicious apples, which seem to be available everywhere all the time, will also work well as long as they have not become too old and mealy.

For the least amount of waste, use a vegetable peeler instead of a knife to peel apples. Apples can be kept from turning brown after they have been sliced or cut by tossing them into a small amount of lemon juice diluted with water.

Baking Powder

Natural food stores sell baking powder that is free of the aluminum compounds that many people consider to be unhealthy. Baking powder has about a one-year shelf life and should be replaced yearly. Store baking powder in an airtight container in a cupboard—not in the refrigerator—to avoid loss of strength due to humidity.

Baking Soda

Used by itself, baking soda has no leavening ability. But used in combination with an acid ingredient, such as a fruit sweetener, as well as baking powder, it creates carbon dioxide bubbles which leaven the batter.

Since baking soda is usually very lumpy in the box, it is important to sift it once before measuring, and then again with the flour. Otherwise the final product will have little dark brown spots scattered throughout which can be quite bitter.

Butter

I prefer to use unsalted butter because of its wonderful flavor and delicious aroma. By using unsalted butter you can easily control both the quantity and the quality of salt in everything you cook or bake. Unsalted butter has a much shorter shelf life than salted butter and can become rancid in a couple of weeks in the refrigerator. However, it may be stored for a couple of months in the freezer.

Unless otherwise stated in the recipe, butter should be used at room temperature for ease in blending with sweetener or other ingredients.

Butter comes in either ¼ pound sticks or 1 pound solids. A stick of butter equals ½ cup, 8 tablespoons, or ¼ pound. Two sticks equal 1 cup, 16 tablespoons, or ½ pound. Three sticks equal 1½ cups, 24 tablespoons, or ¾ pound. And 4 sticks of butter are equivalent to the 1 pound solid, and equal 2 cups, or 32 tablespoons. One ounce of butter is equivalent to 2 tablespoons.

Carob Powder

Carob is also known as Saint John's Bread. It is an ideal substitute for cocoa powder or chocolate, as it is similar in both flavor and color. Carob, a good source of calcium, is free of the detrimental effects of caffeine, theobromine, and calcium oxalate, which are all found in cocoa beans. Carob powder is low in fat and naturally sweet. When you have a choice, choose dark roasted carob powder, which gives a richer flavor and color.

Carob powder can be purchased in natural food stores and should be stored at room temperature. Carob powder has a tendency to form rock-hard clumps, so be sure to sift it before mixing it with other ingredients.

Cornstarch and Arrowroot

These two thickeners create beautiful translucent sauces and glazes. Arrowroot is recommended for use with acid fruits, as it does not break down and thin in their presence.

Dissolve *cornstarch* in some of the cool liquid called for in the recipe. Heat the remaining liquid to the boiling point. Gradually whisk in the dissolved cornstarch, whisking constantly while the mixture returns to a boil. Reduce the heat and simmer for 5 minutes to stabilize the cornstarch. Remove from the heat. Cornstarch-based mixtures will thicken upon cooling and can be reheated to return to the desired consistency.

Dissolve *arrowroot* in some of the cool liquid called for in the recipe. Heat the remaining liquid just to the boiling point and reduce the heat. Whisk in the dissolved arrowroot. As soon as the mixture thickens, remove it from the heat. Don't allow the arrowroot to get too hot (above 175° F.), or it will break down and thin the mixture. Arrowroot-thickened mixtures cannot be reheated and retain their original consistency.

Dried Fruit

Use naturally dried, unsweetened fruit found in natural food stores rather than fruit dried with sulfur dioxide or sweetened with additional sugar.

Eggs

All of these recipes have been formulated using large eggs. When separating eggs, learn to do it cleanly. That means there should be no yolk in the whites and no whites (or very little white) in with the yolks.

The greatest volume can be gotten from eggs that are brought to room temperature before whipping. However, it is preferable to begin with chilled whites when you use the following technique to stiffly whip egg whites.

Egg Whites

To whip whites, place a small portion of the sweetener in the recipe in with the cold whites right from the beginning. Although this will slightly retard the whipping action, it will prevent the whites from over-whipping and becoming dry and difficult to fold into other mixtures.

Begin using a medium-high speed for whipping the whites. Once they have whitened, increase the speed to high. The whites will take a little longer to become stiff this way and there will be less air beaten into them, producing slightly less volume; however, the whites will be stronger and deflate less when folded into the other ingredients.

Salt from the amount in the recipe and/or a squeeze of fresh lemon juice can be added just before the whipping is completed both to tighten the structure and stabilize the whites.

For the best volume when working with a small number of egg whites, it is important that the mixing bowl, the whip or the beaters, and the whites themselves be free of any trace of egg yolk or grease.

Egg Yolks

When preparing cakes, the sweetener and yolks are often whipped together (without additional heat) beyond the formation of a "ribbon," until they are very light and fluffy. This creates greater volume and a finer texture in finished cakes.

Flour

A point of pride in my adopted state: Montana, with its long, hot summer days, cool nights and good soil, is the home of most of the best wheat in the United States. Its wheat is so well known that many professionals specify Montana wheat for their baking.

The following flours are used in the recipes throughout this book. They can be purchased in natural food stores, some gourmet stores, and most supermarkets.

Unbleached White Flour

Bleached by an aging process rather than a chemical process, unbleached white flour is made from a blend of hard wheats, but it is still a good all-purpose flour. When combined with whole wheat pastry flour, it gives unsurpassed flavor and texture to pastries and biscuits.

Whole Wheat Flour

Containing both the bran and the germ,

whole wheat flour is made from hard wheat and is used mainly in breads. It might also be labeled as whole wheat bread flour.

Whole Wheat Pastry Flour

Because this flour still contains the bran and germ, it has a slightly brownish color. It is made from soft wheat and is best used in pastries, biscuits, and cakes. Whole wheat pastry flour may be used interchangeably with white cake flour.

White Cake Flour

Made from soft wheat, this flour makes the whitest, lightest, and most tender cakes.

Brown Rice Flour

For those who are gluten sensitive, brown rice flour, which is available from natural food stores, is a good alternative to wheat in everything but yeasted breads. Brown rice flour often gives a crunchy, crumbly texture. Yet, in most baked goods, the difference in texture is not even noticeable. Brown rice flour should be stored in the refrigerator as it is especially susceptible to rancidity. When rice flour is rancid, it will impart a slightly bitter aftertaste to baked goods.

Oat Flour

Available from natural food stores, oat flour has very little gluten and is best used in combination with other flours. If you would like to make your own oat flour, blend rolled oats, ½ cup at a time, in either a food processor or electric blender. Once ground, oat flour should be stored in the refrigerator as it is especially susceptible to rancidity. When oat flour is rancid, it will impart a slightly bitter aftertaste to baked goods.

To Measure Flour

Measure the quantity of flour called for in the recipe before sifting Do not shake or pack it into the measuring cup. Use a scoop to place the flour in the cup, then cut off the excess evenly with a knife. Or, dip the measuring cup into the flour, and level off the excess with a knife. Never level flour by shaking the measuring cup.

Flour on the Work Surface

When the recipe indicates that a dough should be kneaded or rolled out on a floured surface, sprinkle the surface with a light coating of flour, adding additional flour only as necessary. Dough absorbs flour easily, and too much flour can alter the recipe proportions, affecting both texture and taste.

Frozen Fruit

Use only individually quick-frozen fruits without added sugar.

A number of years ago, I spoke with a gentleman who spent his college summers as a purchasing agent for a frozen fruit company. I asked him to explain to me why frozen fruit, such as raspberries and strawberries, have such a wonderful color, beautiful fragrance, and full flavor. He explained that because the freezing process itself breaks down flavor and smell, the frozen fruit companies have to contract with growers for the best of their crops: the fruit with the best color, flavor, and smell. He said that canned fruit processors have similar contracts, as the canning process is even harder on fruit than freezing. So, unfortunately, the fruit and berries available to the consumer are rarely the top quality, those having already been contracted away.

Fruit-Sweetened Jams

Fruit-sweetened jams come in many delicious flavors. I am especially fond of the jams from Sorrell Ridge because of their consistently high quality of both taste and appearance. Fruit-sweetened jams are available in natural food stores and many supermarkets.

Fruit Sweeteners

These concentrated sweeteners are made from fruit that has been pressed into juice, then reduced for a long time until they have a consistency similar to that of honey. They come in many flavors—apple, white and red grape, and raspberry, to name a few. My very favorite fruit concentrate, and the one used for almost everything we bake at The Ranch Kitchen bakery, we call "3-P," for it is made from the juices of peaches, pears, and pineapples. One of the advantages of 3-P is its well-rounded flavor. It combines the three fruit flavors without any one of them predominating; and because it provides so much flavor along with its sweetness, it is possible to use less sweetener.

We purchase our sweetener, 1,500 pounds at a time, from American Fruit Processors in Pacoima, California. Mystic Lake Dairy in Redmond, Washington, also produces a mixed fruit concentrate from peaches, pears, and pineapples. Mystic Lake Dairy's mixed-fruit sweetener can be purchased in the refrigerator section of most natural food stores. Make sure you also store these fruit sweeteners under refrigeration, but use them at room temperature for best results in blending with other ingredients.

Frozen fruit juice concentrates, such as unsweetened apple and orange juice, are readily available in almost every grocery store. These frozen juice concentrates are less sweet and more liquid than the concentrates used at the bakery. Frozen apple juice concentrate can be placed in a small pan and brought to a boil, then simmered for 10 minutes to evaporate the excess liquid and concentrate the flavor. This form of apple juice concentrate works well in pies, apple butter, sauces, and fillings. Once thawed, these concentrates must be stored under refrigeration, where they will keep for about 2 weeks. Orange juice concentrate is too strongly "orange" to use for general purposes, and is best used in combination with apple juice concentrate.

To adjust recipes calling for sugar, reduce the amount of sugar in a recipe by half, and replace that amount with a concentrated fruit sweetener. You will then have to adjust only your techniques and not the liquid or dry ingredients. If there is a slightly acidic aftertaste in the finished product, you have used too much sweetener and can reduce it more next time.

When creaming butter and fruit sweetener, if either of the two is too cold, they will not come together. You can place the mixing bowl, if it is metal, over direct heat for a few moments to begin to soften the butter. If the mixing bowl is not metal, place the bowl in hot water. Do this for 15 to 30 seconds, just to heat the sweetener and butter long enough for them to come together when returned again to the mixer. (It is still important to cream the butter and sweetener until they are light and fluffy, especially if you heated the butter too long and it melted.)

It is necessary to add a small amount of baking soda to batters and doughs to neutralize the acidity of fruit sweeteners in a proportion of approximately ½ teaspoon baking soda to 2 cups acid ingredients.

Kiwis

Distinctive kiwi fruits have the best texture, least tart flavor, and brightest green color when they are ripe and barely soft to the touch.

Peel kiwis with a small, sharp knife. Be careful to remove only the outer fuzzy brown peel, leaving the shape and size of the fruit intact. Kiwis are round or oval-shaped fruits. Be careful not to peel them into hexagons.

Once peeled and washed, kiwis quickly soften and darken in color. Thus, it is best not to peel or slice them until just before they are to be used.

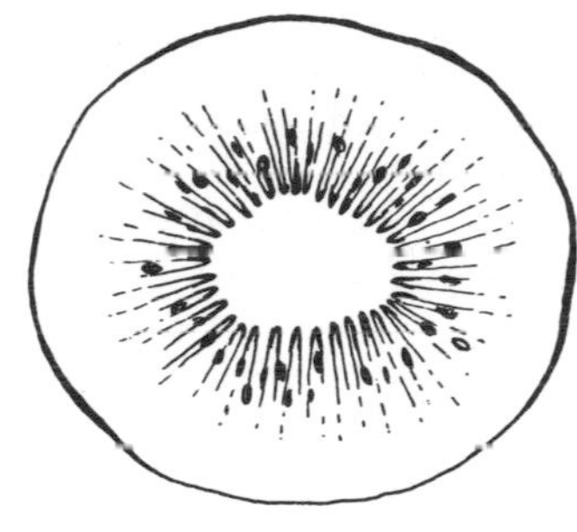

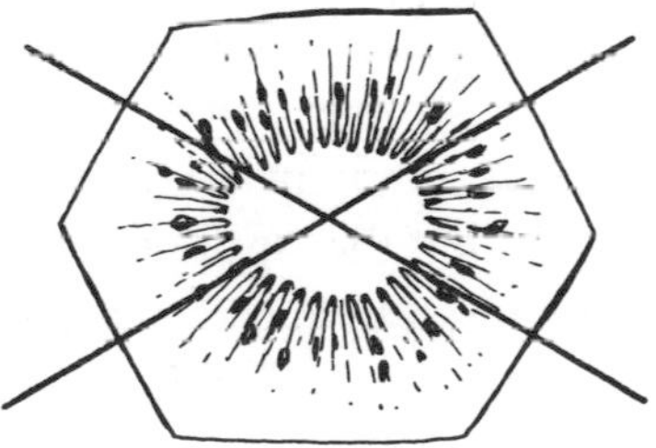

Kuzu

Kuzu is the powdered root of the wild arrowroot plant. The kuzu plant is native to the mountains of Japan and the southern United States (where it is called kudzu). The plant often grows to a height of 30 feet, with tough deep roots. The extraction of the starch from the roots is done by hand in a long and expensive process.

Kuzu can be purchased in natural food stores. It is usually packaged in small, white irregular lumps, which disperse quickly in cold water to make a milky liquid. When heated and stirred over heat, the liquid suddenly becomes clear and thick. Cook kuzu-thickened mixtures at a simmer for another 5 minutes to stabilize the kuzu. At the bakery, we sometimes use kuzu as a thickening agent in place of arrowroot, cornstarch, or eggs.

Kuzu is used medicinally in the Orient in a thickened beverage to soothe and strengthen the intestines.

Lecithin Spray/Nonstick Vegetable Spray

I prefer to use Pam®, a spray-on food release made from lecithin and a small amount of soy oil, for stick-free baking. It is faster, neater, and more convenient than using butter or oil for greasing pans.

The sides of cake pans should not be sprayed with lecithin spray. This I unhappily learned the day I felt inspired to spray the sides of the cake pan for easier cleanup. Instead, my cake was unable to rise and its sides collapsed in on themselves. I can now affirm with certainty that cakes need a nonslippery surface to cling to as they rise in the oven.

Margarine

Margarine is a less expensive, nondairy alternative to butter. Although margarine has been manufactured to be similar to butter, it does fall short of butter's taste and texture. Always use margarine at room temperature unless otherwise directed by the recipe. Unsalted margarine is preferred, so that you can control the amount and quality of salt in the recipe.

Molasses

All molasses is very high in minerals, but contains from 35 to 70 percent sucrose, even though it has only half the sweetening power of white sugar. The molasses called for in these recipes, and the best-tasting, is unsulphured molasses. Unsulphured molasses is made by concentrating the juice of sun-ripened sugar cane.

Sulphured molasses is created as a by-product of refining sugar cane. It contains sulphur dioxide, which may cause allergic reactions. A third kind of molasses is very strong-tasting blackstrap molasses, which is basically a waste product from refining sugar.

The only time I use molasses is in making whole wheat bread and some spice cookies, where a richer color and distinct flavor are desired. Molasses also improves the keeping qualities of breads. If you prefer not to use molasses at all, you can replace it with an equal amount of concentrated fruit sweetener.

Nuts

Walnuts, almonds, pecans, and hazelnuts (filberts)—are all prominently featured in many of these recipes, as nuts enhance the nutritional value as well as the texture, flavor, and appearance of finished baked goods.

I always recommend using toasted nuts unless otherwise specified in the recipe.

To Toast Nuts

Place them in a single layer on a baking sheet. Bake at 350° F for 7 to 10 minutes, stirring occasionally. Taste a nut or two to test for doneness. Over-toasting will make nuts bitter. Cool the nuts before chopping or grinding. Nuts that will not be used immediately store well in the refrigerator for a couple of weeks or for a couple of months in the freezer.

Oats

In these recipes, use only regular rolled oats (also known as old-fashioned oats). Quick-cooking oats absorb liquids more quickly and will alter the texture and moistness of any recipes in which they are used, unless expressly specified.

Oil

Often oil can be substituted for butter to lower the cholesterol in baked goods. Canola oil is recommended. It is a high-quality tasteless oil, high in monounsaturated fats and very low in saturated fat. It should be stored in a cool place.

If you prefer to use unrefined oils, be careful that their taste is mild enough not to overwhelm the other ingredients in the recipe. Many delicate cakes, like the sponge cakes in this book, will be ruined by a too strong-tasting oil (so I once learned, too late). Unrefined oils can easily become rancid and must be stored in the refrigerator once they have been opened.

Peaches, Nectarines, and Apricots

Always use ripe peaches, nectarines, and apricots. If the fruit is not ripe when you begin, it will not ripen after cooking but will remain hard and green-tasting.

Peaches, nectarines, and apricots are usually used peeled. To peel them, bring a pot of water to boil. Add only a few pieces of fruit at a time to the pot so that the water continues to boil. Count to 10 and remove the fruit to a bowl of cold water. Use the point of a small knife to remove the peel. If the peel does not come off easily, return the fruit to the boiling water for another couple of seconds and try again.

Peach Extract

My favorite discovery of 1989! You will find I add a dab of peach extract in many unsuspected places where its use heightens and brightens flavors.

Naturally flavored peach extract is available at many health food stores, or can be purchased directly from Bickford Laboratories in Cleveland, Ohio (800-283-8322). They require no minimum order.

Pears

Highly flavored and very perishable, pears are a wonderful fall and winter fruit. Some of my favorite varieties are Seckels, Bartletts, Anjous, and Winter Nells.

As most pears are overripe and mealy when they are soft, it is good to know that you can press a pear gently at the stem end to see if it is ripe. When it is soft to the touch, the pear is ripe and should be used within the day (or some people say, within the hour!). Do not bake with underripe pears. They will remain unripe and as hard and thoroughly disappointing at the end of the baking time as they were at the beginning.

For the least amount of waste, use a vegetable peeler instead of a knife to peel pears. Tossed in a small amount of lemon juice diluted with water, pears can be kept from turning brown after they have been sliced or cut.

Plumped Raisins

Use plumped raisins in any recipe requiring raisins. They are more tender and more delicious than dried raisins. They can be plumped in a large quantity at a time, or in just the amount you will need for a specific recipe. Raisins measure about the same dry as they do after plumping.

To Make 1 Cup of Plumped Raisins

Bring 2 cups of water to a boil. Add 1 cup of raisins. When the water returns to a boil, turn off the heat. Let the raisins plump in the water for 10 to 30 minutes. Drain the raisins, reserving the "raisin water" for use in place of the same amount of water in breads, cookies, or other recipes. Store both plumped raisins and raisin water (separately) in the refrigerator for 2 or more weeks.

Raisin Water

Raisin water is the liquid remaining after draining plumped raisins. It has a rich, dark brown color and sweet flavor. It can be used in place of an equal amount of water in breads, cookies, or other recipes. Raisin water is often used in whole wheat breads to give them a deeper color and sweeter flavor. Raisin water may be stored for 2 or more weeks in the refrigerator.

Raspberries and Blackberries

As both raspberries and blackberries are more fragile than strawberries, they should not be dipped in water, where they would easily become water-logged and flavorless. It is best to sort through them and discard any spoiled berries, and then to place the good berries on a pan covered with a clean, dry kitchen towel. Shake the pan so that the berries roll around and clean themselves of dirt, leaves, etc. As with strawberries, if the berries are to sit before you use them, be sure they are spaced so as not to touch one another.

Sea Salt

Natural, sun-dried white sea salt contains many trace amounts of minerals that are important to the functioning of the human body. Ordinary table salt has had all but the sodium and chloride removed during the refining process, thus reducing salt from a vital food to a flavoring agent.

I include a small amount of salt in many recipes where it helps heighten and balance flavors, thus reducing the amount of sweetener needed by producing a sweeter taste on the tongue.

As high-quality, natural, sun-dried sea salt is not readily available to most Americans, regular commercial salt should be used only in moderation.

Soy Milk

Rich in protein and low in fat, soy milk is a nondairy alternative to cow's milk. Increasingly popular, it is available in natural food stores in a variety of flavors, although plain or vanilla-flavored are the best for cooking and baking. Once opened, soy milk must be stored in the refrigerator and will keep for up to a week.

Strawberries

Wash fresh strawberries very quickly by placing them in a colander and dipping them in water. This is usually sufficient to remove any soil or leaves clinging to them. Immediately place the wet strawberries on a pan covered with a clean, dry kitchen towel. Shake the pan so that the berries roll around and dry themselves. If the berries are to sit a while before you use them, keep the berries from softening and bruising by spacing them so that they do not touch one another. As strawberries are fragile and delicately flavored, do not remove the hulls until after the strawberries are washed.

Use the point of a sharp knife or the tip of a vegetable peeler to remove the hulls. Remove only the hull; do not cut off the top of the berry with a knife in order to remove the hulls. A strawberry is heart-shaped, not triangular.

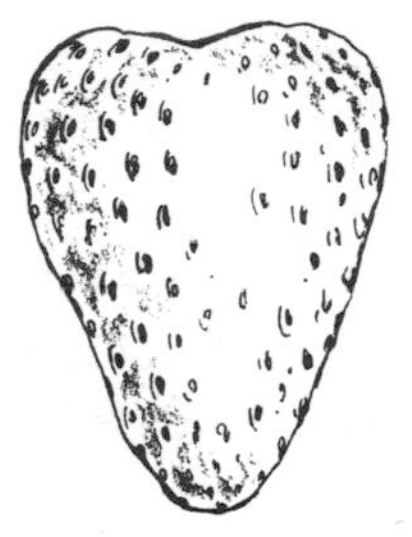

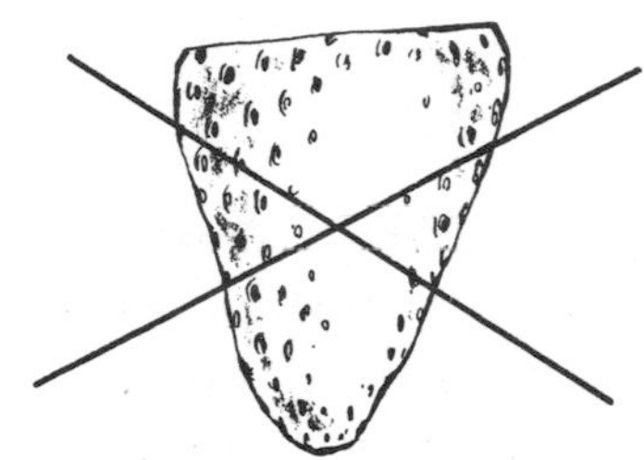

Tahini

Tahini is made from hulled roasted or hulled unroasted sesame seeds. It is rich in calcium, phosphorus, lecithin, iron, vitamins B and E, and protein. Unroasted, or raw, tahini can be purchased in natural food stores, whereas roasted tahini can be purchased in either natural food stores or major supermarkets. Maranatha Foods and Westbrae Natural Foods manufacture and nationally distribute both roasted and raw tahini. Once opened, tahini is best stored in the refrigerator to keep it from becoming rancid.

Roasted tahini is called for in most recipes. However, for both the Apple and Boysenberry Custard Pies (pages 98 and 99) raw tahini is used because of its milder flavor.

Whipping Cream

Whenever you need stiffly whipped cream, heavy cream is recommended. It has a higher percentage of butterfat than regular cream, which makes it whip up more easily and hold a firmer texture longer than regular cream. This is especially important when preparing frostings or whipped cream using fruit sweeteners.

Zest

Zest refers only to the colored part of the citrus peel, not to the white portion, which can be quite bitter. There is a heavy concentration of oil in the colored portion of the peel, which gives it its intense flavor.

The zest of citrus fruits is much easier to remove when the fruit is whole, before it is cut in half and juiced. The zest can be grated with a hand-held grater, or removed in strips with a vegetable peeler, according to the individual recipes.

Recommended Equipment

"Why don't my pies, cakes, muffins, or cookies look like the ones from the bakery?"

One of the answers is equipment. When you use specialized equipment the results are more professional and the whole baking process is more efficient and convenient. For example: High, dome-shaped muffin tops or perfectly round cookies are the result of using ice cream scoops for forming them; an electric knife cuts crisp, clean pieces of cake—it even cuts through raisins and nuts; and an oven thermometer means that you don't have to burn a cake to realize that your oven bakes too hot; a free-standing mixer frees you to make bread at the same time that you chop the vegetables for the soup; a piece of baking parchment lining the pan means you no longer have to grease and flour; and an electric mixer of any kind gives greater volume to egg whites than you can achieve by using a whisk.

While special equipment is more efficient, it is not essential. I've rolled out pie crust using a mason jar turned on its side, and I've cut out biscuits with a blue plastic glass. I've cut up cardboard boxes to make cardboard cake rounds, and, yes, I've even used that special tool on my pocket knife to open a can. None of these was the most efficient or professional method, although in some cases it was the only means to the desired end—and considering the circumstances, the results were perfect.

So please know that you can have acceptable results improvising with the equipment you now have. Then, as you become more serious about baking, you can upgrade your equipment along the following guidelines, beginning with the basics and proceeding to the optional items. Always purchase the best equipment and tools you can afford, preferably professional, commercial quality items.

Electric hand-held mixer

Electric blender

Electric coffee grinder for spices, coconut, poppy seeds, etc.

Oven, well calibrated, either gas or electric

Good knives

Chef's knife, 8-inch or 10-inch blade

Paring knife

Serrated knife for cutting cake layers, bread, etc.

Sharpening steel for keeping your knives sharp

Angled 8-inch spatula for applying frosting and lifting cakes

Mixing bowls—stainless steel or ceramic in graduated sizes

If you have only plastic bowls, which are very hard to keep grease-free, try to have one stainless steel bowl for whipping egg whites.

Measuring cups

For dry ingredients (with smooth rims for leveling off excess): graduated sizes from ⅛ cup to 2 cups

For liquid ingredients (with pouring spout): 1 cup

My favorite glass measuring cup for liquids comes in an extra-large 8-cup size. It is not only beautiful to look at but doubles as a mixing bowl.

Measuring spoons in graduated sizes from ⅛ teaspoon to 1 tablespoon

Strainers for sifting dry ingredients and straining wet ingredients

A fine small-mesh strainer and a medium and large medium-mesh strainer

Vegetable peeler

Apple corer

Cutting board for all chopping and cutting. Use one side of the board for strong-smelling foods like onions and garlic, and reserve one side of the board for neutral-smelling foods like nuts and fruit.

Wire whisks, small and medium, preferably with thick handles for easy gripping

Extra-large wire cooling racks

Wooden spoons

Rubber spatulas, small and large

Stainless steel grater

Saucepans

1 quart, 2 quarts, 1 gallon. Heavy, commercial-quality stainless steel pots with aluminum or copper cores at their bottoms for even heat distribution

Baking pans—choose heavy-weight aluminum pans

Muffin pans, regular and mini

Jelly roll pan: 10½-inch by 15½-inch is standard; 12-inch by 17-inch is the commercial size, available at restaurant-supply stores and some houseware stores

Cookie sheets, as large as your oven will accommodate, 2 or more, insulated if possible, for baking cookies

Cake pans (round), with straight sides, two pans each size: 8-inch by 2-inch, 10-inch by 2-inch

Cake pan (rectangular), 9-inch by 13-inch

Cake pan (square), 9-inch by 9-inch

Tube pan, 10-inch

Bread pans, standard 8¾-inch by 4¼-inch, small 3¼-inch by 5¾-inch

Pie pans, one or two 9-inch by 1¼-inch

Tart pan, 10-inch pan with removable bottom

Tartlet pans, four to six 2-inch and/or 4-inch pans, preferably with removable bottoms

Baker's Tip

• Disposable aluminum pie tins actually work very well. And they have the advantage that you can cut the sides of the pan and fold them down easily to remove the first piece perfectly!

Rolling pin, 15-inch by 3-inch (24 inches long including handles) wood, with ball bearings

Dough scraper (also known as a baker's knife)

Pastry brush, with soft bristles. Have one brush for baking needs and another for general cooking, as brushes pick up odors and colors easily.

Biscuit and cookie cutters—metal cutters work best and last the longest

Pie spatula for serving pies and cakes

Oven thermometer

Cheesecloth

Spray bottle

Kitchen clock

Timer

Kitchen scissors

Baking paper (parchment paper)

Plastic wrap

Aluminum foil

Basic decorating equipment

Pastry bags, 8-inch and 10-inch

Couplers, 2 (one for each pastry bag)

Tips—these numbers refer to Wilton metal decorating tips:
- plain round: #3, #6, and #9
- star: #14, #18, and #21
- multi-opening: #233 (for carrot tops)
- leaf: #65 and #69

Large tips to use without couplers—these numbers refer to Ateco large metal decorating tips:
- round: #6
- star: #4

Food coloring: paste or liquid colors

Optional Equipment

Free-standing heavy-duty mixer; 5-quart capacity is my preference. These mixers come with a paddle, a whip, and a dough hook. If you plan to make many cakes, I suggest you purchase an extra mixing bowl and whip attachment.

Food processor—great for chopping nuts and making pie crusts.

Electric knife—almost nothing works better than an electric knife for cutting beautiful slices of cake. Electric knives cut right through the hardest nuts or the most ornery raisins.

Drum sifter—very efficient when sifting large quantities. Be sure to have a mixing bowl just the right diameter of your sifter, to be the most efficient.

Ice cream scoops—#12, #24, and #40. These are indispensable for well-formed muffins and cookies (as well as for scooping perfect rounds of ice cream).

Apple peeler-corer-slicer—for peeling, coring, and slicing apples. A wonderful hand-operated tool that saves much time and energy and apples. A must if apple pie is your family's favorite.

Marble surface—because marble stays cool in any weather, it is wonderful for rolling out pie dough or for working with puff pastry.

Pastry wheel for cutting lattice strips for pies. Purchase the kind that has 2 cutting wheels, one fluted and one plain.

Ruler for cutting straight lattice strips, or straight puff pastry, or for measuring dough for cinnamon rolls.

Kitchen scale—by far the most accurate method of measuring ingredients, as there is less room for error.

Doilies for placing under pies, tarts, and cakes.

Cardboard cake rounds, 8-inch and 10-inch.

Cake turntable—makes frosting and decorating cakes much easier.

2

BREADS, MUFFINS, AND BISCUITS

There is so much joy in making bread. If the promise of having that wonderful and all-pervading aroma of fresh-baked bread throughout your kitchen is not enough reason to get you started, then consider the unrivaled experience of feeling the alive and vibrant dough in your hands, and the expectancy and comfort of that first soft bite of fresh-baked bread still hot from the oven.

YEASTED . . .

All of these yeast bread recipes have been perfected at The Ranch Kitchen bakery, and many of them have been blue ribbon winners at the local Park County or Montana state fairs. As The Ranch Kitchen is nestled in the Gallatin Mountain Range at over 5,000 feet in elevation, all of our yeast doughs rise very quickly. Therefore, I often suggest giving the dough a second rising before forming it into loaves or rolls. You may or may not choose to do this, though a second rising at any elevation helps produce a fine-textured bread with a more developed flavor.

The yield is given in both the size and number of loaves or rolls and in pounds. When a number of loaves or rolls is given they are for 1½ pound loaves baked in standard 4-inch by 8-inch loaf pans, and for 2-ounce to 3-ounce rolls.

Bread making is easy to master once you know a bit about the principal ingredients and the techniques for working with them. I have included tips for making yeasted breads by hand as well as by machine. If you choose the efficiency of kneading your bread in an electric mixer with a dough hook, you will still have the pleasure of having your hands on the dough when you punch it down after it has risen and when you form your loaves.

The Basic Ingredients

Yeast

Yeast is a living organism with very specific needs for its growth and multiplication. Yeast thrives in the presence of sweetener and warm temperatures between 80° and 115° F. Yeast begins to die with too much heat; thus, the temperature of the ingredients and the warmth of the place for the dough's rising are very important. Salt, oil, and cold temperatures all inhibit the growth of yeast, so you can place your bread dough in the refrigerator overnight without its rising too much, and it will be ready to work with in the morning.

Yeast is available as active dry yeast or compressed yeast. Active dry yeast is called for in all of these recipes. It is available in small, flat foil packets everywhere from supermarkets to natural food stores. Yeast is highly dependable as long as it is fresh, so be sure to check the expiration date on each packet before you use it. If you are at all uncertain of the freshness of the yeast, dissolve it in ¼ cup of the lukewarm water and 1 teaspoon of sweetener called for in the recipe. If it is not bubbly and smelling strongly of yeast after 5 minutes, dispose of it and begin again with yeast that you are sure about.

Flour

Since flours vary in their ability to absorb moisture and to develop gluten, it is hard to specify an exact amount of flour in a bread recipe. Therefore all of the recipes suggest holding back a portion of the flour and adding only the amount necessary to make a well-kneaded dough that is smooth and elastic and no longer sticky to the touch or that comes off both the bottom and sides of the mixing bowl of an electric mixer. In making the dough by hand, be careful not to add too much flour during the kneading process. As you become an efficient kneader, and lift the dough up off the table with each turn, you will use less flour than you did as a beginner.

Mixing and Kneading Bread Dough

The main differences between preparing dough by hand and preparing it by machine are the amount of time needed to properly knead the dough and the amount of effort you will need to expend. Once the dough is in its bowl rising, the rest of the process is the same whether the dough has been kneaded by hand or by machine.

By Hand

When preparing dough by hand, activate the yeast before beginning, by stirring the yeast into ¼ cup of the liquid and 1 teaspoon of sweetener called for in the recipe. The best temperature for this liquid is approximately 105° F, which should feel warm to the touch. Let the yeast activate itself undisturbed for a few minutes until it is bubbly and fragrant, while you prepare the other ingredients.

Combine the dry ingredients in a large mixing bowl, making a well in the center. Pour in the wet ingredients and the yeast mixture. Use a wooden spoon, a rubber spatula, or your hand to begin stirring in a spiral motion from the center, gradually stirring in a wider and wider spiral, incorporating a little more flour with each outward spiral. Once the mixture feels like a thick batter, begin to use your hand to incorporate the remaining flour into it. You will have a soft, very sticky mass in your mixing bowl.

Next, lightly flour your work surface and turn the sticky mass of dough onto it. Before proceeding further, I usually wash my hands to remove any bits of dough clinging to them, and then dry them and lightly dust them with flour.

Now begins the wonderful process of kneading the dough. Until the dough has begun to develop its gluten and come together in a ball, it is helpful to use a dough scraper or baker's knife to help with the kneading. Use the scraper to get under the dough and fold it over itself. Use the palm and heel of your other hand to press into the dough and away from you for the count of 2; then lift your hand away. With the dough scraper, get under the dough and give the entire mass a quarter turn and fold the dough in half. Once again use the heel of your other hand to press into the dough and away from you, again for the count of 2. Continue this process of scraping the dough from underneath, giving it a quarter turn, folding it in half, and pressing in and away, until the dough begins to develop itself into a smoother, more compact whole. You will probably need to sprinkle a little flour under the dough each time you scrape it from underneath to prevent it from sticking to the table.

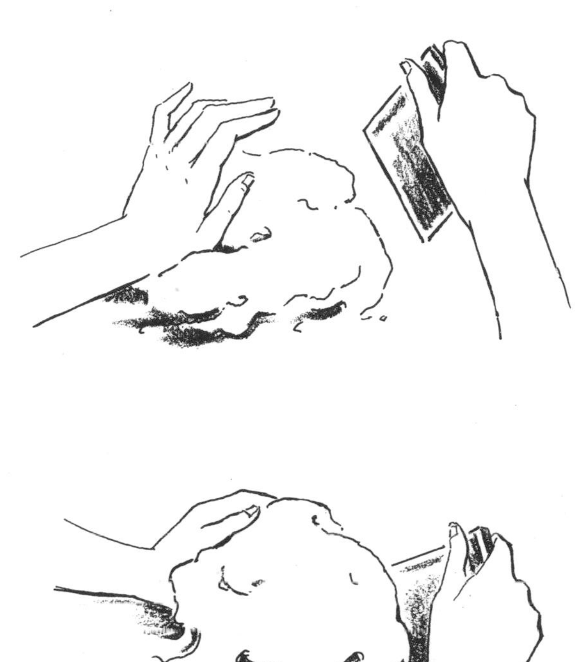

At this point you can stop using the dough scraper and use both of your hands to knead the dough. You will soon develop a very rhythmical motion to your kneading. Remember to lift the dough from the table with each quarter turn and to use a firm touch but not so hard as to break or tear the dough.

This process can take from 10 to 20 minutes or more, depending upon the quantity of dough and your skill as a kneader. The final dough should be smooth and elastic. It will be firm but soft and no longer sticky to the touch. You will be able to pick the dough up and pull it gently apart without its tearing. Dough at this stage is truly beautiful to work with. It feels so alive in your hands and so vital that you may not want to stop working with it.

By Machine

It is very important that you have a heavy-duty mixer with a strong motor if you are going to prepare dough with it. Read the manufacturer's instructions before you begin. The instructions will tell you the maximum amount of flour that your machine's motor is capable of handling. This is very important to the life of your mixer.

You may prefer to activate the yeast first, as described in the section on preparing yeasted dough by hand, and then add the dissolved yeast to the lukewarm liquids in the mixing bowl, along with the flour and salt.

The alternative is to place the liquids in the mixing bowl of your electric mixer. On the lowest speed, use the dough hook to mix the liquids. When they are lukewarm, stir in the undissolved yeast, then the flour and salt to form a soft dough. *Note:* This method should be used only when you know that your yeast is fresh.

With either method of working with the yeast, increase the mixer speed to medium, and knead in additional flour just until the dough forms itself into a ball that comes off both the sides and bottom of the bowl.

Raising, Shaping, and Baking the Bread

The remaining steps of bread making are the same whether you have kneaded your dough by hand or by machine.

Raising the Dough

Let the dough rest a moment while you lightly oil a bowl large enough to allow the dough to rise to double its size. Place your dough in the bowl and turn the dough over, so that the top is lightly coated with oil. Cover the bowl with plastic wrap and place the bowl in a warm, draft-free place. As yeast is susceptible to sudden drafts that could deflate the dough, it is often suggested to put dough to rise in an oven with a pilot light.

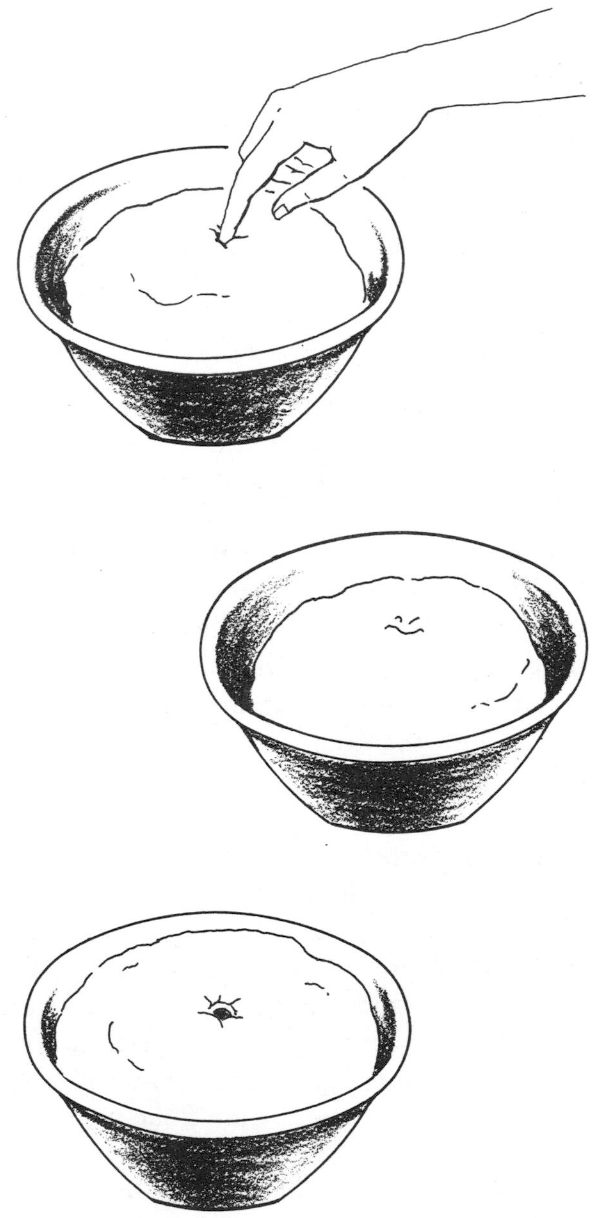

The dough is ready when it has doubled in size. The time needed for this first rising is quite variable; it may take from 45 minutes to 2 hours, depending upon the amount of yeast in the recipe in proportion to the flour and the temperature of the area where the dough is rising. Rather than giving you an exact time, I will tell you what to look for so your bread dough itself will be your guide. Do, however, check the dough's progress after 45 minutes. A good test is to poke it gently with your forefinger. If the space begins to fill back in, cover the dough and let it rise longer. If the space does not fill back in, the dough is perfect and ready for its next step. If the dough collapses when you poke it, it has risen too long and must be worked with immediately. When the dough has over-risen, the resulting bread may be dry, coarse in texture, and heavy (but still suitable for bread pudding or croutons).

Punching the Dough Down

When the dough has doubled, remove the plastic wrap and lightly punch the center of the dough with your fist. This is called "punching the dough down." Now knead the dough 8 to

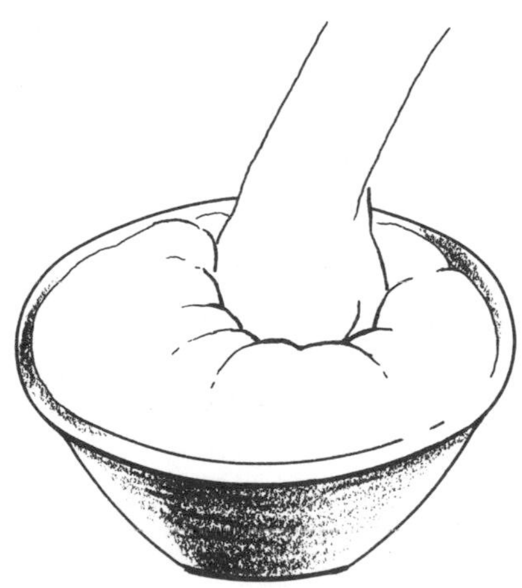

10 times in the mixing bowl. If you are going to give the dough a double rise, cover it again with plastic wrap and place it in the same warm, draft-free spot. This rise will take about half as long as the first rise. Test the dough for readiness after 25 minutes with the same poking test. Punch the dough down again.

Shaping the Dough

Turn the dough out onto a very lightly floured work surface, as the dough should no longer be sticky.

Using the dough scraper as a knife, divide the dough into the size and number of pieces you will need. Lightly knead each piece and put them at the back of your work space, covered loosely with plastic wrap.

Forming Loaves

Lightly oil or spray the bottom of your pans with lecithin spray.

Form your loaves with as little handling as possible. Otherwise you will again activate the gluten, which makes the shaping of loaves very difficult: You push one direction and it pulls itself away. If you have made an unusually shaped loaf and want to redo it, let the dough rest for 10 minutes, lightly covered with plastic wrap, before you try again.

For loaves, I use a very simple technique, similar to kneading the dough. With 4 to 6 movements, shape the dough into a rectangle to fit a loaf pan. With the second knead you seal the dough into itself using the heel of your hand and pressing to form a rectangle. With the next turn fold the dough in about one-quarter. Another turn and fold the dough in half, once again sealing with the heel of your hand. Give the dough one more turn, then roll

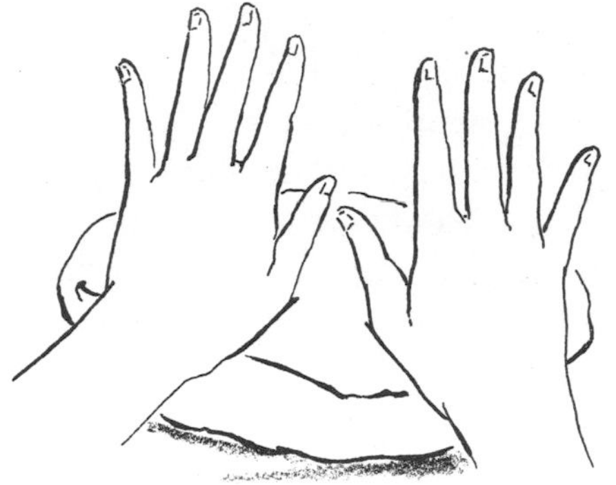

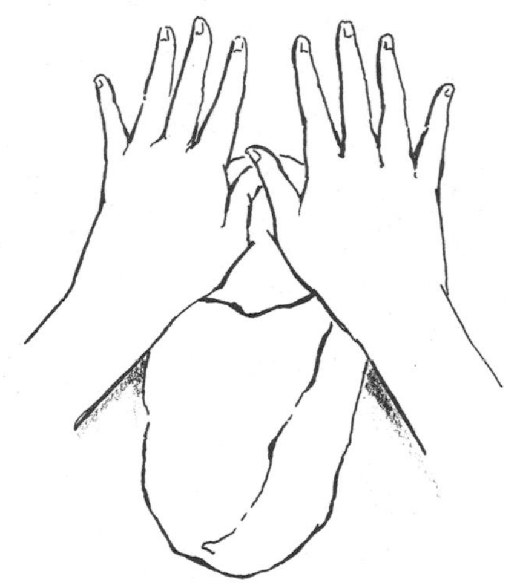

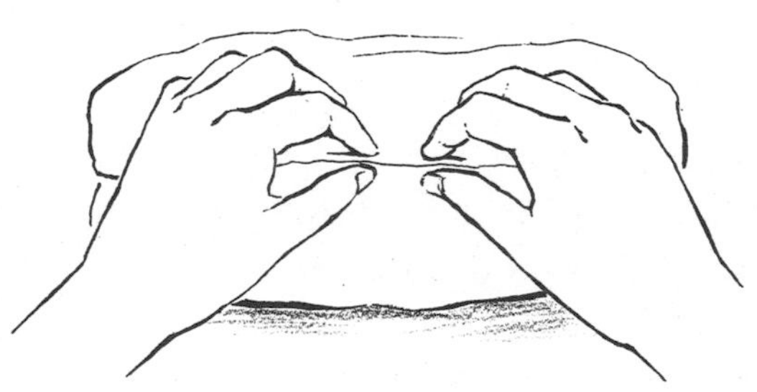

the dough tightly towards you, rounding and shaping the loaf as you roll. Press the ends together to seal them as well as the bottom seam, using your fingertips. Lift the dough into the loaf pan, pressing it if necessary to fill out the pan.

Lightly cover the completed loaves with lightly oiled plastic wrap (so they won't stick to the plastic as they rise). Place the loaves in a draft-free spot to rise. It is best not to use the oven you will be baking in this time, as you would need to remember to remove the loaves when you preheat the oven halfway through their proofing.

To Form Rolls

Line baking sheets with baking paper or lightly spray them with lecithin spray.

Form your rolls with as little handling as possible. Otherwise you will again activate the gluten, which makes further shaping very difficult. If you have made unusually shaped rolls and want to redo them, let the dough rest for 10 minutes, lightly covered with plastic wrap, before you try again.

Rolls come in all shapes and sizes from simple to complex. At the bakery we do a simple shape, our current favorite being a 7-inch rope tied in a knot with the ends concealed in the middle.

It is important when rolling out a rope of dough for shaping to use no flour on the work surface. If there is more than just the flour on your hands, the dough just flops around and refuses to stretch out for more than a couple of inches.

The advantage of simple shapes with rolls (especially with whole wheat bread) is that simple shapes, without intricate turns and twists, minimize the amount of crust and maximize the amount of soft interior.

Place formed rolls on prepared baking sheets. Cover them lightly with a piece of lightly oiled plastic and let them rise in a draft-free spot until almost doubled in size.

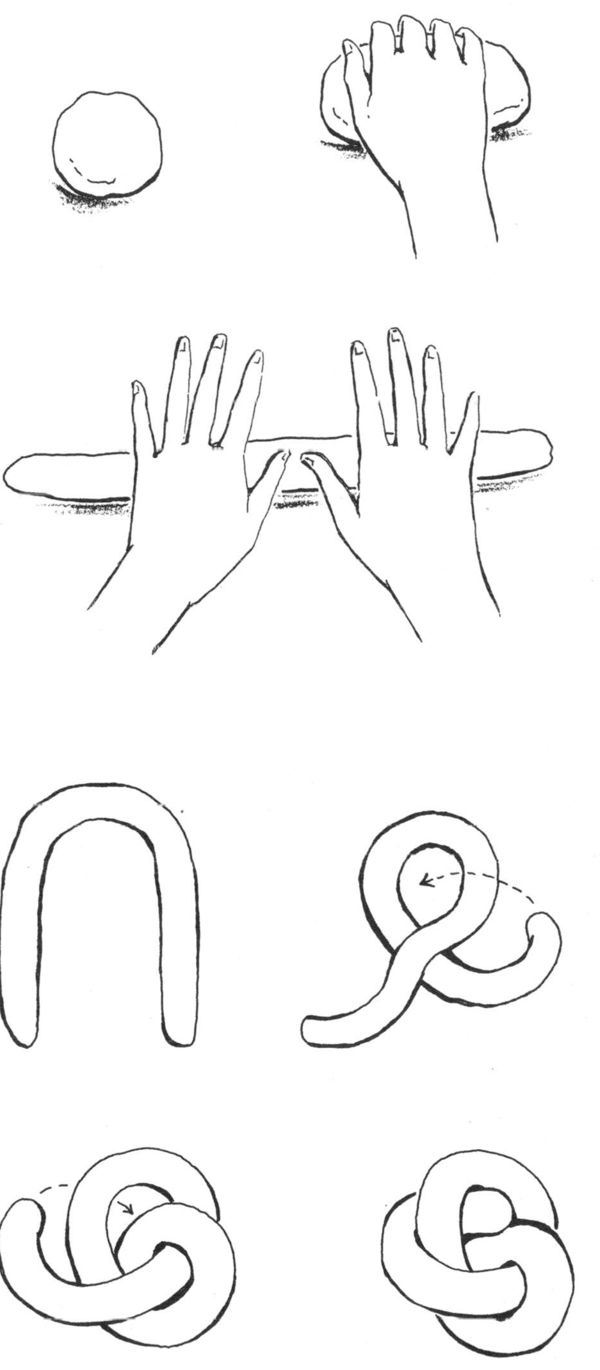

Baking the Bread

Be sure to preheat the oven 15 minutes before you will need it, about halfway through the rising of the shaped loaves or rolls. The loaves or rolls will be ready to be baked when they have a spring to them when touched lightly with your finger. Do not poke the dough this time or you will deflate your loaf and you will need to reshape it. Loaves should also have risen over the edge of the pans, doming in the center.

You may wish to glaze the loaves or rolls with an egg wash (made by combining a whole egg with a pinch of salt and ¼ cup of water) before placing them in the oven. After brushing with the egg wash, you can sprinkle on poppy seeds or sesame seeds for extra flavor, texture, and appearance.

To keep well-kneaded dough from bursting at its sides in the oven, it is wise to use a serrated knife to slash the tops of the loaves on the diagonal.

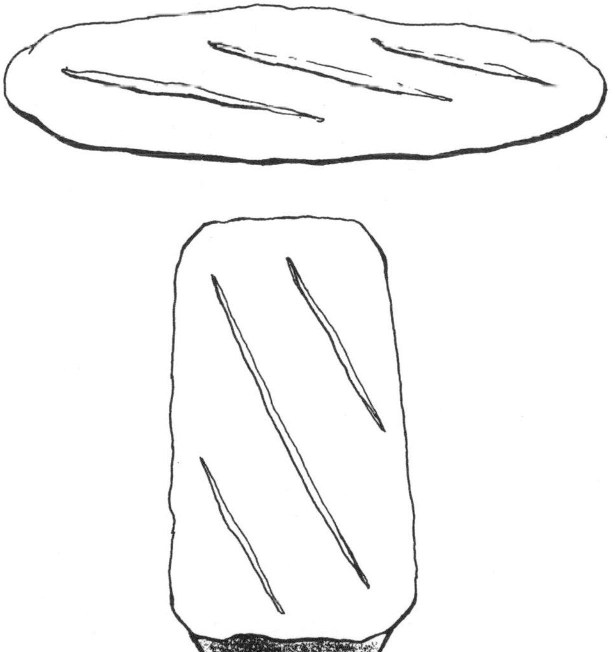

Place the loaves or rolls on the middle shelf in a preheated oven and bake according to the instructions in the individual recipes. Large loaves usually take from 40 to 60 minutes; small rolls require half that amount of time.

You may open the oven door to check on your bread after half of the baking time has elapsed. If your oven cooks unevenly, you may need to adjust the placement of the loaves or rolls for even browning. Close the oven door as soon as possible to minimize the loss of heat.

Your bread is done when it easily slips out of the loaf pans; has a deep, rich-colored crust; feels firm to the touch when you gently squeeze the long sides of the loaf; and responds with a hollow sound when you tap on the bottom of the loaf. Rolls are done when they are golden brown on their tops and slightly more golden on their bottoms.

Place the hot loaves or rolls onto a wire rack for cooling. Be sure to let the bread or rolls cool completely before wrapping them. And, if you can wait, it is much easier to cut fresh bread after it has cooled completely. For the best results, use either a serrated knife or an electric knife for slicing bread.

Some breads, like French bread, are best if served hot from the oven or on the same day they are baked. Other breads, such as egg bread and whole wheat, keep well for a number of days. Most breads freeze well. However, they are best eaten reheated from the oven or as toast, as the freezing process tends to dry them out.

Baker's Tips

- Activating the yeast with a little sweetener and warm water from the recipe before adding it to the other ingredients is very important if you are uncertain about the freshness of your yeast. If the yeast fails to become bubbly and fragrant after 5 minutes and you know that your liquid was not too warm to have killed the yeast, then you have saved yourself from making a brick. Begin again with different, fresher, and, hopefully, more active yeast.

- The rising process for bread can be slowed down considerably by placing the dough in the refrigerator overnight. Weight down the dough, which is still in its lightly oiled bowl and covered with plastic wrap, by placing a couple of heavy cans directly on the plastic wrap. Until the dough has chilled all the way through, it will continue to be active, so it will be necessary to punch the dough down once or twice during the first few hours in the refrigerator. The next day when you are able to work with the dough again, remove the dough from the refrigerator at least a couple of hours before you are ready to begin. Remove the weights and let the dough return to room temperature to reactivate the yeast before you start to work with it.

Crusty French Bread

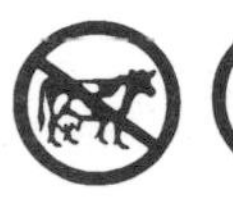 *

Yield:
2 large loaves, 14 inches long
6 small loaves, 6 inches long
2¼ pounds of dough

This is the fabulous recipe for the Crusty French Bread that has been served with dinner at The Ranch Kitchen for the past 10 years. We serve our French Bread right from the oven, so it has the crustiest crust and the softest and chewiest inside. If you can't serve it right away, French Bread can be reheated for 5 minutes at 350° F. However, remember that all French-type breads are at their best when eaten the same day they are baked.

If there is any leftover bread, it can be stored in the freezer for up to 2 months. It can then be sliced for wonderful French toast or garlic bread, or diced for Crisp Croutons (page 45).

½ cup egg whites* ***(replace with water for egg-free)***
1½ cups lukewarm water
¾ tablespoon dry baker's yeast
2 teaspoons salt
4 cups unbleached white flour

For the Baking Pan

¼ cup cornmeal

To Prepare the Dough by Machine

Combine the warm water and egg whites in the bowl of an electric mixer. Mix together until a foam forms, using the dough hook attachment. With the machine on the lowest speed, stir in the yeast, salt, and 3½ cups of the flour. Once the flour is incorporated, increase the mixer speed to medium and knead the dough for about 5 to 10 minutes, adding only enough additional flour to form a soft dough that comes off both the sides and bottom of the bowl.

To Prepare the Dough by Hand

In a small bowl, stir the yeast into ¼ cup of the lukewarm water. Set the bowl aside for 5 minutes, until the yeast is bubbly. In a medium-size bowl, stir the remaining 1¼ cups lukewarm water and the egg whites with a wire whip until the mixture becomes foamy. Stir in the activated yeast, salt, and 3½ cups of the flour to make a soft dough.

Sprinkle a little flour on your work surface. Knead the dough on the work surface, adding additional flour only if necessary to keep the dough from sticking. Knead the dough for 10 to 15 minutes until it becomes smooth and quite elastic.

Raising the Dough and Forming the Loaves

Place the well-kneaded dough into a lightly oiled bowl. Cover the bowl with plastic wrap, and let the dough rise in a warm, draft-free place until it has doubled in size. Remove the plastic from the bowl and, using your fist, gently deflate the dough by punching it down. Turn the dough out onto a very lightly floured work surface.

Line the baking pans with baking paper and sprinkle with cornmeal.

Divide the dough into 2 equal portions for large loaves, or into 6 equal portions for small loaves. Using a rolling pin to roll, or your hands to pat, form each portion into a rectangle 1 inch thick. Form each rectangle into a French loaf by rolling the dough toward you along its length, using your hands to smoothly shape the loaf and to taper the ends. Then roll each loaf back and forth under your hands until it is 14 inches long for the large loaves, and 6 inches long for the smaller loaves. Place the shaped loaves seam-side down on the prepared pans. Put the loaves in a draft-free spot to rise again until they are increased half again in size.

To Bake the Loaves

Preheat the oven to 425° F and place an empty 9-inch-square pan, or its equivalent, directly on the floor of a gas oven, or on the lowest shelf of an electric oven.

When the loaves are ready to be baked, use a serrated knife to slash the tops of the loaves on a diagonal, about ½ to ¾ inch deep, just underneath the crust, not straight down (see illustration on page 31). Use a spray bottle to spray the tops and sides of the loaves with water. Place the loaves on the middle shelf of the preheated oven. As soon as the loaves are in place, pour a couple of cups of boiling water into the empty pan. Shut the door immediately to keep in as much steam as possible. By spraying the loaves with water and steaming the oven, the crust will be crisp, golden brown, and gorgeous.

Bake the small loaves for approximately 20 minutes; bake the large loaves for 25 to 30 minutes. The breads are done when they are a rich golden brown and sound hollow when tapped on the bottom. Spray the loaves again with water after removing them from the oven. Remove the loaves from the baking pan and cool them on a wire rack.

The Best Egg Bread

Yield:
Two 4-inch by 8-inch loaves
24 rolls
3 pounds of dough

Soft and velvet-textured, this is truly the best egg bread I have ever eaten. Its exquisite texture and sensational taste are especially suited for Our Famous Cinnamon Rolls (page 37) and yeasted coffee cakes, for toast and jam, and for sandwiches.

I was given this recipe by one of my college roommates, more than 20 years ago, when we used to bake bread weekly for ourselves and friends. The original recipe included sugar and was for challah (Jewish egg bread). It had been passed down in her family from her mother's South Carolina Jewish grandmother.

In Montana this egg bread has fared well also, bringing in blue ribbons at the local county and Montana state fairs for both Cinnamon Rolls and sandwich loaves.

1½ cups milk
3 tablespoons fruit sweetener
6 tablespoons softened butter
3 eggs
2 teaspoons dry baker's yeast
2 teaspoons salt
5 to 5¼ cups unbleached white flour

Garnish for Rolls

Egg Wash for Bread (page 45)
Poppy or sesame seeds (optional)

To Prepare the Dough by Machine

In a small saucepan, scald the milk with the fruit sweetener over medium heat. Combine the milk, sweetener, and softened butter in the bowl of an electric mixer. With the mixer on the lowest speed, use the dough hook to mix until the butter has melted and the milk and sweetener have cooled to lukewarm. Now that there is no danger of cooking the eggs, add them, the yeast, the salt, and 5 cups of the flour to form a soft dough. Increase the mixer speed to medium and knead the dough for 5 to 10 minutes, adding only enough additional flour to form a medium-stiff dough that comes off both the sides and bottom of the bowl.

To Prepare the Dough by Hand

Scald the milk. Pour ¼ cup of the scalded milk into a small bowl with 1 tablespoon of the sweetener. When the milk has cooled to lukewarm, stir in the yeast. Set the bowl aside until the yeast is bubbly, about 5 minutes.

Meanwhile, pour the remaining 1¼ cups of scalded milk into a medium-size bowl with the softened butter and 2 tablespoons of the sweetener. When the butter has melted and the milk has cooled to lukewarm, use a whisk to stir in the eggs, the salt, and the activated yeast. Switch to a wooden spoon or your hand and stir in 5 cups of the flour to form a medium-soft dough.

Sprinkle a little flour on your work surface. Knead the dough, adding additional flour only if necessary to keep the dough from sticking. Knead the dough for 10 to 15 minutes, until it becomes smooth and quite elastic.

Raising the Dough and Forming the Loaves or Rolls

Place the well-kneaded dough in a lightly oiled bowl. Cover the bowl with plastic wrap, and let the dough rise in a warm, draft-free place until doubled in size. Remove the plastic from the bowl, and using your fist, gently deflate the dough by punching it down. Knead the dough in the bowl about 10 times. Cover the bowl with plastic wrap and again let the dough rise until doubled. Punch the dough down and turn it out onto a very lightly floured surface.

Form the dough into 2 loaves or 24 rolls, or a combination of both. Place the loaves into bread pans and the rolls onto a baking-paper lined baking sheet. Place the rolls 3 inches apart to allow room for them to spread while they rise. Lightly cover the bread and/or rolls with an oiled piece of plastic, and let the formed dough rise until almost doubled in size.

To Bake the Loaves or Rolls

Preheat the oven to 350° F.

For loaves, use a serrated knife to make a diagonal slash across the top of the loaves. Place them on the middle shelf of the preheated oven, and bake for 40 to 45 minutes. The tops will be golden, and the bread will slide easily out of the baking pan when the loaves are done. Give the bottom of the loaf a tap. It should sound hollow. Let the loaves cool out of their pans on a wire rack.

For rolls, prepare the Egg Wash (page 45). Lightly brush the tops of each roll with the Egg Wash and sprinkle them with either poppy or sesame seeds, or leave them plain. Bake the rolls on the middle shelf of the preheated oven for 20 to 25 minutes. The rolls are done when they are a beautiful golden brown on their tops and bottoms. Remove the rolls from the baking pan and cool them on a wire rack.

Baker's Tips

• Scalding milk means to heat it to the point where tiny bubbles form around the edge where the milk touches the pot, and a skin forms on the top of the milk. Scalding milk neutralizes two of its proteins, which would otherwise weaken the gluten. After scalding it is always necessary to cool the milk to lukewarm before adding the yeast.

• Monarch rolls—a Ranch Kitchen exclusive. These fancifully shaped rolls came about the first year of the restaurant. I was asked to make kaiser rolls for a grilled chicken sandwich. Nowhere could I find the technique for forming kaiser rolls. Trying from memory to duplicate them was not exactly working. The closest I came was a "kaiser-like" shape with an extra twist on top. And as kaiser is another name for a

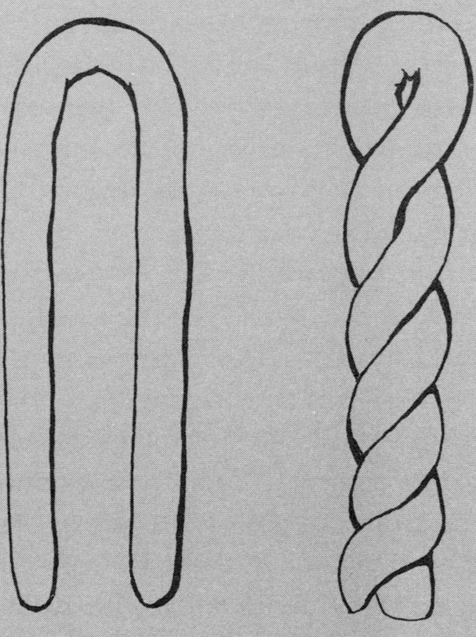

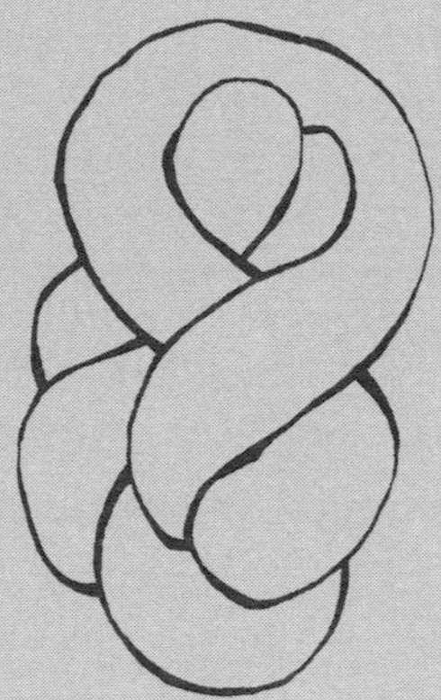

king, I called my creation "monarchs." Somehow the name stuck, and to this day we continue to make monarch rolls exclusively at The Ranch Kitchen.

To form monarch rolls in your own kitchen, use the Best Egg Bread recipe. Divide the dough into 12 portions. Form each portion into a rope 20 inches long. Form a horseshoe shape with the rope and twist the ends around themselves 4 or 5 times. Then bring the two ends up and poke them through the top loop. Place them on a baking sheet to rise. After the monarchs have doubled in size, brush them with egg wash and sprinkle them with sesame seeds. Bake until golden brown, 25 to 30 minutes.

Our Famous Cinnamon Rolls

Yield:
9 huge rolls

These incomparable cinnamon rolls have been famous since before the first day The Ranch Kitchen opened its doors! And they are so lovely, I've been tempted to rename them Cinnamon Roses.

Back in 1982, when I was first shown the proposed menu for The Ranch Kitchen, it had "Our Famous Cinnamon Rolls" listed under breakfast items. I said, "Great. Let me see the recipe." I was told, "They still have to be developed, but we would like to be famous for our cinnamon rolls." So for a week I made a new and improved version daily, until one day, the manager exclaimed, "Now these are famous cinnamon rolls!" The only thing that has changed in the recipe over the years has been the sweetener—from brown and white sugars, to fructose, to maple sugar, and now to fruit sweetener. As liquid fruit sweetener makes a softer filling than a dry sweetener, it is best to prepare the cinnamon roll filling the day before you need it and to refrigerate it overnight. Always use the filling directly from the refrigerator so it is easier to work with.

Locals as well as hunters and tourists from all over North America come to the restaurant to start their day with one of these huge, irresistible cinnamon rolls. So we can truly call them Our Famous Cinnamon Rolls.

Cinnamon rolls are at their most delicious when served hot from the oven.

1 recipe Best Egg Bread (page 34)

Cinnamon Roll Filling

1 cup walnuts
3/4 cup raisins
1 cup fruit sweetener
1/4 cup butter, softened
2 tablespoons cinnamon
3 tablespoons flour

Cinnamon Roll Glaze

1/4 cup non-instant dry milk powder
2 1/2 tablespoons unsweetened apple juice
3/4 cup fruit sweetener
1/4 teaspoon vanilla extract
1/8 teaspoon almond extract

The night before, or up to a couple of weeks before, prepare the Cinnamon Roll Filling. Toast the walnuts in a 350° F oven for 7 to 10 minutes. Allow the nuts to cool, then process them in a food processor, using a pulsing action, until coarsely chopped.

Bring 1 cup of water to a boil and add the raisins. When the water returns to the boil, turn off the heat. Let the raisins plump in the water for 10 minutes. Drain the raisins, saving any raisin water for another use. Store the raisins in the refrigerator until needed.

Use an electric mixer to cream the sweetener and butter until well mixed. Stir in the cinnamon and flour and then the coarsely chopped toasted walnuts. Make sure this mixture is refrigerated before using. Otherwise it is a bit messy to work with.

Prepare the Egg Bread according to the recipe directions. After the dough has risen a second time, roll it into a rectangle that measures 18 inches by 20 inches. Cover the rectangle evenly with the chilled Cinnamon Roll Filling, leaving a 1/2-inch to 3/4-inch space at the top of the rectangle without filling. (This will facilitate rolling and sealing the roll.)

Sprinkle the plumped raisins evenly over the filling.

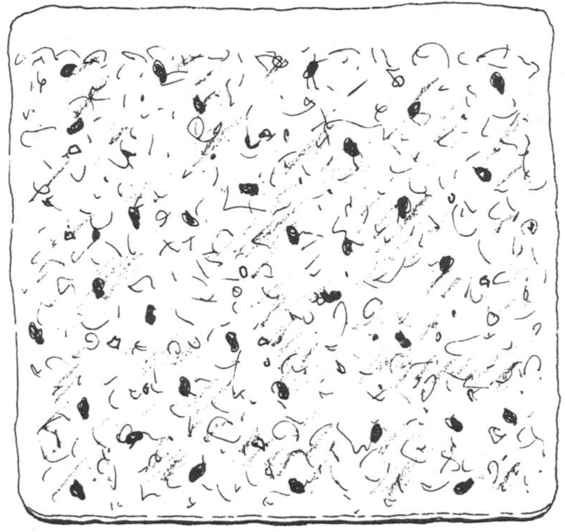

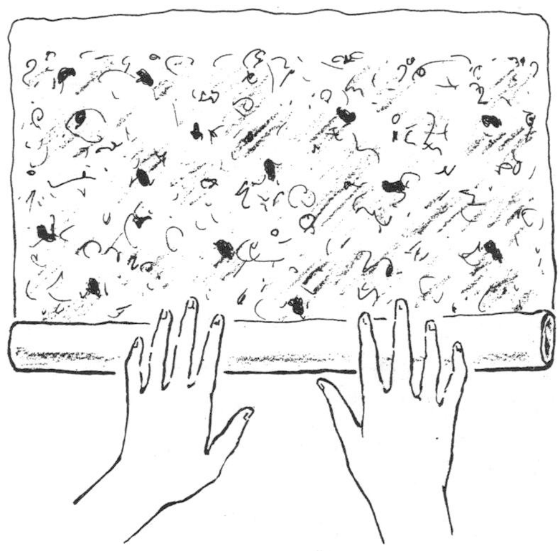

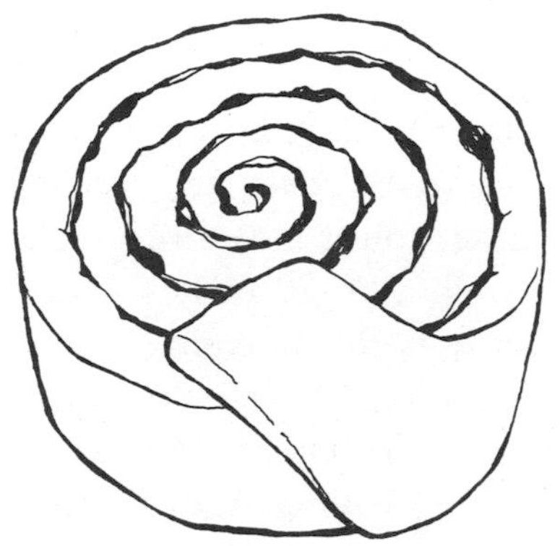

Beginning at the side closest to you, make a very tight roll all along the length of the rectangle to make a well-formed spiral in the center of each roll. Continue to roll the dough tightly, rolling it away from you. When you have finished rolling, move the roll closer to you and place the seam side down. Using a serrated edge knife, cut the roll into 9 equal portions. Lift up each roll and tuck the loose end under the bottom. Place the cinnamon rolls 1 inch apart on a paper-lined baking sheet. If the rolls are farther apart from one another they will spread out too much and lose their compact shape.

Cover the rolls lightly with an oiled piece of plastic and let them rise until almost doubled.

Preheat the oven to 350° F. Bake the Cinnamon Rolls on the middle shelf of the oven for 25 to 30 minutes, until golden brown and slightly crusty.

While the Cinnamon Rolls are baking, prepare the Cinnamon Roll Glaze. Use your food processor or blender to combine the dry milk and apple juice until lump-free. Stir in the fruit sweetener and extracts.

Generously brush the Cinnamon Rolls with the Cinnamon Roll Glaze while they are still hot from the oven.

Cinnamon Rolls are at their absolute best within the first couple of hours after baking.

Baker's Tip

- If you would prefer to make smaller Cinnamon Rolls, roll the dough 24 inches long and 12 inches wide. Follow the instructions for filling and rolling the dough. Then cut the roll into 15 equal portions. Follow the instructions for the final proofing of the rolls and their baking, reducing the baking time to 20 to 25 minutes.

Golden Carrot Bread

 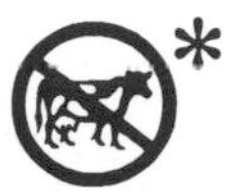*

Yield:
Two 4-inch by 8-inch loaves
20 rolls
3 pounds of dough

This exciting Golden Carrot Bread is not only light, delicious, and beautiful but also dairy-free and egg-free. With its soft, almost cakelike texture, this delectable bread seems to be a universal favorite.

Be sure to make an extra loaf, as Golden Carrot Bread is excellent made into croutons (page 45) for soups and salads.

3 medium-size carrots
2 cups water
2½ teaspoons dry baker's yeast
2 teaspoons fruit sweetener
⅓ cup lukewarm water
½ cup butter* ***(substitute margarine for dairy-free)***
⅓ cup fruit sweetener
⅔ teaspoon salt
5 to 6 cups unbleached white flour

Peel and slice the carrots. Cook them with the 2 cups of water in a small covered pot until soft. Drain the carrots, reserving ¾ cup of the cooking water. Purée the carrots and the reserved cooking water in a blender or food processor.

Stir the yeast and 2 teaspoons of sweetener into the ⅓ cup lukewarm water. Set aside until the yeast is bubbly, about 5 minutes.

To Prepare the Dough by Machine

Melt the butter or margarine and combine it with the remaining ⅓ cup of sweetener, the puréed carrots, and the salt in the bowl of an electric mixer. When the mixture is lukewarm, use the dough hook to stir in the activated yeast and 5 cups of the flour to form a medium-soft dough. Once the flour is incorporated, increase the mixer speed to medium and knead the dough for 5 to 7 minutes, adding only enough additional flour to form a dough that comes off both the sides and bottom of the bowl.

To Prepare the Dough by Hand

Melt the margarine or butter and combine it with the remaining ⅓ cup of sweetener, the puréed carrots, and the salt in a medium bowl. When the mixture is lukewarm, stir in the activated yeast and 5 cups of the flour to form a medium-soft dough.

Sprinkle a little flour on your work surface. Turn out the dough onto your table and knead it, adding additional flour only if necessary to keep the dough from sticking. Knead the dough for 10 to 15 minutes, until it becomes smooth and quite elastic.

Raising the Dough and Forming the Loaves or Rolls

Place the well-kneaded dough in a lightly oiled bowl. Cover the bowl with plastic and let the dough rise in a warm, draft-free place until doubled. Remove the plastic from the bowl and, using your fist, gently deflate the dough by punching it down. Knead the dough in the bowl 8 to 10 times. Cover the bowl with plastic wrap and again let the dough rise until doubled. Punch the dough down and turn it out onto a *very* lightly floured surface.

Form the dough into 2 loaves or 20 rolls, or a combination of both. Place the loaves into standard-size bread pans, and rolls onto baking-paper-lined baking sheets. Place the rolls 3 inches apart to allow room for them to spread as they rise. Lightly cover the bread and/or rolls with an oiled piece of plastic, and let the formed dough rise until doubled in size.

Preheat the oven to 350° F.

For loaves, use a serrated knife to make a diagonal slash across the tops of the loaves. Place them on the middle shelf in the preheated oven, and bake for 45 to 50 minutes. The tops will be a golden brown and the bread will slide easily out of the baking pans when the loaves are done. Give the bottom of the loaf a tap. It should sound hollow. Let the loaves cool out of their pans on a wire rack.

For rolls, bake them for 25 minutes until they are golden brown. Remove the rolls from the baking pan and cool them on a wire rack.

The Ranch Kitchen Whole Wheat Bread

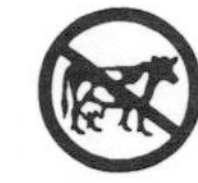

Yield:
Two 4-inch by 8-inch loaves
24 rolls
3¼ pounds of dough

The Ranch Kitchen Whole Wheat Bread is another blue ribbon winner at our local county fair. This full-flavored, well-textured whole wheat bread has been a Ranch Kitchen favorite since 1982. We bake it fresh daily for sandwiches, dinner rolls, and, most recently, for Cinnamon Swirl Raisin Bread (page 42).

⅞ cup cold raisin water (page 19)
⅞ cup hot water
2 tablespoons unsulphured molasses
¼ cup oil
2 tablespoons dry baker's yeast
1 tablespoon salt
3 eggs
5 to 6 cups whole wheat flour

Garnish for Rolls

Egg Wash for Breads (page 45)
Sesame seeds or poppy seeds (optional)

To Prepare the Dough by Machine

Combine the cold raisin water with the hot water so that the mixture is lukewarm. Pour it into the bowl of your electric mixer.

Add the molasses, oil, yeast, salt, and eggs. On the lowest speed, use the dough hook to stir in 5 cups of the whole wheat flour to form a medium-soft dough. Once the flour is incorporated, increase the mixer speed to medium and knead the dough for 5 to 10 minutes, adding only enough additional flour to form a medium-stiff dough that comes off both the sides and bottom of the bowl.

To Prepare the Dough by Hand

Combine ¼ cup of the hot water with 1 tablespoon of the molasses in a small bowl. When the mixture is lukewarm, stir in the yeast. Set the bowl aside until the yeast is bubbly, about 5 minutes.

Meanwhile, mix together the raisin water, the remaining 10 tablespoons hot water, the remaining 1 tablespoon molasses, the oil, salt, and eggs. Stir in the activated yeast and 5 cups of the whole wheat flour to form a medium-soft dough.

Sprinkle a little bit of flour on your work surface. Knead the dough, adding additional flour only if necessary to keep the dough from sticking. Knead the dough for 15 to 20 minutes, until it becomes smooth and elastic.

Raising the Dough and Forming the Loaves or Rolls

Place the well-kneaded dough in a lightly oiled bowl. Cover the bowl with plastic wrap, and let the dough rise in a warm, draft-free place until doubled in size. Remove the plastic from the bowl, and using your fist, gently deflate the dough by punching it down. Knead the dough in the bowl about 10 times. Cover the bowl with plastic wrap and again let the dough rise until doubled. Punch the dough down and turn it out onto a very lightly floured surface.

Form the dough into 2 loaves or 24 rolls, or a combination of both. Place the loaves into standard-size bread pans, and the rolls onto baking-paper-lined baking sheets. Place the rolls 3 inches apart to allow room for them to spread as they rise. Lightly cover the bread and/or rolls with an oiled piece of plastic, and let them rise until doubled in size.

To Bake the Loaves or Rolls

Preheat the oven to 350° F.

For loaves, use a serrated knife to make diagonal slashes across the tops of the loaves. Place them on the middle shelf of the preheated oven, and bake for 40 to 45 minutes. The tops will be a deep brown, and the bread will slide easily out of the baking pan when the loaves are done. Give the bottom of the loaf a tap. It should sound hollow. Let the loaves cool out of their pans on a wire rack.

For rolls, prepare the Egg Wash (page 45). Lightly brush the tops of each roll with the Egg Wash and sprinkle them with either poppy or sesame seeds, or leave them plain. Bake the rolls on the middle shelf of the preheated oven for 20 to 25 minutes. The rolls are done when they are a deep brown on their tops and bottoms. Remove the rolls from the baking pan and cool them on a wire rack.

Whole Wheat Cinnamon Swirl Raisin Bread

*

Yield:
Two 8-inch by 4-inch loaves
Five 6-inch by 3-inch loaves
3¾ pounds of dough

Dramatic Cinnamon Swirl Raisin Bread was my favorite bread as a child. I just loved it toasted, with all those raisins everywhere. And best of all, that delicious spiral of cinnamon in the center of each slice—such a miracle. I always wondered why every loaf of bread didn't have such a swirl in its center. I remember on more than one occasion trying to eat just the spiral, leaving the rest of the bread for the ducks at a nearby pond. . . .

Oh, so delightful to be able to reproduce that spiral and delicious perfume of cinnamon. This bread seems perfect for giving to friends, especially when made into small, individual-size loaves.

Dough

2 cups raisins
⅞ cup hot raisin water
⅞ cup cool water
¼ cup fruit sweetener
¼ cup oil
2 tablespoons dry baker's yeast
3 eggs
1 tablespoon salt
5 to 6 cups whole wheat flour

Cinnamon Swirl

¼ cup fruit sweetener
1½ tablespoons cinnamon

For the Finished Loaves

Softened butter* ***(omit or substitute margarine for dairy-free)***

Begin by plumping the raisins and preparing the raisin water. Bring 2 cups of water to a boil in a small pan. Add 2 cups of raisins and turn off the heat, letting the raisins sit in the water for at least 10 minutes. Drain the raisins, saving the raisin water.

To Prepare the Dough by Machine

Measure the hot raisin water and combine it with the cool water so that the mixture is lukewarm. Pour it into the bowl of your electric mixer. Add the fruit sweetener, oil, yeast, eggs, and salt. Stir in 5 cups of the whole wheat flour. On the lowest speed, use the dough hook to form a medium-soft dough. Once the flour is incorporated, increase the mixer speed to medium and knead the dough for 5 to 10 minutes, adding only enough additional flour to form a medium-stiff dough that comes off both the sides and bottom of the bowl. Reduce the speed to low, and gently knead in the plumped raisins.

To Prepare the Dough by Hand

Combine ¼ cup of the hot raisin water with 1 tablespoon of the fruit sweetener in a small bowl. When the mixture is lukewarm, stir in the yeast. Set the bowl aside until the yeast is bubbly, about 5 minutes.

Meanwhile, mix together the remaining 10 tablespoons of raisin water, the cool water, the remaining 1 tablespoon fruit sweetener, the oil, eggs, and salt. Stir in the activated yeast and 5 cups of the whole wheat flour to form a medium-soft dough.

Sprinkle a little flour on your work surface.

Knead the dough, adding additional flour only if necessary to keep the dough from sticking. After 10 minutes of kneading, gently knead in the plumped raisins. Continue to knead the dough for another 5 minutes until it becomes smooth and quite elastic.

Raising the Dough and Forming the Loaves

Place the well-kneaded dough in a lightly oiled bowl. Cover the bowl with plastic wrap, and let the dough rise in a warm, draft-free place until doubled in size. Remove the plastic from the bowl and, using your fist, gently deflate the dough by punching it down. Knead the dough in the bowl about 10 times. Cover the bowl with plastic wrap and again let the dough rise until doubled. Punch the dough down and turn it out onto a very lightly floured surface.

Divide the dough into the number and size of loaves you want to make. Use a rolling pin to roll each portion of dough into a square ⅓ inch thick.

Combine the Cinnamon Swirl ingredients in a small bowl or cup, stirring with a fork until the cinnamon is totally mixed with the fruit sweetener. Use a pastry brush to spread the cinnamon mixture thickly onto each square of dough. Roll each square up tightly, jelly-roll fashion, pinching the bottom seam and side edges well to seal each loaf. Place the finished loaves in lightly oiled bread pans. Cover the pans lightly with a piece of oiled plastic, and let the loaves rise until they are about 1½ inches above the top of the pans.

To Bake the Loaves

Preheat the oven to 350° F.

Place the loaves on the middle shelf of the preheated oven. Bake the large loaves for 45 to 60 minutes, and the smaller loaves for 30 to 35 minutes. The tops will be a rich brown, and the bread will slide easily out of the baking pan when the loaves are done. Give the bottom of the loaf a tap. It should sound hollow. When the loaves have finished baking, rub their tops with softened butter to tenderize the crust and add shine and flavor. Place the finished loaves on a wire rack to cool.

Squaw Bread

 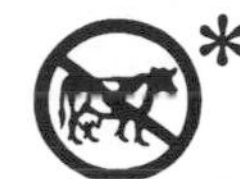*

Yield:
2 round loaves
4 pounds of dough

A few years ago we spent some time developing a few fabulous varieties of bread to serve in our dinner bread basket. This full-bodied classic Squaw Bread is one of our favorites. Multigrained Squaw Bread is a well-balanced, not-too-sweet dinner bread. Adding raisins makes any bread a special treat and Squaw Bread is no exception. It makes excellent toast and sandwiches, as well as dinner rolls.

1¼ cups raisin water (page 19)
½ cup raisins
Approximately 1 cup lukewarm water
2 tablespoons dry baker's yeast
½ cup fruit sweetener
⅓ cup oil
3 cups unbleached white flour
1 tablespoon salt
1 cup rye flour
2 to 3 cups whole wheat flour

For the Baking Pan

¼ cup cornmeal

For the Finished Loaves

Softened butter* ***(omit or substitute margarine for dairy-free)***

First, plump the raisins by bringing 1¼ cups of water to a boil and adding ½ cup raisins. Turn off the heat and let the raisins sit in the water for at least 10 minutes. Drain the raisins, saving the raisin water. Add only enough lukewarm water to the raisin water to make a total of 2¼ cups. Put the raisins aside.

Stir the yeast and sweetener into the 2¼ cups water. Let this mixture sit for 5 minutes, until the yeast is bubbly.

To Prepare the Dough by Machine

Combine the oil, unbleached white flour, salt, rye flour, and 2 cups of the whole wheat flour in the mixing bowl of an electric mixer. Stir in the activated yeast. Once the flour is incorporated, increase the mixer speed to medium. Use the dough hook to knead the dough for about 10 minutes, adding only enough additional flour to form a medium-stiff dough that comes off both the sides and bottom of the bowl. Reduce the speed and gently knead in the raisins.

To Prepare the Dough by Hand

Combine the oil, unbleached flour, salt, rye flour, and 2 cups of the whole wheat flour in a medium-size mixing bowl. Use a wooden spoon to stir in the activated yeast. Mix all together to form a medium-soft dough. Sprinkle a little whole wheat flour on your work surface. Knead the dough, adding additional flour only if necessary to keep the dough from sticking. Knead the dough for 15 to 20 minutes, until it becomes smooth and quite elastic.

Raising the Dough and Forming the Loaves

Place the well-kneaded dough in a lightly oiled bowl. Cover the bowl with plastic wrap, and let the dough rise in a warm, draft-free place until doubled. Remove the plastic from the bowl and, using your fist, gently deflate the dough by punching it down. Knead the dough in the bowl about 10 times. Cover the bowl with plastic wrap and again let the dough rise until doubled in size. Punch the dough down and turn it out onto a very lightly floured surface.

Divide the dough in half. Knead each half 8 to 10 times. Turn the dough over and, by placing your fingers on the bottom of the dough and your thumbs on the top, "cup" each half to form 2 round loaves. Place them on a cornmeal-sprinkled, baking paper-lined pan. Put the loaves in a draft-free spot to proof until doubled in size.

Preheat the oven to 350° F. With a serrated knife, cut a cross on the top of each loaf. Bake the loaves in the preheated oven for 45 to 50 minutes.

When the loaves are removed from the oven, brush their tops with softened butter.

Crisp Croutons

Yield:
4 cups

Crisp Croutons are an excellent use for leftover bread. Their satisfying crunch and distinctive flavor transform salads and soups into textural treats. Cut the bread into ⅜-inch cubes and flavor them with a variety of dried herbs according to your own taste or, as we do at the restaurant, with thyme, basil, and oregano. Croutons freeze very well and defrost in a couple of minutes, so don't be concerned about making too many.

6 tablespoons olive oil or melted butter
1 teaspoon dried ground thyme
1 tablespoon dried basil
1 tablespoon dried oregano
Few twists freshly ground black pepper
Pinch salt
4 cups cubed bread

Preheat the oven to 325° F. Stir the herbs and seasonings into the olive oil or melted butter. In a large bowl, drizzle the oil or butter mixture over the cubed bread, tossing to mix well. Spread the cubes in a single layer on a paper-lined baking pan. Depending on the dryness of the bread, bake for 10 to 30 minutes in the preheated oven. Stir the croutons every 10 minutes so they can brown evenly. Cool the croutons before sprinkling on salads.

Croutons freeze well stored in plastic bags for many months. Stored at room temperature, croutons will keep for a couple of weeks.

Egg Wash for Bread

Yield:
1/4 cup

Egg Wash is the secret of the shiny, golden crust on all of our breads and rolls and the key to keeping sesame and poppy seeds in their place.

1 egg
Pinch salt
¼ cup water

In a small bowl or cup, use a fork to beat the egg and salt together. Stir in the water. Use a soft brush to apply the Egg Wash to rolls or loaves just before baking them.

Egg Wash can be stored in the refrigerator for 2 to 3 days if well covered.

. . . And Not: Quick Breads and Muffins

Delicious, fast, and easy to make, quick breads and muffins always make meals more special. They are often filled with chunky nuts or dates, chopped or mashed fruits, and/or grated or purēed vegetables; and they are often fragrant with spices like cinnamon and ginger. It is just these fruits, nuts, and vegetables that make muffins and quick breads so appealing and versatile. Quick breads are as wonderful hot or toasted for breakfast as they are at afternoon tea or for rounding out a light soup and salad dinner. And muffins have become so popular they now star throughout the day from their first sustaining bite in the morning to their last remaining crumb at midnight.

Quick breads gain a lot in texture by borrowing techniques usually reserved for cakes. I suggest using an electric mixer to cream the sweetener and butter or oil together until light and fluffy, and then adding the eggs one at a time. This provides a strong structure in which to fold in the remaining ingredients. The resulting breads are more tender and close-grained than if made by the muffin method.

Muffins, on the other hand, must be made by hand to give them their characteristic coarse grain and hearty, tender texture. Muffins are made by combining the sifted dry ingredients with the wet ingredients with as few movements as possible, just to moisten the flour. When the muffin batter is half-mixed, the fruit and nuts are quickly folded in. To have tender and light muffins it is important to leave the muffin batter lumpy, rather than smooth and ribbonlike as with cake batters.

Each of these muffin recipes was developed for making beautiful, large muffins in regular-size muffin pans. The muffin batters are just the right consistency for filling each muffin cup completely. This is why ice cream scoops are recommended. They give a wonderful domed top to each muffin. Because of the large size of these muffins, lightly spray the top of the pans as well as the individual muffin cups with lecithin spray to keep the muffins from sticking.

It is important to bake both muffins and quick breads in a completely preheated oven. Quick breads bake well in a 350° F oven and are done when they shrink slightly from the edge of the pan, have a most inviting aroma, and don't stick to a clean toothpick when it is inserted in the center of the loaf.

Muffins do best in a slightly hotter oven, 375° F. The oven must be hot when you put in your muffins in order to get the highest rise and best shaped muffins. Depending upon the efficiency of your oven, you may need to turn the muffin pan halfway through the baking time for even browning. The old-fashioned toothpick test doesn't work well with those muffins that have moist fruit added to them, such as blueberries and cranberries, so you will need to go by rich color and aroma. Another test that works well is to press the tops of the muffins lightly. They should spring back to your touch. If they don't, bake the muffins for another few minutes.

Cool muffins and quick breads in their baking pans for a few minutes before removing them to a wire rack to finish cooling, though both are delicious eaten hot from the oven. However, some quick breads, such as Banana and Cranberry Nut Bread, and Date Nut Bread, taste even better if you can wait at least 12 hours before slicing and eating them.

Irish Soda Bread

Yield:
2 round loaves
3 pounds of dough

It must be the crunchy outside and the tender inside, combined with the well-balanced flavor of the raisins and caraway seeds, that makes Irish Soda Bread almost everyone's favorite. When we serve this exceptional bread on our dinner theater buffet, we can barely make enough of it. And it is remarkable how many people have stories to tell from their past of just what this bread reminds them of. . . .

At The Ranch Kitchen we like to serve Irish Soda Bread hot, cut into 8 to 10 wedges per loaf, as an accompaniment to soups, stews, and salads.

Irish Soda Bread is best stored at room temperature, well wrapped in plastic.

Fruit and Seeds

¾ cup raisins
4 teaspoons caraway seeds

Dry Ingredients

¾ cup cold butter
5 cups unbleached white flour
1 teaspoon baking soda
1½ teaspoons baking powder
¾ teaspoon salt

Wet Ingredients

6 tablespoons fruit sweetener
1⅓ cups buttermilk
2 eggs

Begin by plumping the raisins. Bring 1 cup of water to a boil and add the raisins. When the water returns to the boil, turn off the heat. Let the raisins plump in the water for at least 10 minutes. Drain the raisins, saving any raisin water for another use. Set the raisins aside.

Preheat the oven to 350° F. Lightly spray a baking sheet with lecithin spray, or line it with baking paper.

Cut the cold butter into ½-inch pieces. Sift the dry ingredients together into a medium-size bowl or the mixing bowl for your electric mixer. With the mixer on its lowest speed, use the paddle attachment or your beaters to cut the cold butter into the dry ingredients, until the mixture resembles coarse cornmeal. Stir in the plumped raisins and the caraway seeds.

In a small bowl, whisk together the sweetener, buttermilk, and eggs and add to the flour mixture. Stir together on medium-low speed just until mixed.

Place the dough on a lightly floured work surface. Divide it into 2 equal portions. Knead each portion 8 to 10 times, and form into a round loaf, 8 inches in diameter. Place the loaves on the prepared baking pan. Use a serrated knife to cut a ½-inch-deep cross on the top of each loaf. Place the loaves on the middle shelf in the preheated oven, and bake for 40 to 50 minutes until golden brown and crusty.

Remove the loaves to a wire rack to cool. Irish Soda Bread is wonderful served hot from the oven.

Cornbread

Yield:
9-inch-square pan
9 to 12 servings

Light, fluffy, golden yellow Cornbread is a most welcome and satisfying treat with salads, soups, and stews. In the delicious Ranch Kitchen version, we will sometimes fold in a cup of fresh shucked or defrosted frozen corn for an even livelier taste. Cornbread has the perfect texture when it is eaten hot from the oven. It can be stored for 2 days at room temperature if well wrapped.

Wet Ingredients

5 tablespoons butter, softened
2 tablespoons fruit sweetener
3 eggs
1¼ cups buttermilk

Dry Ingredients

¾ teaspoon baking powder
¾ teaspoon baking soda
¼ teaspoon salt
1 cup unbleached white flour
1⅛ cups cornmeal

Preheat the oven to 350° F. Spray a 9-inch-square pan with lecithin spray.

With an electric mixer on medium-high speed, use the paddle attachment or beaters to cream the softened butter and fruit sweetener until light and fluffy. Beat in the eggs, one at a time, being sure that the first egg is incorporated before the next one is added.

Sift the dry ingredients together.

Reduce the mixer speed to low. Add the sifted dry ingredients, one third at a time, alternating with the buttermilk.

Pour the batter into the prepared 9-inch-square pan. Place the pan on the middle shelf of the preheated oven and bake for 30 to 35 minutes. When done, the cornbread will be a rich golden yellow and will spring back when touched lightly in its center.

Cool the cornbread in its pan on a wire rack. Cornbread is great eaten hot from the oven. It is best stored at room temperature, well wrapped in plastic.

Zucchini Bread

Yield:
9-inch-square pan
9 to 12 servings

A well-balanced, savory bread with a cake-like texture, Zucchini Bread is especially delectable served warm from the oven. Zucchini Bread provides a perfect answer to that familiar query each year during peak zucchini growing season.

Wet Ingredients

2¼ cups grated and drained zucchini (see below)
¼ cup "zucchini water" (see below)
⅓ cup fruit sweetener
¾ cup oil
3 eggs
1 tablespoon vanilla extract

Dry Ingredients

¾ cup walnuts
2⅓ cups unbleached white flour
4 teaspoons cinnamon
¾ teaspoon nutmeg
1 teaspoon baking soda
¾ teaspoon baking powder
½ teaspoon salt

Preheat the oven to 350° F. Lightly spray a 9-inch-square pan with lecithin spray.

Toast the walnuts in the oven for 7 to 10 minutes, stirring occasionally. Allow the nuts to cool. Then coarsely chop them with a knife or with the pulsing action in a food processor, and put them aside.

Grate the zucchini using a medium grater. Place the grated zucchini in a sieve over a bowl and use your hand to press out the extra liquid. This is the "zucchini water." Measure out ¼ cup and set aside.

Sift the dry ingredients together.

Use an electric mixer on medium-high speed to whisk the sweetener and oil together until thickened. Then add the eggs one at a time, beating well after each addition before adding the next. Reduce the speed to low and stir in the vanilla and zucchini water. On the lowest speed, add the sifted dry ingredients alternately with the grated zucchini and the toasted walnuts.

Pour the batter into the prepared pan. Place the pan on the middle shelf of the preheated oven and bake for 45 to 50 minutes. A toothpick inserted in the center of the bread will come out clean when the bread is done.

Cool the bread in its pan on a wire rack, but don't cool it too much, for Zucchini Bread is great served hot from the oven. Store it well wrapped in plastic at room temperature.

Date Nut Bread

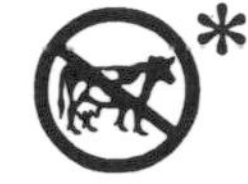
*

Yield:
Two 4-inch by 8-inch loaves

Another moist, quick, delicious tea bread that is sure to please.

1½ cups walnuts
1½ cups date pieces
½ teaspoon baking soda
½ teaspoon baking powder
½ teaspoon salt
1½ cups warm water
½ cup fruit sweetener
½ cup softened butter* ***(substitute margarine for dairy-free)***
2 eggs
3 cups unbleached white flour

Preheat the oven to 350° F. Lightly spray 2 bread pans with lecithin spray.

Toast the walnuts in the preheated oven for 7 to 10 minutes, stirring occasionally. Allow the nuts to cool, then coarsely chop them with a knife or with a pulsing action in a food processor, and put them aside.

Combine the date pieces, baking soda, baking powder, and salt in a small bowl. Stir in the warm water.

On medium speed beat the fruit sweetener and butter together until light and fluffy. Add the eggs, one at a time, beating well after each addition before adding the next. On the lowest speed, stir in the flour and then the date mixture and the toasted walnuts.

Pour the batter into the prepared pans. Place the loaves on the middle shelf of the oven, and bake for approximately 1 hour. A toothpick inserted in the center of the loaf will come out clean when the bread is done.

Cool the loaves slightly before removing them from the pans and cooling them on a wire rack. Wrap the breads in plastic wrap and let them sit for a few hours to overnight at room temperature before slicing.

Banana Nut Bread

Yield:
Two 4-inch by 8-inch loaves

This is a lovely, quick, and easily made bread. At the bakery we found that Banana Nut Bread makes sensational breakfast bread if sliced a little thicker than usual and toasted. Once you try it you will soon be purposefully forgetting your ripening bananas as an excuse to have Banana Nut Bread on hand for breakfast.

Nuts

¾ cup walnuts

Dry Ingredients

2 cups unbleached white flour
2 teaspoons baking soda
½ teaspoon baking powder
1 teaspoon cinnamon
¼ teaspoon salt

Wet Ingredients

½ cup oil
¾ cup fruit sweetener
3 eggs
2¼ teaspoons vanilla extract
¾ cup mashed bananas (1 to 2 medium-size bananas)

Preheat the oven to 350° F. Lightly spray 2 loaf pans with lecithin spray.

Toast the walnuts in the oven for 7 to 10 minutes, stirring occasionally. Allow the nuts to cool. Then coarsely chop them with a knife or with a pulsing action in a food processor. Put them aside.

Sift the dry ingredients together.

Use an electric mixer on medium speed to whisk the oil and the sweetener together until thickened, about 5 minutes. Add the eggs one at a time, beating well after each addition. Reduce the speed and stir in the vanilla and the mashed bananas.

On low speed, slowly add the sifted dry ingredients and the toasted nuts. Mix just until blended, being careful not to over-mix. Pour the batter into the prepared loaf pans. Bake the loaves on the middle shelf of the preheated oven for 45 to 60 minutes, until a toothpick inserted into the center of the loaf comes out clean.

Cool the loaves slightly before removing them from the pans and cooling them on a wire rack. When cool, wrap the breads in plastic wrap and let them sit overnight at room temperature before slicing (if you can wait).

Baker's Tip

• Quick breads, such as Banana Nut Bread, seem to improve in flavor if they are not sliced for a few hours to overnight after baking. They will also store well in the freezer for up to a month.

Cranberry Banana Walnut Bread

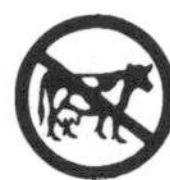

Yield:
Two 4-inch by 8-inch loaves

If you love cranberries as much as I do, you will find Cranberry Banana Walnut Bread a most satisfying quick bread, with its intriguing tart-sweet flavor and bright specks of red throughout.

Easily prepared, Cranberry Banana Walnut Bread freezes well for about a month, making it a great treat to have on hand for expected or unexpected company.

Fruit and Nuts

½ cup walnuts
1½ cups fresh or frozen cranberries

Dry Ingredients

2½ cups unbleached white flour
1 teaspoon cinnamon
1 teaspoon baking soda
1 teaspoon baking powder
½ teaspoon salt

Wet Ingredients

½ cup fruit sweetener
½ cup oil
¼ teaspoon grated orange zest
2 eggs
3 tablespoons unsweetened orange juice
½ teaspoon vanilla extract
1 cup mashed ripe bananas (1 to 2 medium-size bananas)

Preheat the oven to 350° F. Lightly spray the loaf pans with lecithin spray.

Toast the walnuts in the preheated oven for 7 to 10 minutes, stirring occasionally. Allow the nuts to cool. Then coarsely chop them with a knife or with a pulsing action in a food processor, and put them aside.

Wash and sort the cranberries. Coarsely chop them with a knife or with the pulsing action in a food processor, and put them aside.

Sift the dry ingredients together.

Use an electric mixer on medium speed to whisk together the sweetener, oil, and orange zest until thickened, about 5 minutes. Add the eggs, one at a time, beating well after each addition. Reduce the speed and stir in the orange juice, vanilla, and mashed bananas.

On low speed, slowly add the sifted dry ingredients, walnuts, and cranberries. Mix just until blended, being careful not to over-mix. Pour the batter into the prepared loaf pans. Bake the loaves on the middle shelf in the preheated oven for 50 to 60 minutes, until a toothpick inserted in the center of each loaf comes out clean.

Cool the loaves slightly before removing them from the pans and cooling them on a wire rack. Wrap the cool breads in plastic wrap and let them sit for a few hours to overnight at room temperature before slicing.

Cranapple Walnut Muffins

Yield:
10 large muffins
30 mini muffins

Delicious Cranapple Walnut Muffins are the number-one best-selling muffin at The Ranch Kitchen. Their flavor is perfectly balanced between tart and sweet, and their texture is delightfully light and crunchy.

In order to make these exceptional muffins all through the year, we freeze a lot of extra cranberries in November, making for a very special breakfast treat in the middle of July.

Fruit and Nuts

½ cup walnuts
1 cup peeled and diced apples (1 to 2 medium-size apples)
1½ cups fresh or frozen cranberries

Wet Ingredients

½ cup oil
14 tablespoons fruit sweetener
2 eggs
1 teaspoon vanilla extract
⅓ cup unsweetened applesauce

Dry Ingredients

2¾ cups unbleached white flour
1 teaspoon baking powder
1 teaspoon baking soda
1 teaspoon cinnamon
½ teaspoon nutmeg
½ teaspoon salt

Preheat the oven to 375° F. Lightly spray regular-size or mini muffin tins with lecithin.

Toast the walnuts in the oven for 7 to 10 minutes, stirring occasionally. Allow the nuts to cool. Then coarsely chop them with a knife or with a pulsing action in a food processor. Wash and sort the cranberries. Then coarsely chop them in a food processor using the pulsing action.

Whisk the wet ingredients together in the order listed until well blended. Sift together the dry ingredients into a large bowl. Make a well in the center and stir in the wet mix. When half mixed, stir in the diced apples, coarsely chopped cranberries, and toasted walnuts. Do not over-mix. The batter should remain lumpy.

Use a rounded #12 scoop (½ cup) to place the batter into the regular-size muffin pans. Use a #24 scoop (2 to 3 tablespoons) for the mini muffins.

Bake either size muffins on the middle shelf in the preheated oven. Bake the regular-size muffins for 25 to 30 minutes, and the mini muffins for 15 to 20 minutes. Turn the muffin pans once, if necessary, for the muffins to brown evenly.

Let the muffins cool in the pan for 5 minutes before removing them to a wire rack to cool completely.

Baker's Tip

• Cranberries can be frozen without any special handling. Just put them in the freezer right in the bag in which you buy them. It is best to use frozen cranberries while they are still frozen. They need to be washed with warm water (or they will clump together) and sorted for spoiled and discolored berries. Cranberries can be chopped easily in a food processor while they are still partially frozen.

Pineapple Pecan Muffins

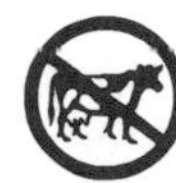

Yield:
10 large muffins
30 mini muffins

Well-balanced flavor and texture describes Pineapple Pecan Muffins perfectly.

During the first few months that we served Cranapple Walnut Muffins, they were so popular that we used cranberries at a fantastic rate. I knew we would need a stopgap measure if we were to continue to offer these muffins through October (it was then June!) when the new crop would be available. So Pineapple Pecan Muffins were created, with the refreshing tartness of crushed pineapple substituting delectably for the tartness of the cranberries. Canned, crushed pineapple must be well drained, but not so well that the fruit becomes dry.

Fruit and Nuts

½ cup pecans
1 cup peeled and diced apples
1⅔ cups canned, crushed unsweetened pineapple

Wet Ingredients

½ cup oil
14 tablespoons fruit sweetener
2 eggs
1 teaspoon vanilla extract

Dry Ingredients

2¾ cups unbleached white flour
1 teaspoon baking powder
1 teaspoon baking soda
1 teaspoon cinnamon
½ teaspoon nutmeg
½ teaspoon salt

Preheat the oven to 375° F. Lightly spray regular-size or mini muffin tins with lecithin spray.

Toast the pecans in the oven for 7 to 10 minutes, stirring occasionally. Allow the nuts to cool. Then coarsely chop them with a knife or with a pulsing action in a food processor. Drain the crushed pineapple, reserving the juice for another use.

Whisk together the wet ingredients in the order listed until well blended. Sift together the dry ingredients into a large bowl. Make a well in the center; and stir in the wet mix. When half mixed, stir in the diced apples, drained pineapple, and toasted pecans. Do not overmix. The batter should remain lumpy.

Use a rounded #12 scoop (⅓ cup) to place the batter into the regular-size muffin pans. Use a #24 scoop (2 to 3 tablespoons) for the mini muffins.

Bake either size muffins on the middle shelf in the preheated oven. Bake regular-size muffins for 25 to 30 minutes, and mini muffins for 15 to 20 minutes. Turn the muffin pans once, if necessary, for the muffins to brown evenly.

Let the muffins cool in the pan for 5 minutes before removing them to a wire rack to cool completely.

Blueberry Muffins

Yield:
12 large muffins
36 mini muffins

Not just your ordinary blueberry muffin. These are power-packed, flavor-packed, exceptional blueberry muffins: wheatless because they are made with rice flour and rolled oats instead of wheat flour; rich with sour cream and buttermilk (which could both be replaced with unsweetened applesauce for a dairyless muffin that is lower in fat and cholesterol); chunky with toasted walnuts; and fruity and flavorful with loads of blueberries, apple butter, and a bit of spice. These are extraordinary Blueberry Muffins!

Fruit and Nuts

1 cup walnuts
2 cups frozen blueberries

Wet Ingredients

1½ cups sour cream
¾ cup fruit sweetener
¼ cup apple butter
2 eggs
1 teaspoon vanilla extract
7 tablespoons buttermilk
1½ cups rolled oats
2 tablespoons butter

Dry Ingredients

2½ cups brown rice flour
1⅛ teaspoons baking soda
1⅛ teaspoons baking powder
½ teaspoon salt
1 teaspoon cinnamon

Preheat the oven to 375° F. Lightly spray regular-size or mini muffin tins with lecithin spray.

Toast the walnuts in the oven for 7 to 10 minutes, stirring occasionally. Allow the nuts to cool. Then coarsely chop them with a knife or with a pulsing action in a food processor. Set aside.

Whisk the sour cream, fruit sweetener, apple butter, eggs, vanilla, and buttermilk together in the order listed until well blended. Stir in the rolled oats. Let this mixture sit for a minimum of 5 minutes while you prepare the rest of the ingredients.

Sift together the dry ingredients into a large bowl; make a well in the center.

Melt the butter and stir it into the wet mix. Stir the wet mix into the dry mix. When half mixed, stir in the frozen blueberries and toasted walnuts, folding and stirring just until mixed. The batter will be lumpy.

Use a well-rounded #12 scoop (⅔ cup) to place the muffin batter in the regular-size pans, and use a #24 scoop (2 to 3 tablespoons) for the mini muffins.

Place either size muffins on the middle shelf in the preheated oven. Bake regular muffins for 30 to 35 minutes, and mini muffins for 15 to 20 minutes. Turn the muffin pans once, if necessary, for the muffins to brown evenly.

Let the muffins cool in the pans for 5 minutes before removing them to a wire rack to cool completely. However, don't be shy about eating Blueberry Muffins right from the oven.

Variation

Dairy-free Blueberry Muffins. Replace the sour cream and buttermilk with 1⅞ cups unsweetened applesauce. Replace the melted butter with vegetable oil. Increase the baking time to 35 to 40 minutes for the regular-size muffins.

Baker's Tip

• In order to avoid making lavender blueberry muffins, it is necessary to stir the blueberries into the batter while they are still solidly frozen. Break up any clumps of frozen blueberries, and stir them in quickly and gently.

Irish Soda Bread Muffins

Yield:
15 large muffins

All of the exceptional qualities of perfectly balanced flavor and texture in Irish Soda Bread are also found in Irish Soda Bread Muffins. The unique combination of raisins and caraway seeds makes you want to take another bite to determine just what the flavor is.

These muffins were developed as the result of a mistake. I misread the Irish Soda Bread recipe while testing recipes for this book, and put in an extra cup of liquid. Looking at the unbelievably wet mixture in the mixing bowl, I decided my only solution was to make muffins. And what muffins they were! I wish all my mistakes could be so delicious. Irish Soda Bread Muffins quickly became the Muffin of the Year for 1991 at The Ranch Kitchen.

Fruit and Seeds

¾ cup raisins
4 teaspoons caraway seeds

Dry Ingredients

5 cups unbleached white flour
1 teaspoon baking soda
1½ teaspoons baking powder
¾ teaspoon salt

Wet Ingredients

¾ cup cold butter
6 tablespoons fruit sweetener
1⅓ cups buttermilk
1 cup unsweetened applesauce
2 eggs

Begin by plumping the raisins. Bring 1 cup of water to a boil and add the raisins. When the water returns to the boil, turn off the heat. Let the raisins plump in the water for 10 minutes. Drain the raisins, saving any raisin water for another use. Set the raisins aside.

Preheat the oven to 350° F. Lightly spray a regular-size muffin tin with lecithin spray.

Cut the cold butter into ½-inch pieces. Sift the dry ingredients together into a medium-size bowl or the mixing bowl of an electric mixer. With the mixer on its lowest speed, use the paddle attachment or your beaters to cut the cold butter into the dry ingredients, until the mixture resembles coarse cornmeal. Stir in the plumped raisins and the caraway seeds.

In a small bowl, whisk together the sweetener, buttermilk, applesauce, and eggs, and add to the flour mixture. Stir together on medium-low speed just until mixed.

Use a rounded #12 scoop (½ cup) to place the batter into the prepared muffin tins.

Bake the muffins on the middle shelf of the preheated oven for 30 to 35 minutes. Turn muffin tins once, if necessary, for the muffins to brown evenly.

Let the muffins cool in the pan for 5 minutes before removing them to a wire rack to cool completely.

Peach Oat Bran Muffins

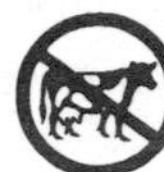

Yield:
12 large muffins

This is one of my favorite breakfast muffins. Pecans, oat bran, and rice flour give them a wonderful crunchy texture, and chopped peaches, dates, and cinnamon give Peach Oat Bran Muffins a very delicious and fruity taste.

These satisfying muffins were developed in response to a customer's request for another wheat-free muffin. Because Peach Oat Bran Muffins are made using rice and oat flours, rolled oats, and oat bran, they are a fragile muffin and must be handled only after they have cooled in the muffin tins.

Fruit and Nuts

¾ cup pecans
½ cup date pieces
2½ cups chopped fresh or frozen peaches*

Wet Ingredients

½ cup fruit sweetener
2 eggs
½ cup oil
1 teaspoon vanilla extract
2 teaspoons peach extract
1¼ cups unsweetened applesauce
1 cup oat bran
¾ cup rolled oats

Dry Ingredients

2⅛ cups brown rice flour
⅓ cup oat flour
2½ teaspoons baking powder
1 teaspoon baking soda
½ teaspoon salt
2 teaspoons cinnamon
½ teaspoon nutmeg

Preheat the oven to 375° F. Lightly spray a regular-size muffin tin with lecithin spray.

Toast the pecans in the oven for 7 to 10 minutes, stirring occasionally. Allow the nuts to cool. Then coarsely chop them with a knife or with a pulsing action in a food processor.

Coarsely chop the peaches.

In a medium-size bowl, mix together the fruit sweetener, eggs, oil, vanilla, peach extract, and applesauce. Stir in the oat bran and the rolled oats. Let this mixture sit for a minimum of 10 minutes while you prepare the rest of the ingredients.

Sift the dry ingredients into a large bowl, and stir in the pecans and the date pieces.

Make a well in the center of the dry ingredients, and stir in the wet mix. When half mixed, stir in the chopped peaches. Be careful not to over-mix. The muffin batter should remain lumpy.

Use a #12 scoop (⅓ to ½ cup of batter) to place the batter into the prepared muffin tins.

Bake the muffins in the preheated oven for 35 to 40 minutes. Let the muffins cool in the muffin pans before removing them. Be extra careful in handling these muffins because they are very fragile when warm.

**Note:* Fresh or unsweetened frozen peaches can be used in these muffins. If you are using frozen peaches, chop and measure the peaches while they are still half-frozen, for once they defrost they compact and then measure only about two-thirds of their full measurement when frozen. If using fresh peaches, peel them before chopping.

Raisin Oat Bran Muffins (Cholesterol-Free)

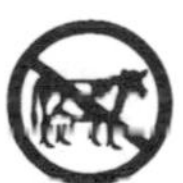 

Yield:
14 muffins

Raisin Oat Bran Muffins are just what the doctor ordered.

One of our customers presented us with a note from her doctor stating that she had to eat a certain amount of oat bran daily. She asked us to make a muffin that she could eat a couple of times a day. We obliged her by developing this pure and simple recipe. We would then make Raisin Oat Bran Muffins in quantity for her about once a month and then present them to her in a big pink bakery box. She would freeze them and take out daily just the number she needed, according to her doctor's prescription.

This recipe makes a thinner batter than our other muffin recipes, so you will not be able to use a scoop to fill the muffin pans. Because it is a thin batter, fill the muffin cups just to the top.

Fruit and Nuts

⅓ cup walnuts
⅜ cup raisins

Wet Ingredients

¾ cup fruit sweetener
¾ cup water
3 tablespoons oil
¼ teaspoon apple cider vinegar
2 cups plus 2 tablespoons oat bran
4 egg whites

Dry Ingredients

1 cup whole wheat flour
1 tablespoon baking powder
1 teaspoon baking soda
1 teaspoon cinnamon
¼ teaspoon salt

Preheat the oven to 375° F. Lightly spray the muffin tins with lecithin spray.

Toast the walnuts in the oven for 7 to 10 minutes, stirring occasionally. Allow the nuts to cool. Then coarsely chop them with a knife or with a pulsing action in a food processor.

Bring ¾ cup of water to a boil in a small pot. Add the raisins. When the water returns to the boil, turn off the heat. Let the raisins plump in the water for at least 10 minutes. Drain the raisins, saving the raisin water. The raisin water can be used to replace part or all of the ¾ cup water.

In a medium-size bowl, combine the fruit sweetener, water, oil, and vinegar. Then stir in the oat bran.

Sift the dry mix ingredients together into a large bowl and make a well in the center. In a small bowl, whip the egg whites until frothy. Then stir them into the oat bran mixture. Stir the oat bran mixture into the dry ingredients. When half mixed, stir in the raisins and walnuts. Spoon the batter into the prepared pans just to the top of each muffin cup.

Bake the muffins on the middle shelf of the preheated oven for 20 to 25 minutes. Turn the muffin tins once, if necessary, to allow the muffins to brown evenly.

Let the muffins cool in the pan for 5 minutes before removing them to a wire rack to cool completely.

Spicy Pumpkin Muffins

Yield:
12 large muffins

Moist, spicy, and delicious, Spicy Pumpkin Muffins were the first egg-free muffin developed at The Ranch Kitchen, back in 1988.

Fruit and Nuts

1½ cups pecans
¾ cup raisins

Wet Ingredients

3 cups canned pumpkin (29-ounce can)
10 tablespoons fruit sweetener
½ cup oil
¾ cup raisin water

Dry Ingredients

3¾ cups brown rice flour
2 tablespoons cinnamon
1 teaspoon nutmeg
¾ teaspoon cloves
¾ teaspoon allspice
3½ teaspoons baking powder
¾ teaspoon baking soda
1 teaspoon salt

Preheat the oven to 375° F. Lightly spray a regular-size muffin tin with lecithin spray.

Toast the pecans in the oven for 7 to 10 minutes, stirring occasionally. Allow the nuts to cool. Then coarsely chop them with a knife or with a pulsing action in a food processor.

Bring 1½ cups of water to a boil in a small pot. Add the raisins. When the water returns to the boil, turn off the heat. Let the raisins plump in the water for at least 10 minutes. Drain the raisins, saving the raisin water. If necessary, add additional water to the raisin water to equal ¾ cup.

Combine the wet ingredients in a medium-size bowl. Sift together the dry ingredients into a large bowl. Make a well in center and stir in the wet mix. When half mixed, fold in the toasted pecans and plumped raisins. Do not over-mix; the batter should remain lumpy.

Use a rounded #12 scoop (½ cup) to place the batter in the prepared muffin tin.

Bake the muffins on the middle shelf of the preheated oven for 30 minutes. Turn the muffin tin once if necessary for the muffins to brown evenly. Turn off the heat and leave the muffins in the oven with the door closed for another 15 minutes.

Let the muffins cool in the tin for 5 minutes before removing them to a wire rack to cool completely.

Very Banana Nut Muffins

*

Yield:
10 large muffins

These are a banana-lover's banana muffins. Very Banana Nut Muffins were developed to make the best use of ripe bananas. They became so popular at the restaurant that we had to buy extra bananas just so we would have ripe ones to make into muffins. If you happen to have more bananas than called for in the recipe, just replace part of the applesauce with bananas. Similarly if you have fewer bananas than called for in the recipe, add more applesauce.

As an extra plus, Very Banana Nut Muffins are wheat-free, dairy-free and low in cholesterol.

Nuts

1 cup walnuts

Wet Ingredients

1⅔ cups mashed ripe bananas (3 to 4 medium-size bananas)
⅔ cup unsweetened applesauce
3 tablespoons apple butter
½ cup oil
⅓ cup water or 2 eggs* *(use water for egg-free)*
½ cup fruit sweetener
¾ teaspoon vanilla extract

Dry Ingredients

3½ cups brown rice flour
1¾ teaspoons baking soda
1¾ teaspoons baking powder
¾ teaspoon salt
1½ teaspoons cinnamon
¼ teaspoon nutmeg

Preheat the oven to 375° F. Lightly spray a regular-size muffin tin with lecithin spray.

Toast the walnuts in the oven for 7 to 10 minutes, stirring occasionally. Allow the nuts to cool. Then coarsely chop them with a knife or with a pulsing action in a food processor.

Whisk the wet ingredients together in the order listed until well blended. Sift together the dry ingredients into a large bowl. Make a well in the center, and stir in the wet mix. When half mixed, stir in the toasted walnuts. Be careful not to over-mix; the batter should remain lumpy.

Use a rounded #12 scoop (½ cup) to place the batter into the prepared muffin tin.

Bake the muffins on the middle shelf of the preheated oven for 25 to 30 minutes. Turn the muffin tin once, if necessary, for the muffins to brown evenly.

Let the muffins cool in the pan for 5 minutes before removing them to a wire rack to cool completely.

Southern-Style Buttermilk Biscuits

Yield:
14 biscuits

These are flaky, buttery, melt-in-your mouth biscuits. This recipe was brought to The Ranch Kitchen one summer by a young cook from South Carolina. The biscuits were her family's recipe passed down by her grandmother.

Serve them hot from the oven for breakfast, lunch, or dinner. Buttermilk Biscuits are also the perfect base for Strawberry Shortcake (page 156).

Dry Ingredients

2 cups unbleached white flour
2 cups whole wheat pastry flour
1 tablespoon baking powder
1 teaspoon baking soda
½ teaspoon salt

Wet Ingredients

10 tablespoons cold butter
1⅞ cups buttermilk
2 tablespoons fruit sweetener

Preheat the oven to 375° F and line a baking sheet with parchment paper.

Sift the dry ingredients into a large bowl. Cut the cold butter into ½-inch pieces. Use the fingers and thumb of each hand to rub in the butter until the mixture resembles coarse cornmeal. Be sure to lift your hands out of the bowl while simultaneously using your thumbs to rub the flour and butter across your fingers. Make a well in the center.

In a small bowl, combine the buttermilk and the fruit sweetener. Pour them into the center of the dry ingredients. Form a rough dough, mixing quickly and gently with your hand or a wooden spoon.

Place the biscuit dough on a lightly floured work surface, and knead it no more than 10 times. Use a rolling pin or your hands to form it into a ¾-inch-thick rectangle.

Lightly dust a plain 2-inch or 3-inch round cutter with flour. Cut the biscuits with a straight cutting motion, being careful not to twist the cutter. To reuse the scraps, do not knead them. Instead, use your fingers to lightly press them together and pat them out again to ¾-inch thickness.

Place the cut biscuits on a baking-paper-lined or ungreased baking sheet. Leave at least 1 inch of space around each biscuit for crusty, evenly browned biscuits.

Bake the biscuits in the preheated oven for 20 to 22 minutes, until golden brown.

Let the biscuits cool on the baking sheet before removing them.

Angel Biscuits

Yield:
15 biscuits

Angel Biscuits combine a little bit of yeast with a little bit of baking powder and baking soda to form flaky, buttery, pillow-soft buttermilk biscuits. Having the dough in your refrigerator just waiting for you to grace your table with freshly baked biscuits is like having an angel in the kitchen. Once the dough is made it can be kept in the refrigerator for as long as a week, while you scoop out just the amount you need each day to form and bake. Besides being great breakfast biscuits, Angel Biscuits are delicious in Strawberry Shortcake (page 156).

2 tablespoons warm water
1 tablespoon dry baker's yeast
1 tablespoon fruit sweetener
2 cups whole wheat pastry flour
3 cups unbleached white flour
1 teaspoon baking powder
1 teaspoon baking soda
1 teaspoon salt
1 cup cold butter
2 cups buttermilk
1 tablespoon fruit sweetener

Place the warm water in a small bowl with the yeast and 1 tablespoon of the sweetener. Stir until the yeast is moistened. Then set the bowl aside until the yeast is bubbly, about 5 minutes.

Sift the flours, baking powder, baking soda, and salt together into a medium-size bowl. Cut the butter into ½-inch pieces. Use the fingers and thumb of each hand to rub in the pieces of butter until the mixture resembles coarse cornmeal. Be sure to lift your hands out of the bowl while simultaneously using your thumbs to rub the flour and butter across your fingers. Make a well in the center.

In a small bowl, combine the buttermilk with the remaining 1 tablespoon fruit sweetener and the activated yeast. Pour them into the center of the dry ingredients. Form a rough dough, mixing quickly and gently with your hands. Cover the bowl with plastic and refrigerate for 1 hour.

Preheat the oven to 375° F. Line a baking pan with baking paper.

Remove from the refrigerator that portion of the dough that you want to make into biscuits and knead it until smooth, 10 to 15 kneads. Roll the dough out ¾ inch thick. With a lightly floured cutter, cut out 2-inch to 3-inch biscuits. Place the biscuits on the prepared pan.

Bake until golden brown, about 15 to 20 minutes. Serve Angel Biscuits hot from the oven.

Baker's Tip

- After the first day, the Angel Biscuit dough should sit for 10 minutes at room temperature before you knead it smooth. After the biscuits are formed, let them sit for another 10 minutes before placing them in the oven.

3

Cookies

Everybody loves cookies. With a crunchy or chewy texture and a burst of flavor in every bite, cookies are great—whether as a snack, as a dessert, or as a gift from home. And best of all, cookies are absolutely simple to prepare and require a minimum of equipment and work space. They are a great way to introduce children to the joys of the kitchen.

Butter-rich or cholesterol-free, here are the cookie recipes for everyone and for every occasion. There are recipes for cookies from Valentine's Day to Christmas and almost every day in between, as well as cookies to meet every dietary requirement from gluten-free to dairy-free to egg-free. There are recipes for cookies in a variety of colorful shapes and sizes to brighten tea trays or gift boxes or even Christmas trees.

Here are a few pointers for success with cookies any time of the year:

- Be sure to preheat your oven before you begin and have all of your ingredients at room temperature.
- Form perfectly shaped cookies using a #24 or #12 ice cream scoop. Scoops can be purchased in restaurant supply and kitchenware shops.

- Whatever method is used for forming the cookies, for them to bake and brown evenly they must be uniform in thickness and size on each baking sheet.
- When cutting out cookie shapes with cookie cutters, be careful to cut them very close to one another, to have as few scraps as possible. If you are careful not to use too much flour when rolling out the dough, you can reroll and cut more cookies from the scraps. However, each time you do this, the cookies will become tougher in texture.
- For ease in clean-up, line baking pans with baking paper. It is not necessary to grease either the pan or the paper. And when making a large batch of cookies, you can reuse the baking paper a number of times.
- Place cookies 1 to 2 inches apart, depending upon how much the cookies will spread.
- Depending upon how evenly your oven bakes, you may find it helpful to bake cookies on one pan inside another pan (referred to as "double pan" in the recipes) to keep the bottoms of the cookies from browning too quickly. This may also increase the baking time a minute or two, depending upon your oven. Many stores sell insulated cookie sheets which are comparable to double pans.
- Also, depending upon your oven (its size and efficiency), it is best to place only one pan of cookies in the oven at a time. This limit ensures good heat circulation so that the cookies cook and brown evenly from top to bottom.
- Bake according to the recipe's directions, but keep a close watch during the baking of the first batch. The actual baking time will vary with the size of the cookies, the thickness of the dough, the quality of the ingredients, and the efficiency of the oven.
- As cookies are usually quite fragile when they are hot from the oven, minimize breakage by letting them cool before removing them from the baking pans to a wire rack.
- To keep cookies crisp, store them in a container with a loose cover.
- To keep cookies soft, store them in an airtight container.
- Frozen cookies keep beautifully for 2 to 3 months. They require just a few minutes to thaw. (Some people even prefer them while still frozen.)

Old-Fashioned Oatmeal Raisin Cookies

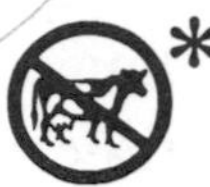*

Yield:
1 dozen giant cookies
3 dozen regular-sized cookies

Delicious, moist, and chewy oatmeal cookies that are especially irresistible when made into giant cookies. I originally found this recipe for "Delicious Oatmeal Cookies" in a magazine during my college years. With a few adjustments, these cookies are just as delicious now, fruit-sweetened, as they were then.

¾ cup walnuts or pecans
¾ cup raisins
1 cup (½ pound) butter* ***(substitute margarine for dairy-free)***
¾ cup fruit sweetener
2 eggs
1 teaspoon vanilla extract
1 teaspoon cinnamon
1 teaspoon baking soda
Pinch salt
1½ cups unbleached white flour
1½ cups rolled oats

Preheat the oven to 350° F.

Toast the walnuts or pecans in the preheated oven for 7 to 10 minutes, stirring occasionally. Allow the nuts to cool. Then process in a food processor, using the pulsing action, until they are coarsely chopped.

Bring 1 cup of water to a boil and add the raisins. When the water returns to the boil, turn off the heat. Let the raisins plump in the water for at least 10 minutes. Drain the raisins, saving any raisin water for another use.

Cream the butter and sweetener together. When light and fluffy, add the eggs one at a time, beating well after each addition. Stir in the vanilla, cinnamon, baking soda, and salt. When mixed, add the flour, oats, chopped nuts, and plumped raisins. Cover the dough and refrigerate it for 30 minutes to make it easier to handle.

Preheat the oven to 325° F. Line baking pans with parchment paper.

Using a #12 scoop (or a ½-cup measure) for giant cookies or a #24 scoop (2 tablespoons) or a spoon for regular-size cookies, scoop out the dough and place the balls 1 inch apart on insulated baking pans. With lightly moistened fingers, flatten the cookies to a thickness of ⅓ inch.

Bake until a light golden brown. Giant cookies bake for 20 to 24 minutes, and regular-size cookies bake for 12 to 15 minutes. Remove the cookies to wire racks to cool.

Crunchy Almond Oatmeal Cookies

Yield:
22 cookies

These are wonderful cookies. They are a delicious variation on the oatmeal cookie theme, with toasted almonds giving them a special crunchiness. I have one friend who makes a triple batch of these cookies monthly as gifts for her many happy friends. She substitutes spelt flour (see Baker's Tip) for the wheat flours in the recipe and adds unsweetened carob chips.

Fruit and Nuts

1½ cups almonds
½ cup raisins

Dry Ingredients

¾ cup whole wheat pastry flour
¾ cup unbleached white flour
1 teaspoon cinnamon
½ teaspoon cardamom
½ teaspoon baking soda
½ teaspoon salt
1¾ cups rolled oats

Wet Ingredients

⅔ cup fruit sweetener
⅓ cup raisin water
½ cup oil
1 egg
1 teaspoon vanilla extract
½ teaspoon almond extract

Preheat the oven to 350° F and line baking sheets with baking paper.

Toast the almonds in the preheated oven for 7 to 10 minutes, stirring occasionally. Allow the nuts to cool. Then process in a food processor, using the pulsing action, until they are medium chopped.

Bring 1 cup of water to a boil and add the raisins. When the water returns to the boil, turn off the heat. Let the raisins plump in the water for at least 10 minutes. Drain the raisins, saving the raisin water.

Sift the flours, spices, baking soda, and salt into a large mixing bowl. Stir in the rolled oats.

Whisk the wet ingredients together until thickened. Stir the wet mixture into the dry ingredients, mixing until well combined. Then stir in the chopped almonds and plumped raisins.

Using a #24 scoop (2 tablespoons) or a spoon, place the balls 1 inch apart on the prepared baking sheets.

Bake until golden brown, approximately 10 to 12 minutes. Let the cookies cool on the pans before removing.

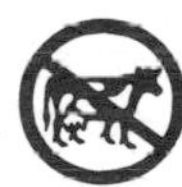 

Variation

Crunchy Carob Almond Cookies. Add ½ cup unsweetened carob chips.

Baker's Tip

• Spelt is an ancient grain first cultivated in Asia. Spelt is a complete protein, and some people consider it more easily assimilated than any other grain. Wheat has been hybridized from spelt. Spelt is widely used in Europe, especially in Germany, where it grows almost wild. In America, spelt can be purchased at some natural food stores.

Cholesterol-Free Oatmeal Cookies

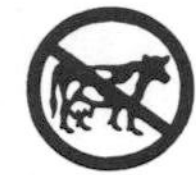 

Yield:
16 cookies

These crisp, chewy, cholesterol-free Oatmeal Cookies are a treat for everyone, and especially for people on a reduced-cholesterol diet.

Fruit and Nuts

⅓ cup walnuts
⅓ cup raisins

Dry Ingredients

½ cup whole wheat pastry flour
1 teaspoon baking powder
2 teaspoons cinnamon
¼ teaspoon nutmeg
⅛ teaspoon salt
1½ cups rolled oats

Wet Ingredients

⅓ cup oil
¼ cup fruit sweetener
¼ cup raisin water

Preheat the oven to 350° F and line baking sheets with baking paper.

Toast the walnuts in the preheated oven for 7 to 10 minutes, stirring occasionally. Allow the nuts to cool. Then process in a food processor, using the pulsing action, until they are coarsely chopped.

Bring ⅔ cup of water to a boil and add the raisins. When the water returns to the boil, turn off the heat. Let the raisins plump in the water for at least 10 minutes. Drain the raisins, saving the raisin water.

Sift the flour, baking powder, spices, and salt into a large mixing bowl. Stir in the rolled oats. In a medium-size bowl, whisk the wet ingredients together until thickened. Stir the wet mix into the dry ingredients, mixing for 1 minute until the oats begin to break down. Stir in the chopped walnuts and the plumped raisins.

Using a #24 scoop (2 tablespoons) or a spoon, scoop out the dough and place the balls 1 inch apart on the baking sheets. With lightly moistened fingers, flatten each cookie to a thickness of ⅓ inch.

Bake until golden brown, 15 to 18 minutes. Remove the cookies to wire racks to cool.

Sesame Raisin Cookies

Yield:
8 giant cookies

As giant cookies, cholesterol-free Sesame Raisin Cookies provide an unbeatable lunch box treat. The toasted sesame seeds give these cookies a full, rich, and well-balanced flavor. And by chopping the plumped raisins, you'll receive a little burst of sweetness in every bite.

Fruit and Seeds

½ cup raisins
½ cup sesame seeds

Dry Ingredients

1 cup brown rice flour
1¼ cups rolled oats
½ teaspoon cinnamon
¼ teaspoon salt

Wet Ingredients

1⅛ cup unsweetened apple juice
2 tablespoons oil
1 teaspoon vanilla extract

Bring ¾ cup of water to a boil and add the raisins. When the water returns to the boil, turn off the heat. Let the raisins plump in the water for at least 10 minutes. Drain the raisins, saving the raisin water for another use. Chop the raisins coarsely.

Toast the sesame seeds by stirring them with a wooden spoon in a heavy sauté pan over medium heat, until the seeds begin to crackle and pop and smell toasted, about 10 minutes.

Preheat the oven to 350° F and line baking sheets with baking paper.

Combine the dry ingredients and stir in the sesame seeds until well distributed.

In a small bowl, combine the wet ingredients. Stir the wet ingredients and the raisins into the dry ingredients, mixing until blended.

Use a #12 scoop (or a ½-cup measure) for each cookie. Place the balls 1 inch apart on the prepared baking pans. With lightly moistened fingertips flatten each cookie to a thickness of ½ inch.

Bake until golden brown, approximately 25 minutes. Let the cookies cool on the pans before removing.

Maple Walnut Cookies

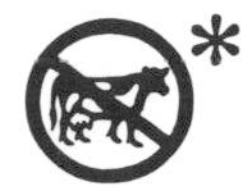

Yield:
3½ dozen

Crunchy, buttery, and maple flavored, these exceptional Maple Walnut Cookies or the delicious variations quickly become everyone's favorite.

3 cups walnuts
1½ cups (¾ pound) butter* ***(substitute margarine for dairy-free)***
¾ cup pure maple syrup
1 egg
½ teaspoon vanilla extract
¾ teaspoon almond extract
1½ cups unbleached white flour

Preheat the oven to 350° F.

Toast the walnuts in a preheated oven for 7 to 10 minutes, stirring occasionally. Let the nuts cool. Then process in a food processor, using the pulsing action, until they are finely ground. Do not overprocess or you will end up with a paste.

Cream together the butter and maple syrup. When light and fluffy, add the egg and beat well for 1 minute. Stir in the extracts, then the flour, and the finely ground nuts. Cover the dough and refrigerate it for 20 minutes to make it easier to handle.

Preheat the oven to 350° F. Line baking sheets with baking paper.

Using a #24 scoop (2 tablespoons) or a spoon, scoop out the dough and place the balls 1 inch apart on the baking sheets. With lightly moistened fingers, flatten each cookie to a thickness of ½ inch.

Bake the cookies until golden brown, for 15 to 18 minutes on an insulated or double pan.

Let the cookies cool on the pans before removing.

Variations

Maple Almond Cookies. Substitute almonds for the walnuts.

Maple Hazelnut Cookies. Substitute hazelnuts for the walnuts.

Maple Pecan Cookies. Substitute pecans for the walnuts.

Almond Cookies. Substitute almonds for the walnuts and fruit sweetener for all or part of the maple syrup.

Hazelnut Cookies

 *

Yield:
2½ to 3 dozen

Toasted hazelnuts give these lovely, crisp cookies a delicate and sophisticated taste.

1½ cups hazelnuts
¾ cup butter* ***(substitute margarine for dairy-free)***
⅓ cup fruit sweetener
¼ teaspoon vanilla extract
Pinch salt
1½ cups unbleached white flour

Preheat the oven to 350° F.

Toast the hazelnuts in the preheated oven for 7 to 10 minutes, stirring occasionally. Let the nuts cool. Then process in a food processor, using the pulsing action, until they are finely ground. Do not overprocess or you will end up with a paste.

Cream together the butter and sweetener until light and fluffy. Stir in the vanilla and salt, then the flour and the finely chopped hazelnuts. Mix just enough to form a dough. Cover the dough and refrigerate it for 20 minutes to make it easier to handle.

Preheat the oven to 350° F. Line baking sheets with parchment paper.

Use a #24 scoop (2 tablespoons) or a spoon to scoop out balls of dough. Place them 1 inch apart on the baking sheets. With lightly moistened fingertips, flatten each cookie to a thickness of ¼ inch.

Bake until golden brown, for 12 to 15 minutes. Let the cookies cool on the pans before removing.

Baker's Tip

• Hazelnuts, also known as filberts, can be purchased with their skin still on, or "blanched" with the skin removed. Hazelnuts' dark brown skins can be bitter, so it is better to remove them before baking with the nuts. If the hazelnuts do have their skins, remove the skins after the nuts have been toasted by rubbing together a few nuts at a time in a kitchen towel.

Basic Shortbread Cookies

 *

Yield:
30 to 35 (2-inch) cut-outs

Old-fashioned Basic Shortbread—rich, crumbly, and delectable—the essence of what a "plain" cookie should be. But you can make them anything but plain by tinting them—depending on the time of year—pink for hearts, green for trees, or yellow for stars.

½ cup nuts (almonds, walnuts, pecans, hazelnuts, or any combination)
1 cup (½ pound) butter* ***(substitute margarine for dairy-free)***
9 tablespoons fruit sweetener
⅛ teaspoon salt
2 teaspoons vanilla extract
2 cups plus 2 tablespoons unbleached white flour

Garnish

2 cups finely ground nuts (optional)

Preheat the oven to 350° F.

Toast the nuts in the preheated oven for 7 to 10 minutes, stirring occasionally. Let the nuts cool. Then process in a food processor, using the pulsing action, until they are finely chopped.

Cream together the butter and sweetener. When light and fluffy, add the remaining ingredients in the order listed, mixing just to blend. Stir in the nuts. Cover the dough and refrigerate it for 20 minutes to make it easier to handle.

Preheat the oven to 350° F and line baking sheets with parchment paper.

Shortbread cookies can be formed in 2 different ways:

1. Form the dough into walnut-size balls. Roll the balls in finely ground nuts and flatten them to ⅓-inch thickness; or
2. Roll the dough out ¼-inch thick and cut it into different shapes with cookie cutters.

Place the cookies 1 inch apart on insulated baking sheets. Bake until lightly brown around the edges, approximately 15 to 20 minutes. Remove the cookies to a wire rack to cool.

Variation

Wheat-less Shortbread Cookies. Substitute brown rice flour for unbleached white flour.

Baker's Tip

- To avoid overmixing the flour and toughening the cookies, color the cookies before adding the flour, just after creaming the butter and sweetener. At this stage, the color should be a little darker than you want the finished cookies to be.

Raspberry Thumbprint Cookies

 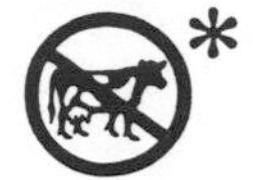*

Yield:
32 cookies

The raspberry jam centers help to make these crisp and delicate rice flour Thumbprint Cookies a delicious treat. Try varying the jam flavor and color by substituting apricot jam, orange marmalade, or even blueberry conserves for the raspberry jam.

1½ cups walnuts
1¼ cups butter* ***(substitute margarine for dairy-free)***
⅝ cup fruit sweetener
3 egg yolks
1¼ teaspoons vanilla extract
2½ cups brown rice flour
½ teaspoon salt
3 egg whites
¾ cup fruit-sweetened raspberry jam

Preheat the oven to 350° F.

Toast the walnuts in the preheated oven for 7 to 10 minutes, stirring occasionally. Let the nuts cool. Then process in a food processor, using a pulsing action, until they are finely ground. Do not overprocess or you will end up with a paste.

Cream together the butter and sweetener until light and fluffy. Add the egg yolks one at a time, beating well after each addition. Stir in the vanilla, flour, and salt. Cover the dough and refrigerate it for 20 minutes to make it easier to handle.

Preheat the oven to 350° F. Line baking pans with baking paper.

Use a #24 scoop (2 tablespoons) or a spoon to scoop out the dough and form it into balls. In a small bowl, stir the egg whites with a fork just to break them down. Roll the cookie balls in the egg whites. Then drain the cookies and roll them in the ground walnuts. Place the cookie balls 2 inches apart on the prepared baking pans. Flatten each ball to ⅓-inch thickness. Then press a "thumbprint" in the center of each cookie. Fill each indentation with 1 teaspoon of raspberry jam.

Bake the cookies in the preheated oven on an insulated or double pan for 15 to 18 minutes, until the cookies are golden around their edges.

Let the cookies cool completely on the pans before removing them. As these are especially fragile cookies when they are warm, handle them with care.

Baker's Tip

- If you prefer a less fragile cookie, prepare Raspberry Thumbprints with unbleached white flour instead of brown rice flour.

Pecan Butter Cookies

 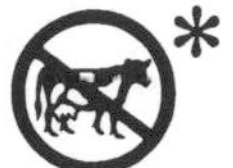*

Yield:
30 cookies

These crisp, pecan-bountiful, and butter-rich cookies are a fruit-sweetened version of a traditional French favorite.

4 cups pecans
1½ cups (¾ pound) butter* ***(substitute margarine for dairy-free)***
½ cup fruit sweetener
3 egg whites
1 teaspoon vanilla extract
2½ cups whole wheat pastry flour

Preheat the oven to 350° F.

Toast the pecans in the preheated oven for 7 to 10 minutes, stirring occasionally. Let the nuts cool. Then process in a food processor, using the pulsing action, until they are finely ground. Do not overprocess or you will end up with a paste.

Cream the butter and fruit sweetener. When light and fluffy, add the egg whites one at a time, beating well after each addition. Stir in the vanilla, then the flour and the finely chopped pecans. Cover the dough and refrigerate it for 20 minutes to make it easier to handle.

Preheat the oven to 350° F. Line baking pans with baking paper.

Using a #24 scoop (2 tablespoons) or a spoon, scoop out the dough and place the balls 1 inch apart on the prepared baking pans. With lightly moistened fingers, flatten each cookie to a thickness of ⅓ inch.

Bake until golden brown, for 15 to 18 minutes. Let the cookies cool on the pans before removing.

Jan Hagels

*

Yield:
9-inch by 13-inch pan
3½ dozen 1-inch diamonds

Jan Hagels are a traditional bar cookie from Holland. They are as rich as shortbread and satisfyingly crunchy with their toasted almond topping.

For easier cutting, it is best to cut Jan Hagels when they are just out of the oven.

1 cup (½ pound) butter* ***(substitute margarine for dairy-free)***
⅔ cup fruit sweetener
1 egg, separated
1 teaspoon cinnamon
¾ teaspoon vanilla extract
2 cups unbleached white flour
½ cup sliced almonds

Preheat the oven to 350° F. Lightly spray a 9-inch by 13-inch rectangular baking pan with lecithin spray or line it with baking paper.

In a medium-size bowl, cream together the butter and sweetener. When light and fluffy, add the egg yolk and beat for 1 minute. Stir in the cinnamon and the vanilla. When mixed, add the flour. Use a rubber spatula to spread the dough evenly in the prepared pan.

In a small bowl, lightly beat the egg white. Carefully brush the surface of the dough with the egg white and sprinkle with the sliced almonds.

Bake until golden brown, approximately 25 minutes.

While the Jan Hagels are still hot, cut them into 1-inch diamonds. Jan Hagels are quite fragile while they are still warm, so it is best to let them cool in the pan.

Carob-Almond Pinwheel Cookies

*

Yield:
50 cookies

These cookies are as fun to make as they are to eat. My great-grandmother made these old-fashioned pinwheel cookies (using chocolate and sugar) each year until she was almost 100 years old. How happy I was to have developed an equally wonderful recipe for making fruit-sweetened and carob-flavored Pinwheel Cookies, thus carrying on her tradition.

These cookies are a bit tricky to prepare, but with patience you and your family and friends will be deliciously rewarded.

Almond Cookie Layer

⅔ cup butter* *(substitute margarine for dairy-free)*
½ cup fruit sweetener
¾ teaspoon almond extract
¼ teaspoon vanilla extract
1 egg
2 cups unbleached white flour

Carob Cookie Layer

⅔ cup butter* *(substitute margarine for dairy-free)*
½ cup fruit sweetener
1 teaspoon vanilla extract
1 egg
1¾ cups unbleached white flour
¼ cup carob powder

Prepare the almond cookie layer first by creaming the butter and sweetener. When light and fluffy, add the extracts and the egg and beat until smooth. Fold in the flour. Roll the dough out between 2 sheets of baking paper or waxed paper to form a 12-inch by 16-inch rectangle. Transfer the dough to a baking pan and refrigerate while preparing the carob cookie layer.

Prepare the carob cookie layer by creaming the butter and sweetener. When light and fluffy, add the extracts and the egg and beat until smooth. Sift together the flour and carob powder. Then fold them into the cookie mixture.

Roll the dough out between 2 sheets of baking paper or waxed paper to form a 12-inch by 16-inch rectangle.

Remove the top sheet of paper from both the carob and almond cookie layers, and invert the whole carob layer onto the chilled almond cookie layer.

Refrigerate both layers for 10 minutes.

To prepare the pinwheels, remove the top sheet of paper. Starting on the long side of the dough, roll it up tightly, jelly-roll fashion. If the layers are too cold to roll easily, let them sit at room temperature for a few minutes, until they will roll without breaking. Wrap the roll in the bottom sheet of paper, and refrigerate it for 1 hour before slicing into cookies.

Preheat the oven to 375° F. Line baking sheets with baking paper.

Cut the chilled roll into ¼-inch-thick slices. Place the cookies ½ inch apart on baking pans.

Bake until a pale golden brown, for about 12 minutes. Let the cookies cool on the pans before removing them.

Gingerbread Girls and Boys

Yield:
36 to 40 cookies

These snappy gingerbread cookies are wonderfully crisp and spicy. The dough is very easy to work with and fun to prepare with children during the holiday season. One year at The Ranch Kitchen we trimmed our Christmas tree with hand-painted Gingerbread Girls and Boys, with each employee and many a customer decorating their own cookies. We had cowboys, farmers, a runner with headphones, a nurse, and even a ballerina on our tree.

Gingerbread cookies can be made 2 to 3 weeks in advance, and their flavor and texture will just keep improving.

Wet Ingredients

1½ cups (¾ pound) butter* *(substitute margarine for dairy-free)*
1½ cups fruit sweetener
3 eggs
2 teaspoons vanilla extract

Dry Ingredients

6 cups unbleached white flour
3 tablespoons cinnamon
2 tablespoons ginger
1 tablespoon nutmeg
1 tablespoon carob powder
2 teaspoons baking soda
2 teaspoons baking powder
¾ teaspoon salt

Garnish

Royal Icing (page 185) *(optional)*

Cream together the butter and sweetener. When light and fluffy, add the eggs one at a time, beating well after each addition. Stir in the vanilla.

Sift the dry ingredients together 3 times and stir them into the wet ingredients, mixing just enough to form a dough. Cover the dough and refrigerate it for 20 minutes to make it easier to handle before rolling out.

Preheat the oven to 350° F. Line the baking sheets with baking paper.

Roll the dough out to a ¼-inch thickness on a lightly floured surface. Dip the cookie cutters in flour before cutting out gingerbread girls and boys or other shapes. Place the cookies on the baking sheets, leaving ½ inch around each cookie.

Bake until a light golden brown, 15 to 16 minutes. Let the cookies cool on the pans before removing.

When the cookies are cool, they can be fancifully decorated with an icing that will dry hard, such as Royal Icing (made with powdered sugar—sorry, I have not yet found a substitute).

Spice Cookies

Yield:
32 cookies

These are lovely cookies with their puffed, round, and crackly tops, and their delicious spicy taste. These Spice Cookies are crisp on the outside and moist and chewy on the inside.

1¾ cups walnuts
¾ cup butter* *(substitute margarine for dairy-free)*
½ cup fruit sweetener
2½ tablespoons unsulphured molasses
1 egg
1 teaspoon cinnamon
¾ teaspoon cloves
½ teaspoon ginger
½ teaspoon nutmeg
2 teaspoons baking soda
⅛ teaspoon salt
2 cups unbleached white flour

Preheat the oven to 350° F.

Toast the walnuts in the preheated oven for 7 to 10 minutes, stirring occasionally. Let the nuts cool. Then process in a food processor, using the pulsing action, until they are finely ground. Do not overprocess or you will end up with a paste.

Cream the butter with the fruit sweetener and the molasses. When light and fluffy, add the egg and beat together for 3 minutes. Stir in the spices, baking soda, and salt. When mixed, add the flour and 1 cup of the finely ground walnuts. Cover the dough and refrigerate it for 20 minutes to make it easier to handle.

Preheat the oven to 350° F. Line baking pans with baking paper.

Use a #24 scoop (2 tablespoons) or a spoon to form the dough into balls. Roll each ball into the remaining ground walnuts and place balls 1 inch apart on the baking pans. Bake until lightly colored, approximately 15 minutes. Let the cookies cool on the pans before removing them.

Carob Chip Cookies

Yield:
45 cookies

A crispy, "unchocolate" version of America's favorite cookie.

1 cup walnuts
1 cup (½ pound) butter,* softened *(substitute margarine for dairy-free)*
½ cup plus 2 tablespoons fruit sweetener
2 eggs
1 teaspoon vanilla extract
¾ teaspoon baking soda
¾ teaspoon salt
3 cups unbleached white flour
2 cups carob chips

Preheat the oven to 350° F.

Toast the walnuts in the preheated oven for 7 to 10 minutes, stirring occasionally. Let the nuts cool. Then process in a food processor, using the pulsing action, until they are coarsely chopped.

Cream the butter and sweetener until light and fluffy. Add the eggs, 1 at a time, beating well after each addition. Stir in the vanilla, baking soda, and salt. When mixed, add the flour, carob chips, and coarsely chopped walnuts. Cover the dough and refrigerate it for 20 minutes to make it easier to handle.

Preheat the oven to 325° F. Line baking sheets with baking paper.

Using a #24 scoop (2 tablespoons) or a spoon, scoop out the dough and place balls 1 inch apart on the prepared baking sheets. With lightly moistened fingers flatten each cookie to a thickness of ⅓ inch.

Bake the cookies until golden brown, for 15 to 18 minutes. Remove the cookies to a wire rack for cooling.

Almond Macaroons

Yield:
48 cookies

Almond Macaroons are delightful, chewy cookies with the crunch and taste of almonds. They are made from a base of almond paste.

It is very difficult to make almond paste as smooth as the commercially prepared paste, but the flavor is wonderful, and you can adjust the sweetener and the sweetness to your own taste.

Almond Paste

1 cup blanched almonds
2 tablespoons fruit sweetener
1 teaspoon almond extract
½ teaspoon vanilla extract
2 tablespoons butter

Macaroons

1 cup almond paste
¼ cup fruit sweetener
1 egg white
2 to 3 tablespoons unbleached white flour

To prepare the almond paste, process the almonds in a food processor, using a pulsing action, until very finely ground. Mix in the sweetener and extracts. Cut the butter into 6 pieces. While the food processor is running, add the butter pieces and process for 30 seconds until well combined.

Preheat the oven to 325° F. Line baking sheets with baking paper.

Use an electric mixer or food processor to blend the almond paste with the ¼ cup of sweetener until smooth. Beat in the egg white, and then fold in the flour. Macaroon batter should be soft, but not runny.

Drop the batter by teaspoonfuls (or pipe through a pastry bag fitted with a plain ½-inch round tip) onto baking sheets, leaving 1 inch around each cookie. Bake for 10 to 15 minutes on insulated or double pans, until lightly browned. Let the cookies cool on the pans before removing.

Baker's Tip

• If the macaroons are difficult to remove from the baking paper, dampen the underside of the paper. Wait a couple of minutes. Then peel the paper away from the backs of the cookies.

4

Pies, Tarts, and Pastries

Pies and Tarts

For many Americans, dessert *is* a piece of pie. Pies and tarts are beautiful to behold, easy to prepare, and a great way to take good advantage of every fresh fruit as it comes into season. With delicious frozen fruit readily available, it is possible to make many of these recipes all year long.

Pie Crusts

Included in this chapter are the recipe and detailed instructions for a tender and flaky Basic Pie Crust that is suitable for almost every pie, tart, or tartlet you make. This basic crust can be made with either butter or margarine and prepared very quickly by hand or in a food processor. You will enjoy great success with this crust if you follow the recipe exactly, measure accurately, prepare the dough quickly, roll it out carefully, and bake the crusts on the lowest shelf in a preheated oven.

I have also included recipes for more specialized crusts and instructions for working with puff pastry to form a number of different sizes of free-standing tart shells. During the spring and summer months when fresh fruit is at its peak, I often use purchased puff pastry as the base for some of the most delicate and wonderful tarts imaginable. Once the tart shell is prepared, it is just a matter of assembling the tart with its filling, using whichever fresh fruit is at its best.

Nutty-Oat Crust, made with oil and sweetened with amazake, is a delicious textural treat with its cookie-like crispness, especially when used in the no-egg custard pies. The special crust for Linzertorte, an integral part of this classic recipe, is presented here in a healthier version. And the Granola Crust (a fruit-sweetened version of the classic graham cracker crust) is perfect with cheesecake or any other pie that needs a completely prebaked crust.

Whether you are making pies, tarts, or tartlets, here are a few important points to remember for rolling out and baking the Basic Pie Crust.

Rolling Out the Crust

The pie dough can be rolled out after it has rested in the refrigerator for at least 20 minutes. If the dough has been refrigerated longer, it should sit at room temperature until it is just barely soft to the touch. Lightly flour your work table, your hands, and your rolling pin. Gently form the dough into a patty 3½ inches in diameter by 1 inch in height. If the dough is hard, beat it with the rolling pin a few times to soften it. Begin each roll across the pastry ½ inch in from the edge closest to you, and end each roll ½ inch in from the edge farthest from you. Roll the pastry out quickly and with even pressure, turning the dough so that each roll is done at right angles to the previous roll. To do this, roll the dough in one direction. Gently slide a long-bladed spatula underneath the pastry to see if it is sticking to the table. If the dough begins to stick, lightly spread a little flour underneath it. Turn the dough 45 degrees and roll again, in one direction only. Continue until you have rolled your pastry into a large square, ⅛ inch thick. Use a saucepan lid or a pan to cut out a circle of dough to fit your pie, tart, or tartlet pans:

- 10 inches for the plain bottom crust in a double-crusted 9-inch deep pie pan

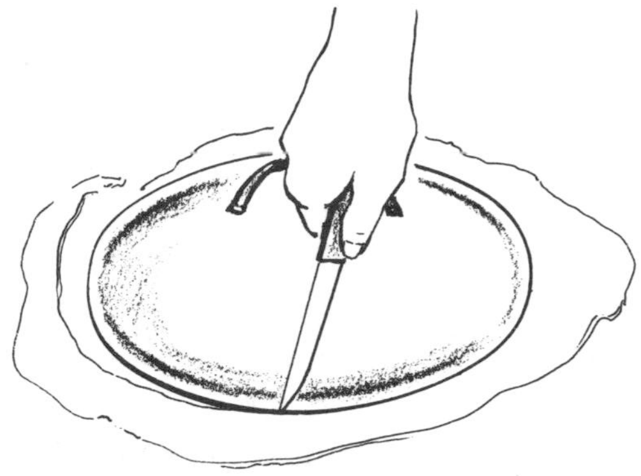

- 11 inches for the top crust in a double-crusted 9-inch deep pie pan
- 12 inches for the fluted bottom crust in a single-crusted 9-inch deep pie pan
- 12 inches for the bottom crust in a 10-inch tart pan
- 5 inches for the bottom crust in a 3-inch tartlet pan
- 4 inches for the bottom crust of tartlets made in standard-size muffin tins

Transfer the pastry to the pie or tart pan by rolling it onto the rolling pin and then unrolling it centered over the pan. With lightly floured

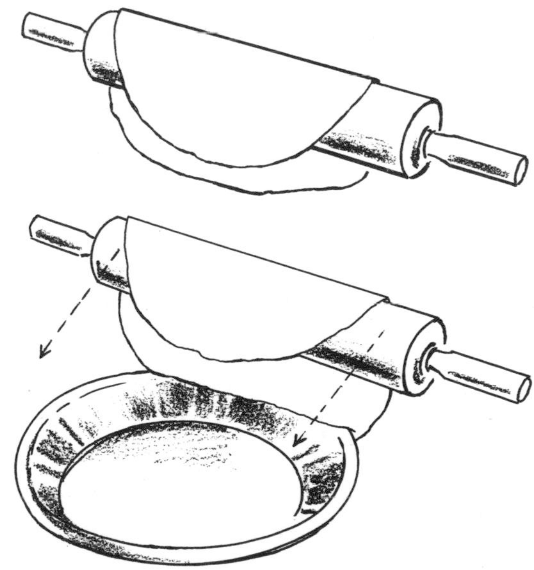

fingers, gently ease the pastry into place, being especially careful to push it into the inside corners. Depending on how the bottom crust is to be finished, either trim the pastry with a pair of kitchen scissors to be ½ inch to ¾ inch larger than the edge of the pie or tart pan, or use the dull side of a small knife to trim the pastry even with the outer edge of the pan. Chill the prepared crust for at least 15 to 20 minutes before filling and/or baking. The top crust or lattice strips can be refrigerated on a flat surface (such as a cookie sheet) and covered with plastic wrap. This chilling period is to relax the gluten in order to minimize shrinkage, and to harden the butter to ensure a flaky crust.

Here are some methods for finishing single-crusted pies, tarts, tartlets, and double-crusted and lattice pies.

Fluted Crust

You must have a ½-inch to ¾-inch edge of pastry extending beyond the pie pan. Turn this edge of pastry under itself to build up the edge. Flute the edge by placing the tip or knuckle of the index finger of your right hand on the inside of the edge, and the tips or knuckles of the index finger and middle finger of your left hand on the outside of the edge on either side of the right finger. Push dough into a "U" shape and continue around the pie.

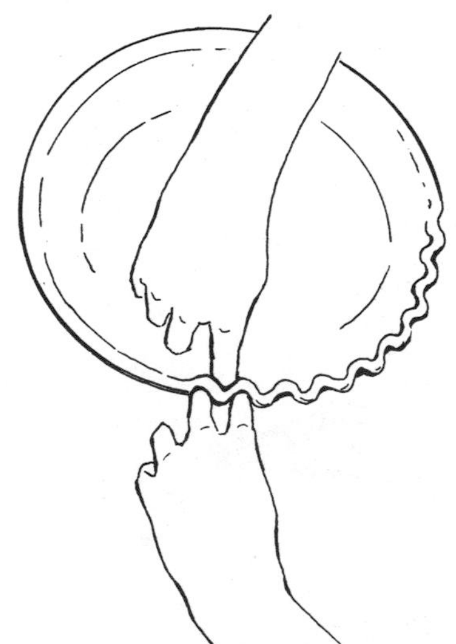

Fork-Edged Crust

Use the dull side of a small knife to trim the pastry even with the outer edge of the pan. Then press the tines of a fork, lightly dusted with flour, around the top edge to decorate the edge and to seal the pie if it is a double-crusted or lattice-topped pie.

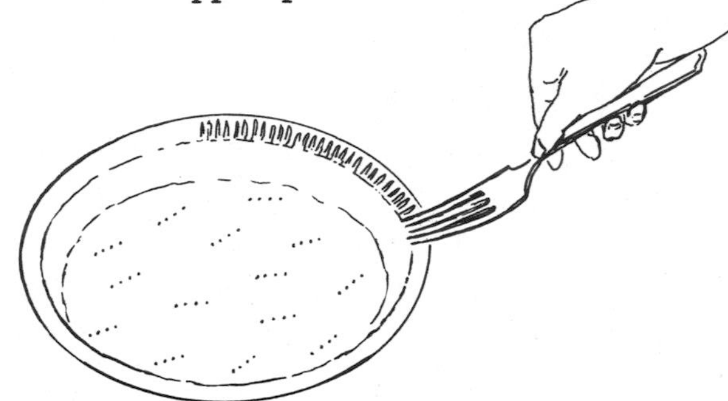

Tart Pan Crust

You must have a ¾-inch edge of pastry extending beyond the tart pan. Fold this pastry to the inside of the tart, building strength into the sides of the tart. Use your fingers to press the dough against the side, both to seal the pastry and to form an even top edge.

Crusts for Tartlet Pans

Line each pan with a round of pastry, easing it into the corners. The pastry should reach,

and be even with, the top of the pan. Use the tines of a fork to prick the bottom of each tartlet shell a couple of times.

Crusts for Tartlets in Muffin Tins

Line each muffin cup with a round of pastry, easing it into the corners and around the sides of each cup. The pastry will not reach the top of the muffin cups, so use your finger tip to pat and slightly extend the top edge of the pastry to make it even. Use the tines of a fork to prick the bottom of each tartlet shell a couple of times.

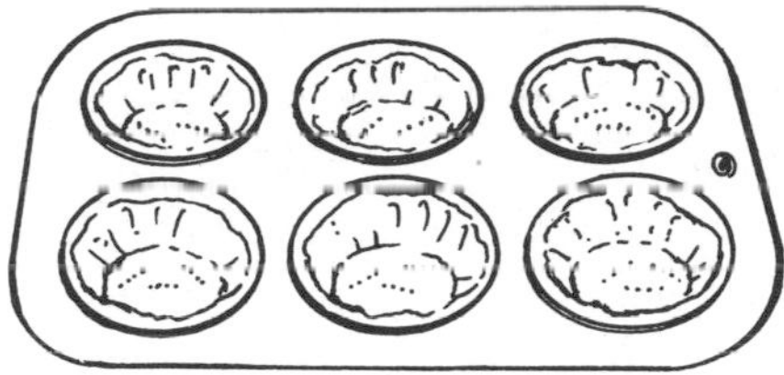

Bottom of a Double-Crusted Pie

Use the dull side of a small knife to trim the pastry even with the outer edge of the pan.

Double-Crusted Pie

Fill the pie with 5 to 8 cups of filling. Then brush Egg Wash (p. 84) on the edge of the bottom crust. Unroll the pastry for the top crust over the pie and press it onto the edge

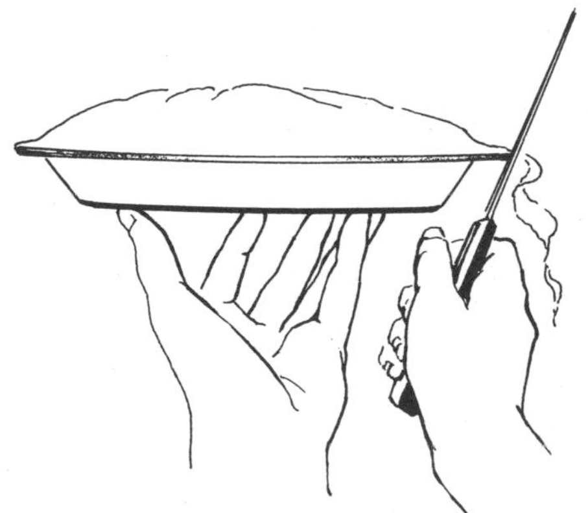

with your fingers. Use the tines of a fork to seal the top and bottom crusts together at the edge. Use the dull side of a small knife to trim off any pastry extending beyond the pie pan.

Lattice-Crust Pie

Roll the dough out to form a 10-inch by 12-inch rectangle. Cut even strips ½ inch to 1¼ inches wide along the length of the pastry rectangle. Beginning in the center of the filled pie, interweave the lattice strips, leaving a space between the strips equal to the width of the strips you are using. Brush Egg Wash on the rim of the pie. Cover the rim all the way around (on top of the ends of the lattice strips) with more strips, placed end to end and cut to fit, as necessary. Seal the pastry together with the tines of a fork. Use the dull side of a small knife to trim off any pastry extending beyond the pie pan.

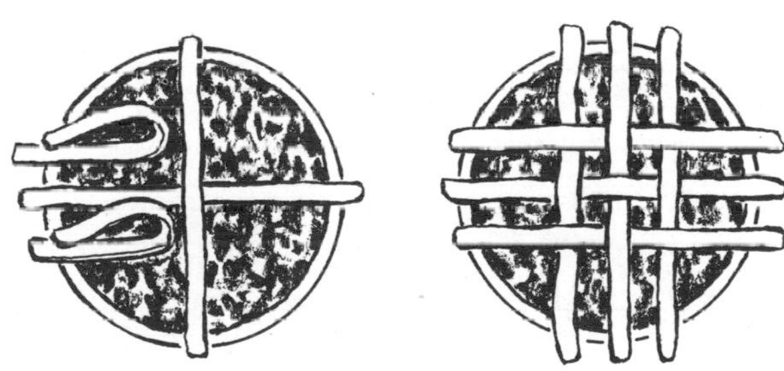

Partially Baking Pie, Tart, or Tartlet Crusts

I have found from baking thousands of pies that partially baking single-crusted pies (and tarts) is a must in avoiding soggy bottom crusts, especially when using custard fillings. Line the unbaked crust with a piece of baking paper, aluminum foil, or a coffee filter, then fill with uncooked beans, rice, or purchased aluminum pie weights. Bake the crust in a preheated

350° F oven for 20 minutes. The crust is ready when you can lift the baking paper and the pastry does not stick to it. Remove the weights (they can be used over and over again for weighting crusts). Then fill the pie shell and bake according to the recipe's instructions.

For tartlets made in muffin tins, place another standard-size muffin tin directly on top of the pastry-lined tin. Turn both pans upside down and use light pressure to push the bottom pan into the dough of the top pan. Bake the pans upside down in the preheated 350° F oven. Alternatively, the individual tarts can be filled with baking paper and pie weights, as with regular-size tart pans.

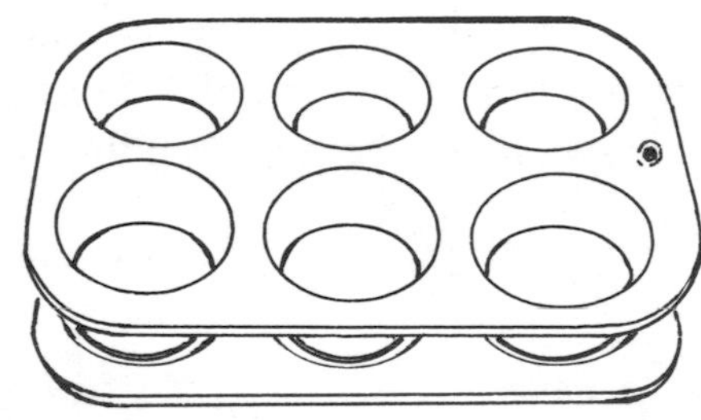

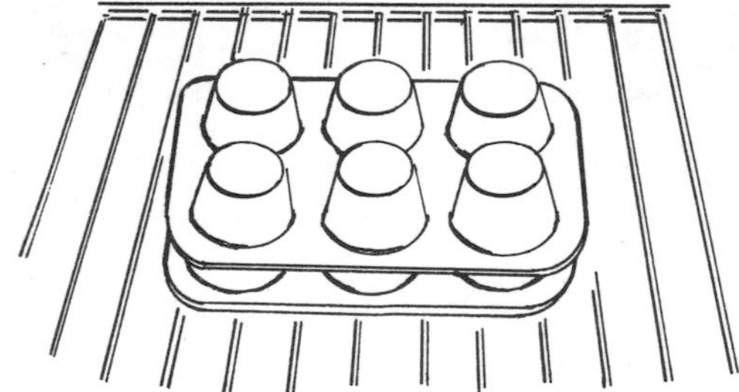

Prebaking (or Blind Baking) Pie, Tart, or Tartlet Crusts

Any pie that has a completely precooked filling, such as cream pies and fresh fruit tarts, should have a completely prebaked crust. Let the pie, tart, or tartlet shells cool completely before filling them.

Follow the directions for partially baked crusts. Once you have removed the pie weights and baking paper, return the crust to the oven. Continue to bake for another 15 to 20 minutes until the crust is golden brown.

With tartlets, once you have removed the pie weights and baking paper, or the top muffin pan, bake them for another 5 to 10 minutes, until the tartlet shells are golden brown.

Baking Filled Pies

A fully baked bottom crust requires sufficient bottom heat to bake the crust thoroughly (so it does not become soggy and almost inedible). With both single- and double-crusted pies, it is very important to position the pie on a baking sheet directly on the floor of a gas oven, or on the lowest shelf of an electric oven. The baking sheet catches any drips, makes the hot pie easier to handle when removing it from the oven, and helps deflect the bottom heat. If your oven has excessive bottom heat, which is unfortunately true of many home ovens, you may need to experiment a bit to find the best way to get enough bottom heat to cook the crust without burning it. Try baking your pies on two baking sheets or in two pie pans, or bake them on the second-lowest shelf in an electric oven or on the lowest shelf in a gas oven. (Don't try everything at once, or you will end up with just what you are trying to avoid, a soggy bottom crust!)

Baker's Tips

• Because pie dough contains a large amount of fat, its temperature when it is rolled out is very important. Very cold dough just out of the refrigerator is too hard to be easily rolled out. Warm, sticky dough is not only difficult to roll out, but the resulting baked crust will not be as flaky or tender.

Pie dough should be firm, yet it should give slightly when you press it with your finger, but it should not stick to your finger.

• When you are comfortable working with the basic pie dough, you can add another step in rolling it out. Every time you turn the dough 45 degrees for the next roll, flip it over as well, so that the bottom becomes the rolling surface, and the rolling surface becomes the bottom. This will help keep the dough from ever sticking to the work table, as you will always know its condition, top and bottom.

• Use a commercial-quality rolling pin for ease in rolling out crusts evenly and quickly. My favorite rolling pin has ball bearing action for ease in handling. It is made from a beautiful piece of maple and is 15 inches in length (25 inches in length including the handles) and 3 inches in diameter. To properly care for a wooden rolling pin, never immerse it in water. When water is necessary to clean it, be sure to dry the rolling pin immediately. This will prevent warping and splitting of the wood.

• When you have time, it is a good idea to make enough pie dough so you can form extra crusts and freeze them for later use. These crusts can be stacked and stored frozen for 2 to 3 months. In fact, they are flakier when frozen before baking. Bottom crusts can be frozen and then stacked together. They should then be used directly from the freezer without thawing. Top crusts and lattice strips can be frozen on a flat surface between pieces of plastic wrap. To prevent them from cracking and for ease in handling them, top crusts and lattice strips must be defrosted in the refrigerator just until slightly softened, before putting them in place.

• Lining pie crusts with baking paper and pie weights for prebaking lessens any shrinkage of the crusts at the sides, and weights the bottom to keep it from puffing up unevenly. When lining crusts with baking paper, crumple the paper first, and then uncrumple it and place it on the crust. Once it is filled with pie weights, the softened paper will then fit more easily into the corners, curves, and fluted sides, thereby more efficiently performing its job.

Basic Pie Crust

 *

Yield:
1, 2, and 4 to 5 9-inch or 10-inch crusts

Exceptionally tender, flaky, and buttery good. This basic crust is suitable for almost every pie or tart you might want to make. It can be made with all butter, all margarine, or half butter and half margarine, and can be prepared very quickly in a food processor, an electric mixer, or by hand. Follow the instructions closely for your own success.

Quantity Crusts			Ingredients
1 Crust	**2 Crusts**	**4 to 5 Crusts**	
½ cup (¼ pound)	**1 cup (½ pound)**	**2 cups (1 pound)**	**cold butter* (or half butter and half margarine)** ***(substitute all margarine for dairy-free)***
⅔ cup	**1⅓ cups**	**2⅔ cups**	**unbleached white flour**
⅓ cup	**⅔ cup**	**1⅓ cups**	**whole wheat pastry flour**
⅛ teaspoon	**⅜ teaspoon**	**¾ teaspoon**	**salt**
2 tablespoons	**¼ cup**	**½ cup**	**cold water**

Cut the cold butter and/or margarine into ½-inch squares. Place the flours, salt, and cold butter into the bowl of your food processor or a medium-size mixing bowl. Use the pulsing action on the food processor to cut the butter into the flour until it resembles coarse cornmeal, or use the electric mixer on low speed to do the same. It is important with either machine not to overmix, not to whip air into the mixture, and not to mix until large clumps begin forming. Add the water all at once and mix just until the dough comes together. This is just a matter of a couple of seconds in the food processor, and to the count of ten with an electric mixer.

When mixing by hand, use the fingers and thumb of each hand to "rub" in the butter until the mixture resembles coarse cornmeal. Be sure to lift your hands out of the bowl while simultaneously using your thumbs to rub the flour and butter across your fingers. Pour the cold water into the center of the flour mixture and mix quickly with your hand to form the dough.

Form the completed dough into a cylinder and wrap in plastic wrap. Place in the refrigerator for at least 20 minutes before rolling out. Then roll and shape according to the directions on pages 77–79.

Nutty-Oat Crust

Yield:
9-inch pie crust

Delightfully crisp and crunchy just like a cookie, Nutty-Oat Crust is the perfect textural complement to creamy Apple Custard Pie (page 98) or Boysenberry Custard Pie (page 99).

¼ cup walnuts
2 cups rolled oats
Pinch salt
¼ cup oil
1½ tablespoons fruit sweetener
½ teaspoon vanilla extract
¼ teaspoon almond extract
¼ cup vanilla amazake

Glaze

1 tablespoon fruit sweetener
1 tablespoon water

Preheat the oven to 350° F.

Toast the walnuts in a preheated oven for 7 to 10 minutes, stirring occasionally. Allow the nuts to cool. Then process them in a food processor, using a pulsing action, until they are finely ground.

Use an electric mixer to mix all the crust ingredients until the oats soften enough for the mixture to hold itself together when squeezed in your hand. Press the dough into a pie tin, forming a rounded edge.

Bake the crust in the preheated over for 20 minutes. Remove the crust from the oven.

In a small bowl combine the fruit sweetener and water for the glaze, and brush on the hot crust. Return the crust to the oven and bake for another 10 to 15 minutes until the crust is evenly browned.

Let the crust cool before filling.

Baker's Tip

• Nutty-Oat Crust, when well wrapped, can be successfully frozen for up to 2 months.

Granola Crust

  *

Yield:
10-inch crust

This Granola Crust is our alternative to graham cracker crust (as I have not yet found sugar-free graham crackers that I like). It can be used with cheesecake or in any other pie which needs a fully prebaked crust before filling. In my early days of baking, before attending cooking school, I specialized only in pies that could be made in graham cracker crusts, as they were the only kind I knew how to make. Fortunately, crumb crusts are delicious, and this Granola Crust is exceptionally so.

½ cup almonds
1¼ cups fruit-sweetened granola (to equal 1⅛ cups crushed)
5 tablespoons (2½ ounces) melted butter* ***(substitute margarine for dairy-free)***
3 tablespoons fruit sweetener
¾ teaspoon cinnamon
2 tablespoons brown rice flour

Preheat the oven to 350° F. Lightly spray a 10-inch pie pan with lecithin spray.

Toast the almonds in a preheated oven for 7 to 10 minutes, stirring occasionally. Allow the nuts to cool. Then process them in a food processor, using a pulsing action, until they are finely ground. Remove the almonds and add the granola. Process the granola until finely crushed.

Use an electric mixer or a food processor to combine all the ingredients together. Press the crust into the prepared pan while the crust mixture is still warm from the melted butter.

Bake the crust in the preheated oven for 10 minutes.

Baker's Tip

• If your granola has raisins in it, be sure to remove them first, as they won't grind up in the processor or soften up during baking.

Egg Wash for Pies and Tarts

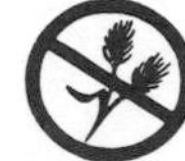

Yield:
¼ cup

Cream is often used in the Egg Wash for Pies and Tarts as it helps the crusts turn a wonderful golden brown as they bake. Milk can be substituted for the cream, and two egg yolks for the whole egg with similar results.

1 egg or 2 yolks
Pinch salt
¼ cup cream or milk

In a cup or small bowl, mix the egg and salt together with a fork until well mixed. Stir in the cream or milk. Apply Egg Wash to the crust using a brush.

Egg Wash can be stored in the refrigerator for a couple of days if kept well covered.

Bakers Tip

• Egg Wash may be omitted for egg-free pies. In double-crusted and lattice-crusted pies, replace the Egg Wash with water for brushing on the edge of the bottom crust, to insure a good seal between it and the top crust. Do *not* brush the top crust with water.

American Beauty Apple Pie

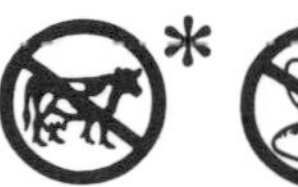

Yield:
9-inch pie
6 to 8 servings

We began serving this favorite American pie at The Ranch Kitchen the very first summer we opened. I decorated the top with pastry rosebuds and then named it American Beauty Apple Pie. The rosebuds, leaves, and stems are made from the pie crust trimmings. My first rosebuds were a bit thick and not cooked all the way through, but the pie was so beautiful and delicious that it was worth the effort to perfect them. Perfected they were, and this incomparable American Beauty Apple Pie has won blue ribbons at the local county fair both years it was entered and continues to earn kudos from our customers.

By experimenting with hundreds of apple pies, we were able to solve the usual problem of air space between the apples and the baked crust in the finished pie. Tossing the sliced raw apples with the sweetener the day before we make the pie draws the juices out of the apples, reducing the volume of the sliced raw apples and making it closer to the volume of the cooked apples. Then, when the top crust is put in place it is just about where it will be when the pie is cooked, with little or no air space in the baked pie. This step is not essential. However, if you have the time and want to serve your pie in picture-perfect slices, give our method a try.

Crust

Basic Pie Crust* (page 82): 9-inch bottom crust and 10-inch top crust
Trimmings for leaves, rosebuds, and stems
Egg Wash for Pies and Tarts* (page 84) ***(omit for egg-free)***

Filling

6 to 7 tart green apples
1 tablespoon fresh lemon juice
1½ teaspoons water
7 tablespoons fruit sweetener
¾ teaspoon cinnamon
¼ teaspoon nutmeg
2⅔ tablespoons unbleached white flour
1 tablespoon butter* ***(substitute margarine for dairy-free)***

The day before you plan to bake the pie, peel, core, and slice the apples ⅛ inch thick. You should have 9 cups of sliced apples. Toss the sliced apples with the lemon juice, water, and sweetener in a medium-size bowl. Cover the bowl of apples with plastic wrap and refrigerate overnight.

Prepare the bottom and top crusts according to the directions on pages 77–79.

On baking day, preheat the oven to 350° F.

Combine the spices and flour in a small bowl. Stir ⅓ cup of the liquid from the apple slices into the flour and spices to make a smooth mixture. Pour this mixture back over the apples and toss well to thoroughly coat them. Pile the apple slices with their juices into an unbaked pie crust. Cut the butter into 4 or 5 pieces, and dot them over the apples.

Prepare the Egg Wash and brush it onto the rim of crust. Cover the pie with the top crust. Seal the edges by pressing lightly with the tines of a fork. Use the dull side of a small knife to trim off any pastry extending beyond the edge of the pie pan.

To prepare the rosebuds, leaves, and stems from the pastry trimmings, roll the pastry trimmings out very thin. Use the point of a small knife to cut 6 rectangles measuring ⅔ inch by 2 inches for the rosebuds. Cut 12 ovals with pointed ends measuring 1½ inches to 2 inches

in length for the leaves. Use some of the remaining trim to make a thin, ⅛-inch-wide rope that measures 12 inches in length. Cut the rope into 6 lengths to form 6 stems.

Use the top of the knife to press a leaf pattern on each of the ovals.

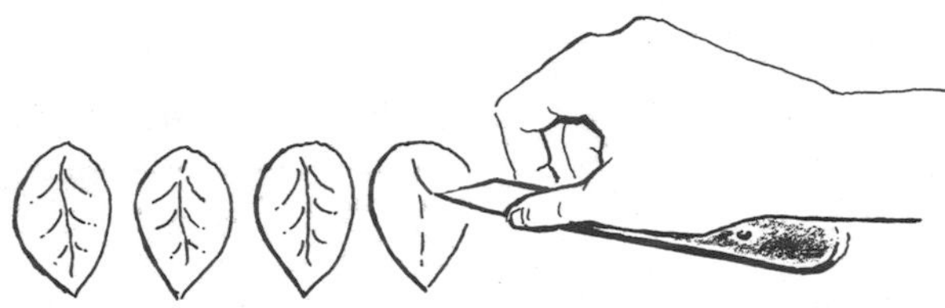

For the rosebuds, flatten a rectangle between your thumb and forefinger. Start at the right side of the rectangle and fold the top corner down to form a loose triangle. The top

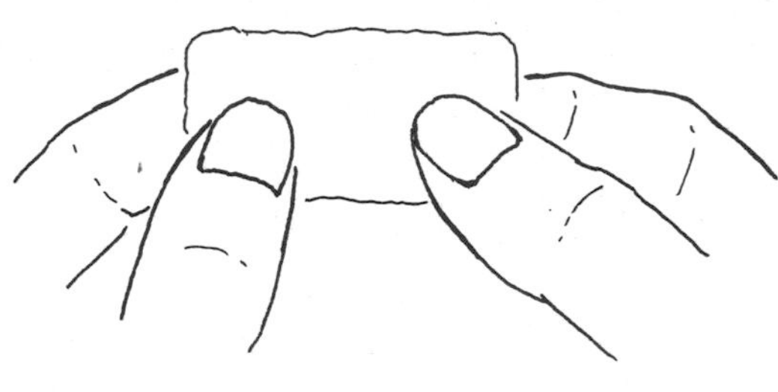

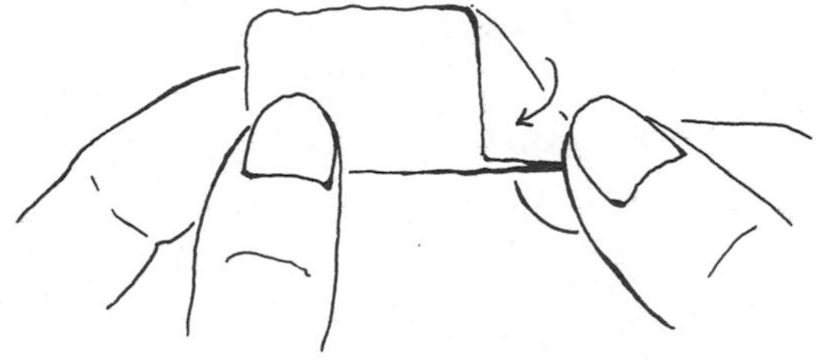

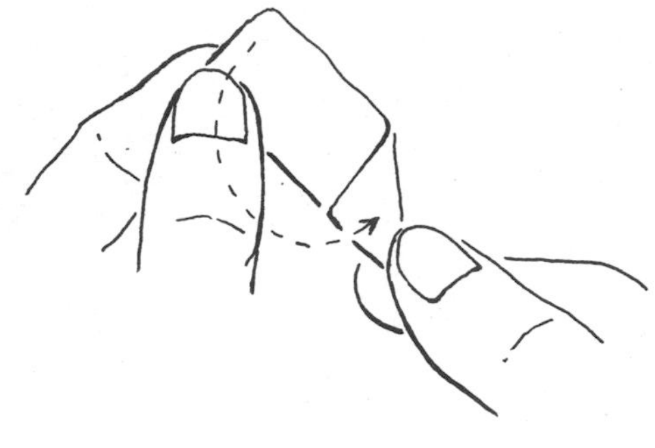

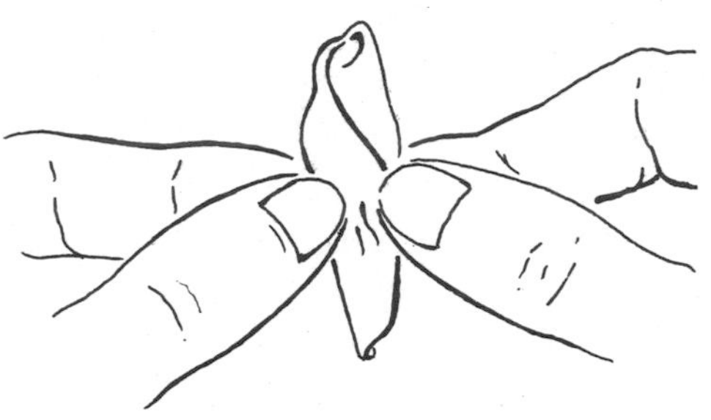

of the triangle now becomes the center of the bud, so angle it straight up and wrap the rest of the rectangle around it loosely, plumping and shaping the bottom to resemble a rosebud.

Brush the top crust with Egg Wash. Dip each stem, bud, and leaf in the Egg Wash, drain the excess, and attach them decoratively to the crust. At The Ranch Kitchen we place 1 bud, 2 leaves, and 1 stem on each portion of pie.

Make 6 small slits towards the center of the top crust for steam to escape during baking. Place the pie on a baking sheet in the preheated oven. Place the pie on the lowest shelf of an electric oven or directly on the floor of a gas oven. Bake for approximately 1½ hours. After an hour, check the apples with a toothpick through the steam slits. The apples are done when they have some resistance, but still feel tender.

For the best appearance on the plate, let the pie cool thoroughly before serving; however, this pie is most delicious hot from the oven, topped with French vanilla ice cream.

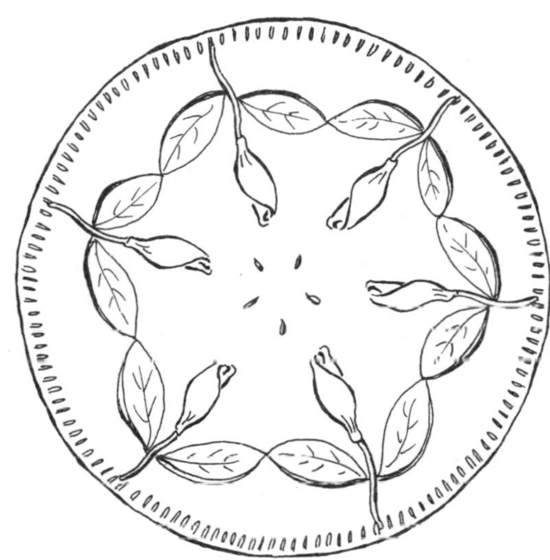

Cranberry Apple Pie

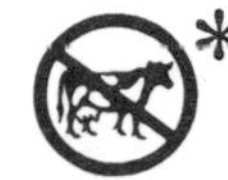*
*

Yield:
9-inch pie
6 to 8 servings

Bright red cranberries and crisp, juicy apples are deliciously complementary to one another with the natural sweetness of the apples mellowing the natural tartness of the cranberries. Cranberry Apple Pie is a fabulous pie to make and enjoy in the late fall, when cranberries and apples are at their peak of flavor and abundance.

Crust

Basic Pie Crust* (page 82): 9-inch bottom crust, unbaked
¾-inch-wide lattice strips for top crust
Egg Wash for Pies and Tarts* (page 84) ***(omit for egg-free)***

Filling

4 to 5 tart apples
½ cup fresh orange juice
½ cup fruit sweetener
2 tablespoons cornstarch
¼ teaspoon salt
2 tablespoons grated orange zest
1 teaspoon cinnamon
¼ teaspoon nutmeg
2½ cups fresh or frozen cranberries
3 tablespoons butter* ***(substitute margarine for dairy-free)***

Prepare the bottom crust according to the recipe directions on pages 77–78. The lattice strips (see page 79) can be cut in advance and refrigerated, covered with plastic. For ease in handling remove them 10 minutes before they are needed.

Peel, core, and dice the apples into small (¼-inch to ½-inch) cubes. You should have 4 cups of diced apples. Cook the apples in the fresh orange juice over medium heat in a medium-size covered saucepan, stirring occasionally. Cook just until the apples are softened. Stir in the remaining filling ingredients, except for the cranberries and butter. Cut the butter into walnut-size pieces. When the apple mixture is well blended, stir in the cranberries and butter. Continue to simmer for about 5 more minutes, until the cranberries pop. Remove the pan from the heat. Place the apple/cranberry filling in a bowl and refrigerate until cool.

Preheat the oven to 350° F. When the apple cranberry filling is well chilled, pile it into the unbaked crust. Prepare the Egg Wash and brush it onto the rim of the crust. Top the pie with interwoven lattice strips. Trim the edge of the pie of any pastry extending beyond the edge of the pie pan, and seal by pressing lightly with the tines of a fork. Brush the lattice top with Egg Wash.

To bake the pie, place it on a baking sheet in the preheated oven, directly on the oven floor of a gas oven or on the lowest shelf of an electric oven. Bake until the crust is golden and the filling is bubbling to within 3 inches of the center of the pie, 1 to 1¼ hours.

Serve Cranberry Apple Pie hot from the oven or at room temperature.

Baker's Tip

• Cranberry Apple Pie turns a lovely shade of pink when it is prepared with frozen cranberries. Freezing breaks down the cell structure of the cranberries so that they release their cranberry-hued juices, in this case turning the apples pink.

Crimson Pie

*
*

Yield:
9-inch pie
6 to 8 servings

Cranberries and blueberries make an incomparable combination, giving me a sense of tradition and comfort in this very beautiful and elegant ruby-colored pie with its accompanying deep, rich flavor. This is a pie to be served in a dark wood-paneled dining room with hunter green walls, patterned china plates, and sparkling crystal—with cabbage roses from the garden everywhere.

However, Crimson Pie goes equally well with very modern Chinette plates, plastic forks, and a green and white checked tablecloth.

Crust

Basic Pie Crust* (page 82): 9-inch bottom crust, unbaked
10-inch top crust
Egg Wash for Pies and Tarts* (page 84) ***(omit for egg-free)***

Filling

½ orange, seeded (do not peel)
4 cups fresh or frozen blueberries
12-ounce bag (3¼ cups) fresh or frozen cranberries
¾ cup fruit sweetener
3 tablespoons cornstarch
1 tablespoon butter* ***(substitute margarine for dairy-free)***

Prepare the bottom and top crusts according to the directions on pages 77–79.

Coarsely grind the half orange (peel included) in a processor or blender. Put the ground orange in a saucepan along with the blueberries, cranberries, and ¼ cup of the sweetener. Cook over medium heat until the mixture comes to a boil.

Meanwhile, dissolve the cornstarch in the remaining ½ cup of sweetener. When the berry mixture is boiling, whisk in the dissolved cornstarch, stirring constantly. When the mixture returns to a boil, reduce the heat and simmer for 5 minutes. Remove from the heat. Place the filling in a bowl and cool it thoroughly before pouring it into an unbaked crust. The filling can be prepared up to a week in advance and refrigerated.

Preheat the oven to 350° F.

Pile the filling into the unbaked pie crust. Cut the butter into 4 or 5 pieces, and dot them over the filling. Prepare the Egg Wash and brush it on the rim of the crust. Cover the pie with the top crust. Seal the edges by pressing lightly with the tines of a fork. Use the dull side of a small knife to trim off any pastry extending beyond the edge of the pie pan. Brush the top crust with Egg Wash. Use a sharp knife to make a few slits in the top crust to release steam during baking.

To bake the pie, place it on a baking sheet in the preheated oven, directly on the oven floor of a gas oven or on the lowest shelf of an electric oven. Bake the pie for about 1 hour, until the crust is golden and the filling is bubbling.

Serve Crimson Pie hot from the oven or at room temperature.

Blueberry Lattice Pie

Yield:
9-inch pie
6 to 8 servings

Another blue-ribbon winner and Ranch Kitchen perennial favorite. Our Blueberry Pies are irresistible because they are loaded with blueberries. The pies are really full and luscious looking. The filling is juicy and yet it holds together so that when the pies have cooled you can cut a perfect piece.

We have found that Blueberry Pies can be prepared in advance and then frozen unbaked. To avoid a layer of gelatin-like cooked cornstarch just above the bottom crust in the baked pie, the frozen blueberries must remain solidly frozen while you prepare the pie. When the blueberries are frozen, the cornstarch and spices stick to them, providing thickening throughout the whole pie.

Crust

Basic Pie Crust* (page 82): 9-inch bottom crust, unbaked
5/8-inch-wide lattice strips
Egg Wash for Pies and Tarts* (page 84) ***(omit for egg-free)***

Filling

1¼ teaspoons cinnamon
3/8 teaspoon nutmeg
3½ teaspoons cornstarch
2 teaspoons lemon zest
1½ teaspoons fresh lemon juice
3 tablespoons cold water
⅔ cup fruit sweetener
5¾ cups frozen blueberries

Prepare the bottom crust according to the directions on pages 77–78. The lattice strips (page 79) can be cut in advance and refrigerated, covered with plastic. For ease of handling, remove them 10 minutes before they are needed.

Preheat the oven to 350° F.

In a small bowl, thoroughly mix together all the filling ingredients, except the blueberries. Remove the blueberries from the freezer to a large bowl. Add the cornstarch/spice mixture and toss to coat the berries evenly. Pile the blueberry filling into the unbaked pie crust.

Prepare the Egg Wash and brush it onto the rim of the crust. Top the pie with interwoven lattice strips. Use the dull side of a small knife to trim off any pastry extending beyond the edge of the pie pan. Seal the edge by pressing lightly with the tines of a fork. Brush the lattice top with Egg Wash. Place the pie directly into the freezer if it is not to be baked immediately.

To bake the pie, place it on a baking sheet in the preheated oven, directly on the oven floor of a gas oven or on the lowest shelf of an electric oven. Bake until the crust is golden and the filling is bubbling to within 3 inches of the center of the pie, 1¾ to 2 hours. Cool the pie before cutting and serving.

Baker's Tips

• Blueberry pies can be frozen unbaked for up to two months. When ready to bake, put them directly from freezer into the preheated oven. *Do not defrost before baking.*

• The "bubbling to within 3 inches of the center" test for doneness ensures a juicy and moist pie. If you let your pie bake longer, you may have drier and less delicious results.

• I prefer and suggest baking berry and other fruit pies at a constant 350° F for their entire baking time. I find that pies baked this way brown evenly and always seem to be the perfect color at the same time the filling is ready. Some bakers suggest baking at a very high temperature for the first 10 minutes, then lowering the temperature after that. This method has not worked well for me, as the pies always seem to brown too much, too quickly.

Fresh Cherry Pie

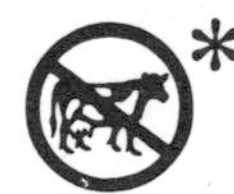**

Yield:
9-inch pie
6 to 8 servings

We use the incomparable dark, sweet cherries from Flathead Lake, Montana, at The Ranch Kitchen. They are unbelievably flavorful and juicy, and they make great pies, with just the right combination of sweet, tart, and delicious. Pitting cherries is admittedly not much fun, but a fragrant, bubbling pie brimming with beautiful red cherries makes it worth all the effort.

Crust

Basic Pie Crust* (page 82): 9-inch bottom crust, unbaked
¾-inch-wide lattice strips
Egg Wash for Pies and Tarts* (page 84) *(omit for egg-free)*

Filling

6 cups fresh dark sweet cherries
1⅔ tablespoons cornstarch
¾ cup fruit sweetener
1 tablespoon fresh lemon juice
½ teaspoon vanilla extract
¼ teaspoon almond extract

Prepare the bottom crust according to the directions on pages 77–78. The lattice strips (page 79) can be cut in advance and refrigerated, covered with plastic. Remove them 10 minutes before they are needed for ease in handling.

Preheat the oven to 350° F.

Pit the cherries. In a medium-size bowl, mix all the filling ingredients except the pitted cherries. Toss the cherries in the mixture to coat them evenly. Pile the cherry mixture into the unbaked crust.

Prepare the Egg Wash and brush it onto the rim of the crust. Top the pie with interwoven lattice strips. Trim from the edge of the pie any pastry extending beyond the edge of the pie pan, and seal by pressing lightly with the tines of a fork. Brush the lattice top with Egg Wash.

To bake the pie, place it on a baking sheet in the preheated oven, directly on the oven floor of a gas oven or on the lowest shelf of an electric oven. Bake at 350° for 1 to 1¼ hours, until the crust is golden and the filling is bubbling to within 3 inches of the center of the pie. Cool the pie before cutting and serving.

Fresh Peach Pie

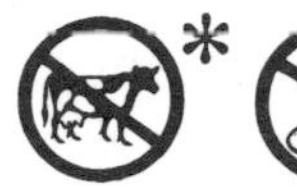*
*

Yield:
9-inch pie
6 to 8 servings

What I love best about Peach Pie is the way it looks. With its golden peach juices bursting out of its wide-lattice top, this pie is a portrait of summertime. A Fresh Peach Pie will just encourage your love affair with peaches, especially if it's midsummer and the peaches are ripe, fragrant, and delicious.

If your peaches are exceptionally juicy, use the greater amount of cornstarch to thicken your pie. If they are a bit less juicy, use the lesser amount of cornstarch.

Crust

Basic Pie Crust* (page 82): 9-inch bottom crust, unbaked
¾-inch-wide lattice strips
Egg Wash for Pies and Tarts* (page 84) *(omit for egg-free)*

Filling

6 to 8 medium-size peaches
¼ cup fruit sweetener
1/8 teaspoon salt
1½ to 2½ tablespoons cornstarch
¼ teaspoon cinnamon
⅛ teaspoon nutmeg
1 teaspoon vanilla extract
1 tablespoon lemon juice
½ teaspoon lemon zest

Prepare the bottom crust according to the directions on pages 77–78. The lattice strips (page 79) can be cut in advance and refrigerated, covered with plastic. For ease of handling remove them 10 minutes before they are needed.

Preheat the oven to 350° F.

Place the peaches in a pot of boiling water for 5 to 10 seconds to loosen their skins. Peel the peaches. Then slice them into ¼-inch slices. You should have 6 cups of sliced peaches.

In a medium-size bowl, mix together all the filling ingredients, except the peaches. Add the sliced peaches and toss to coat them evenly with the cornstarch and spice mixture. Pile the fruit into the unbaked pie crust.

Prepare the Egg Wash and brush it onto the rim of the crust. Top the pie with interwoven lattice strips. Trim from the edge of the pie any pastry extending beyond the edge of the pie pan, and seal by pressing lightly with the tines of a fork. Brush the lattice top with Egg Wash.

To bake the pie, place it on a baking sheet in the preheated oven, directly on the floor of a gas oven or on the lowest shelf of an electric oven. Bake for 1 to 1¼ hours, until the crust is golden and the filling is bubbling to within 3 inches of the center of the pie. Cool the pie before cutting and serving.

Frozen Peach Pie

Yield:
9-inch pie
6 to 8 servings

Using frozen peaches you can prepare Peach Pie in minutes, and enjoy it any time of the year.

Crust

Basic Pie Crust* (page 82): 9-inch bottom crust, unbaked
1¼-inch-wide lattice strips
Egg Wash for Pies and Tarts* (page 84) ***(omit for egg-free)***

Filling

7 cups frozen sliced peaches
3 tablespoons fruit sweetener
2 teaspoons lemon juice
½ teaspoon grated lemon zest
7 teaspoons cornstarch
½ teaspoon cinnamon
⅛ teaspoon nutmeg
¾ teaspoon vanilla extract
Pinch salt

Prepare the bottom crust according to the directions on pages 77–78. The lattice strips (page 79) can be cut in advance and refrigerated, covered with plastic. For ease of handling, remove them 10 minutes before they are needed.

Preheat the oven to 350° F.

Sort through the frozen peaches for extra-thick slices. Cut them so that all of the slices are approximately ¼ inch thick. In a medium-size bowl, mix together all the filling ingredients, except the peaches. Add the sliced peaches and toss to coat them evenly with the cornstarch mixture. Pile the fruit into the unbaked crust.

Prepare the Egg Wash and brush it onto the rim of the crust. Top the pie with interwoven lattice strips. Use the dull side of a small knife to trim off any pastry extending beyond the edge of the pie pan. Seal the edge of the pie by pressing lightly with the tines of a fork. Brush the lattice top with Egg Wash. Place the peach pie directly into freezer if it is not to be baked immediately.

To bake the pie, place it on a baking sheet in the preheated oven, directly on the oven floor of a gas oven or on the lowest shelf of an electric oven. Bake for 1 to 1¼ hours, until the crust is golden and the filling is bubbling to within 3 inches of the center of the pie.

For the nicest presentation, cool the pie to room temperature before cutting and serving.

Baker's Tip

• Peach pies can be frozen unbaked for up to 2 months. When ready to bake, put them directly from the freezer into the preheated oven. *Do not defrost them before baking.*

Fresh Pear Ginger Pie

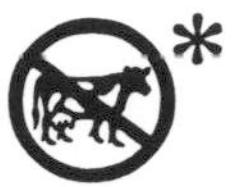
*

Yield:
9-inch pie
6 to 8 servings

This is a fabulous pie—light, not too sweet, and nondairy. Its taste and texture are rich, fruity, and creamy, with the pears enveloped in an almond milk custard. For contrast in texture, the fruit custard is topped with a crunchy streusel crust. I learned the hard way that unless the streusel is put in place after the custard has been partially baked, the bottom part of the streusel will cook with the custard and become soggy and very unappealing in the chilled pie.

Serve Pear Ginger Pie at room temperature or still warm from the oven, when its flavor and texture are the most delicate.

Ripe pears should be used for the fullest flavor and fragrance. Replace the pears with fresh peaches for a delicious summertime variation.

Crust

Basic Pie Crust* (page 82): 9-inch bottom crust, partially baked

Filling

1 cup almond milk (3:1) (page 12)
3 pears
½ teaspoon ginger
⅛ teaspoon nutmeg
⅛ teaspoon salt
⅓ cup fruit sweetener
2 eggs
¼ teaspoon vanilla extract
¼ teaspoon almond extract
½ teaspoon grated lemon zest

Streusel Topping

1¼ cups unbleached white flour
3 tablespoons fruit sweetener
¼ teaspoon cinnamon
⅛ teaspoon nutmeg
¼ teaspoon ginger
¼ teaspoon grated lemon zest
½ cup cold margarine

Preheat the oven to 350° F. Prepare and partially bake the pie crust according to the directions on pages 77–79.

Prepare the almond milk by blending ⅓ cup blanched almonds with 1 cup of water for 5 minutes in a blender. Strain the liquid through a piece of dampened cheesecloth. Measure, and add additional water, if necessary, to make 1 cup of almond milk.

Peel the fresh pears with a vegetable peeler and cut them in thirds, lengthwise. Remove the cores, then slice the pear sections into ¼-inch slices along the width of each section.

Place the sliced pears in the bottom of the partially baked crust. In a small bowl, mix the filling ingredients together in the order listed, mixing in the almond milk last. Pour this mixture over the pears.

To bake the pie, place it on a baking sheet in the preheated oven, directly on the oven floor of a gas oven or on the lowest shelf of an electric oven. Bake for 35 to 40 minutes, until the custard has set slightly.

Meanwhile, prepare the streusel topping. Use either an electric mixer or a food processor to combine all the topping ingredients, except the butter or margarine, until crumbly. Cut the cold butter or margarine into ½-inch pieces. Add them to the topping, mixing with a pulsing action of the food processor or on medium speed of an electric mixer, just so the topping stays crumbly. Do not make a smooth mixture.

Remove the pie from the oven. Cover the custard lightly and evenly with the streusel. Return the pie to the oven and continue to bake for another 20 to 25 minutes, until the streusel is brown.

Variation

Fresh Peach Ginger Pie. Substitute 3 ripe peaches for the pears. Peel the peaches and slice them into ¼-inch slices.

Baker's Tips

• Pears ripen best in a paper bag at room temperature. To tell if a pear is ripe, press gently at the stem end with your forefinger. The pear will give slightly to your touch when it is ripe. This is very important with pears, for they are at their best for a very short period of time. When they are at their best, there is nothing like a creamy, fresh, and juicy pear.

• For the most efficient use of time and movement, I have found it helpful to cut pears or apples into thirds instead of quarters for peeling and coring them. This way you have only 3 portions to work with versus 4; for example, with 4 apples, you need to handle only 12 sections versus 16.

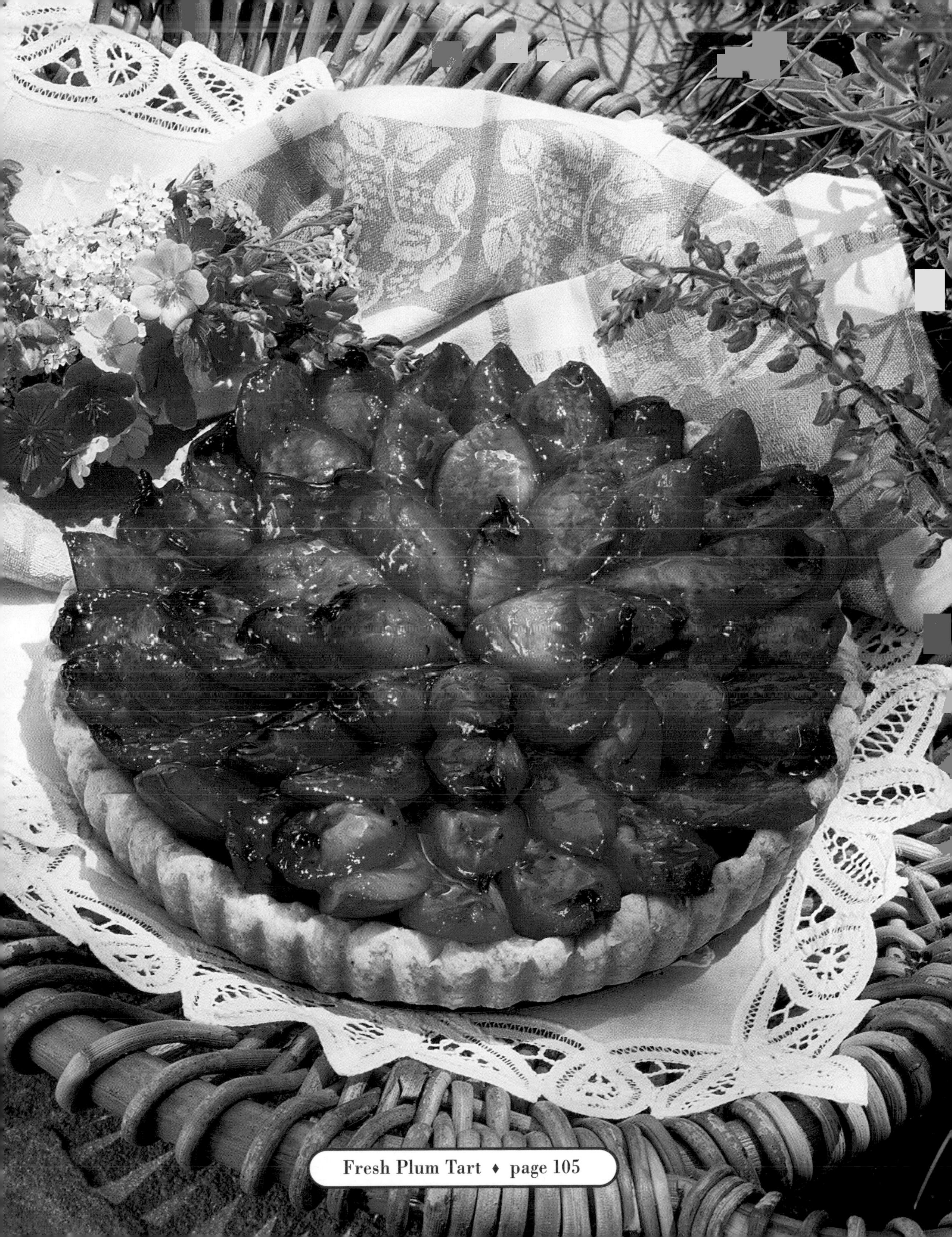

Fresh Plum Tart ♦ page 105

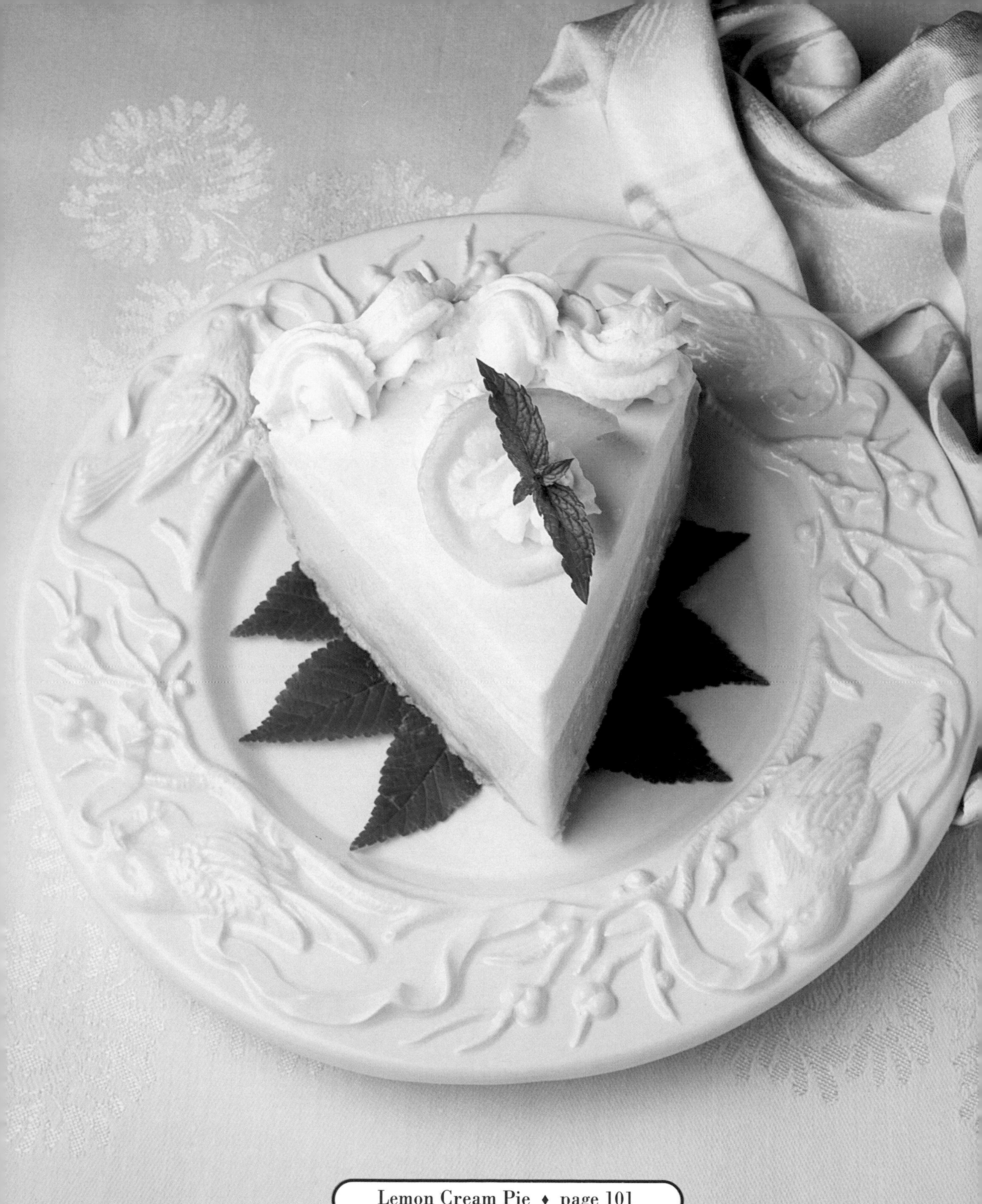

Lemon Cream Pie ♦ page 101

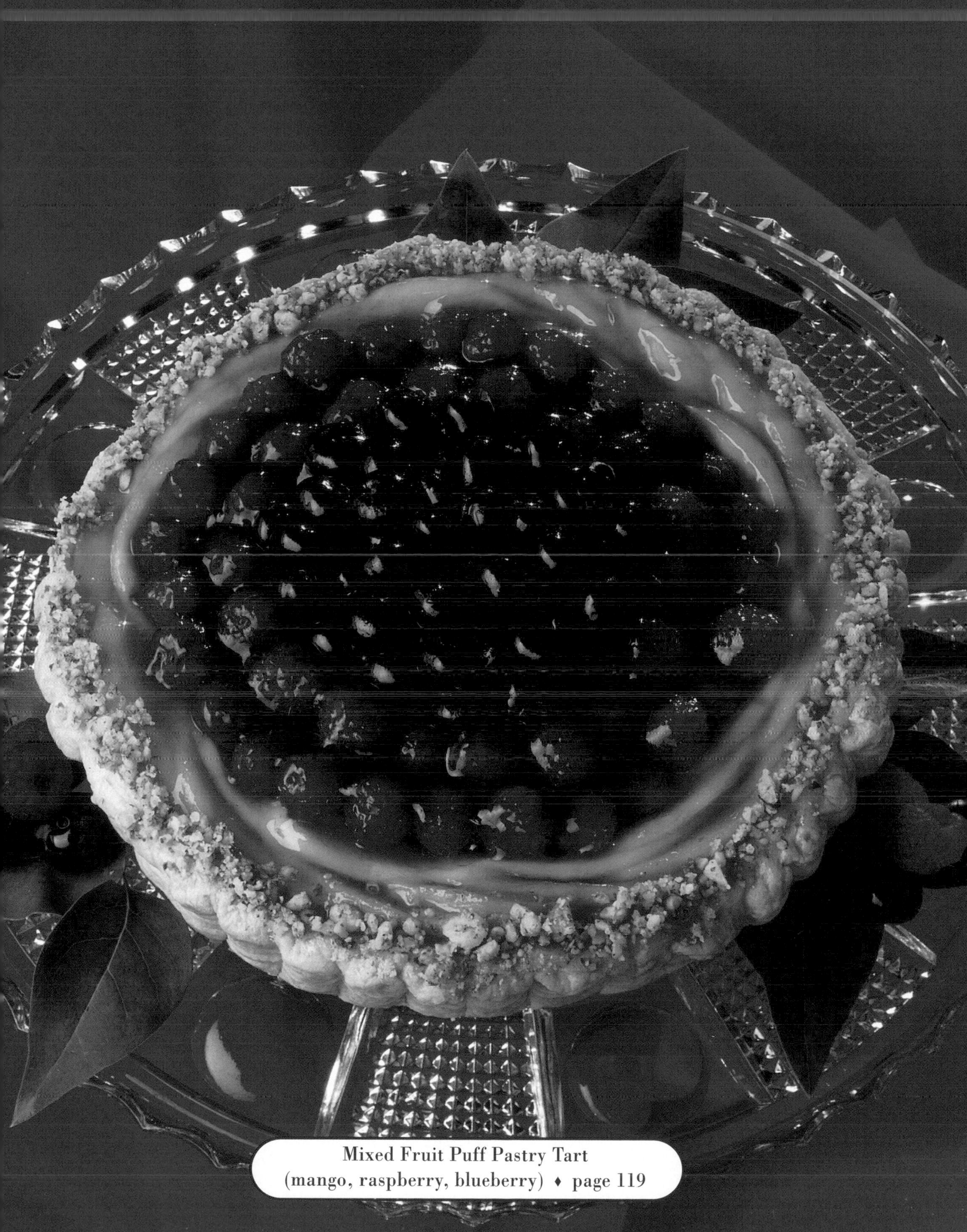

Mixed Fruit Puff Pastry Tart
(mango, raspberry, blueberry) ♦ page 119

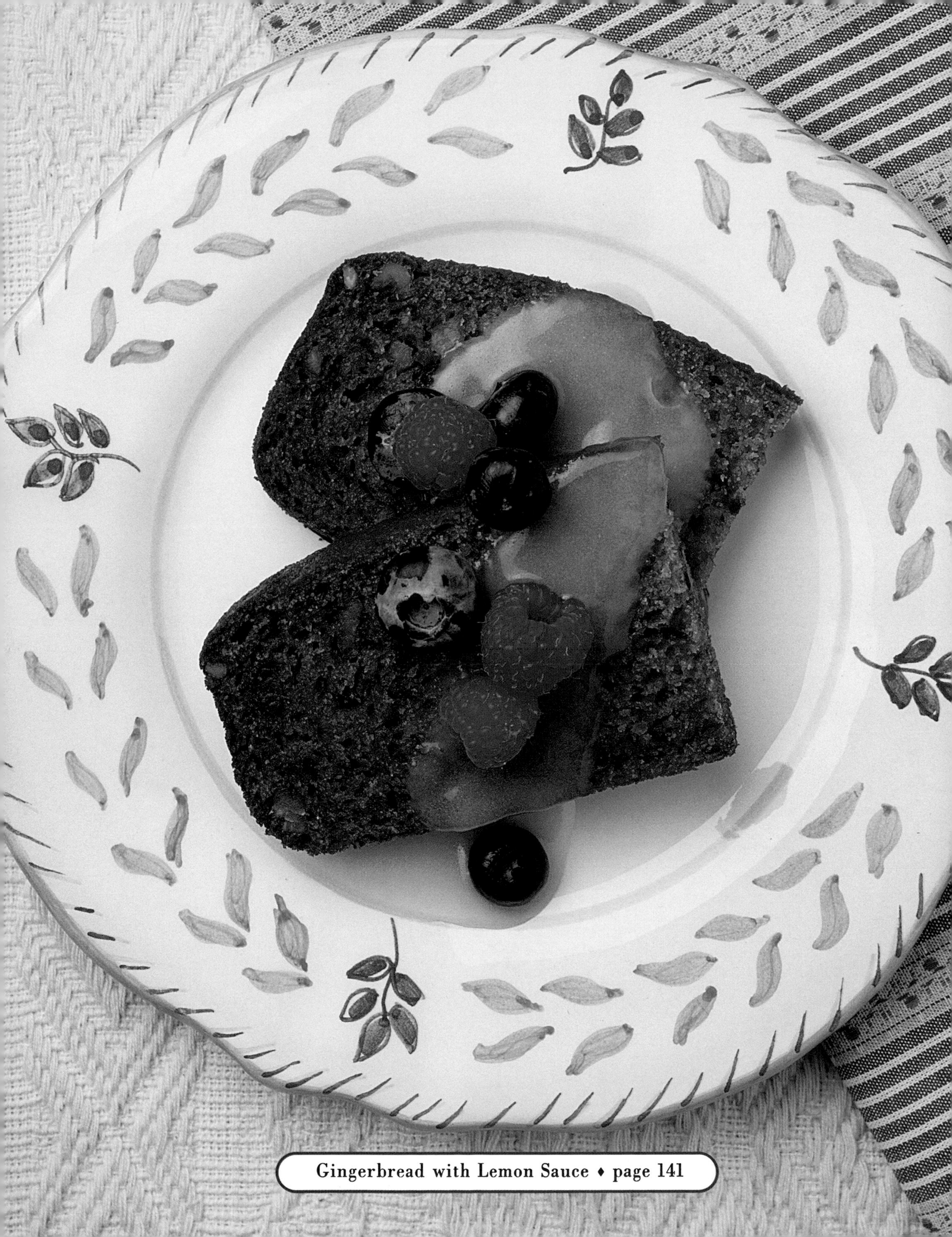

Gingerbread with Lemon Sauce ♦ page 141

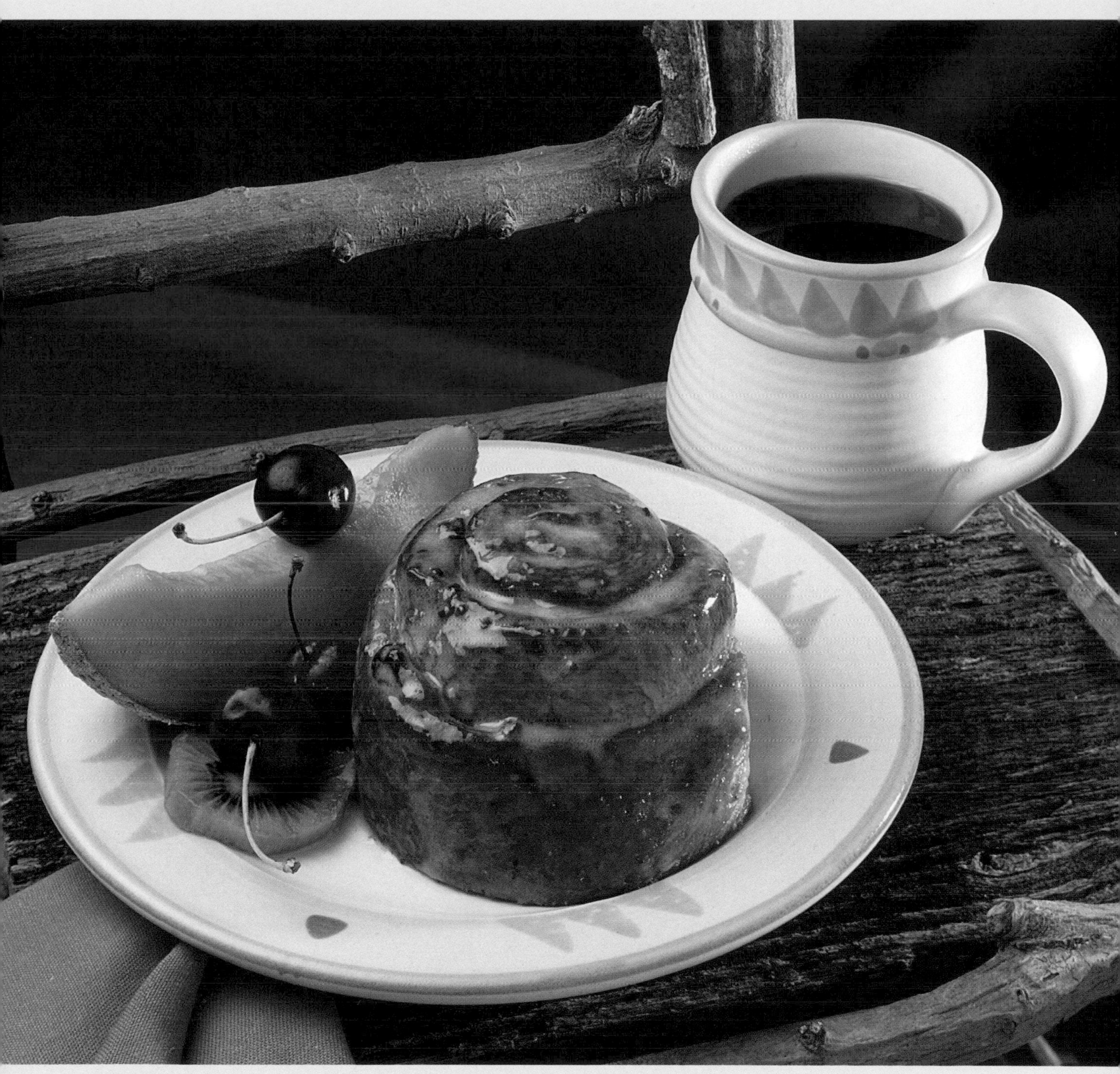

Our Famous Cinnamon Roll ♦ page 37

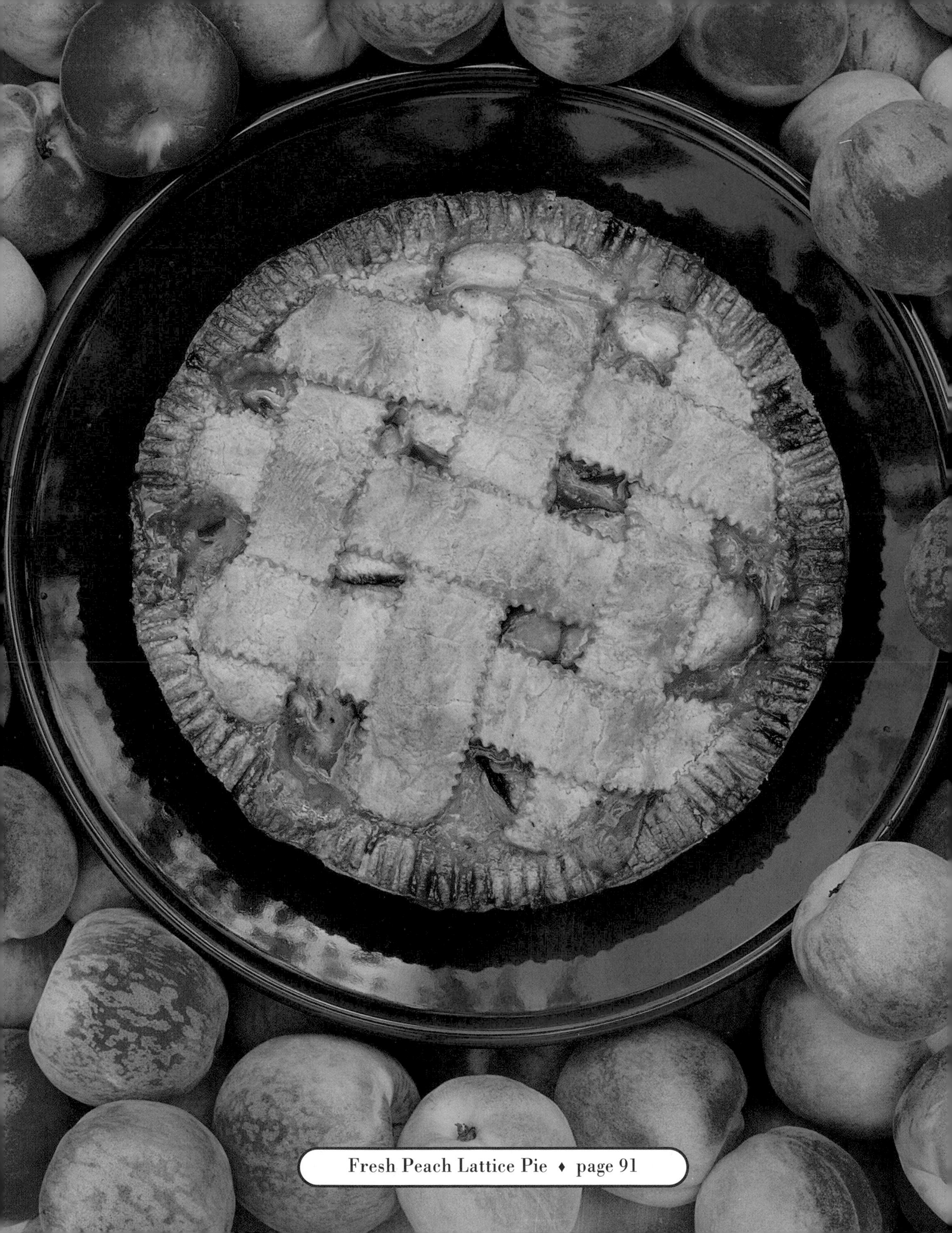

Fresh Peach Lattice Pie ♦ page 91

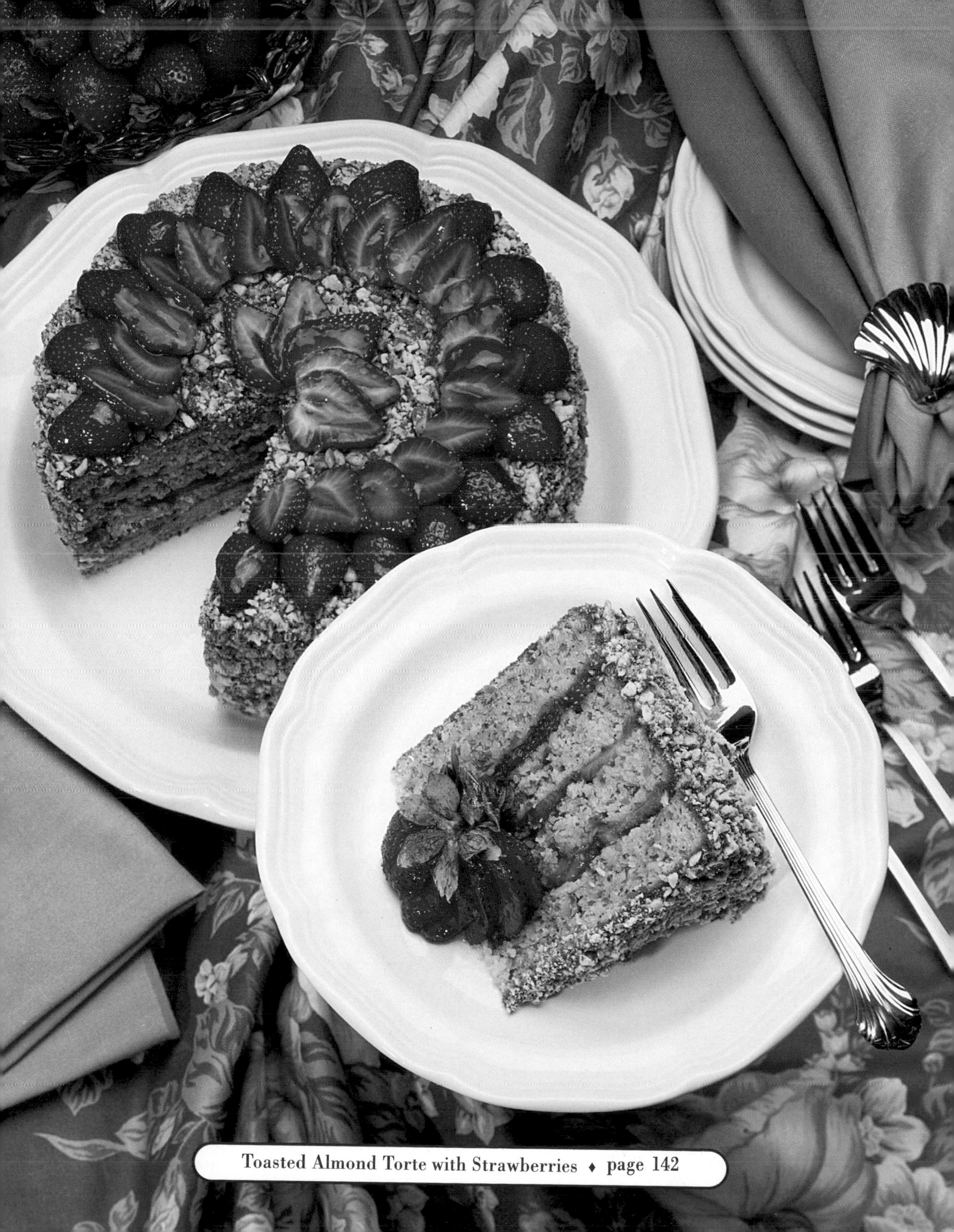

Toasted Almond Torte with Strawberries ♦ page 142

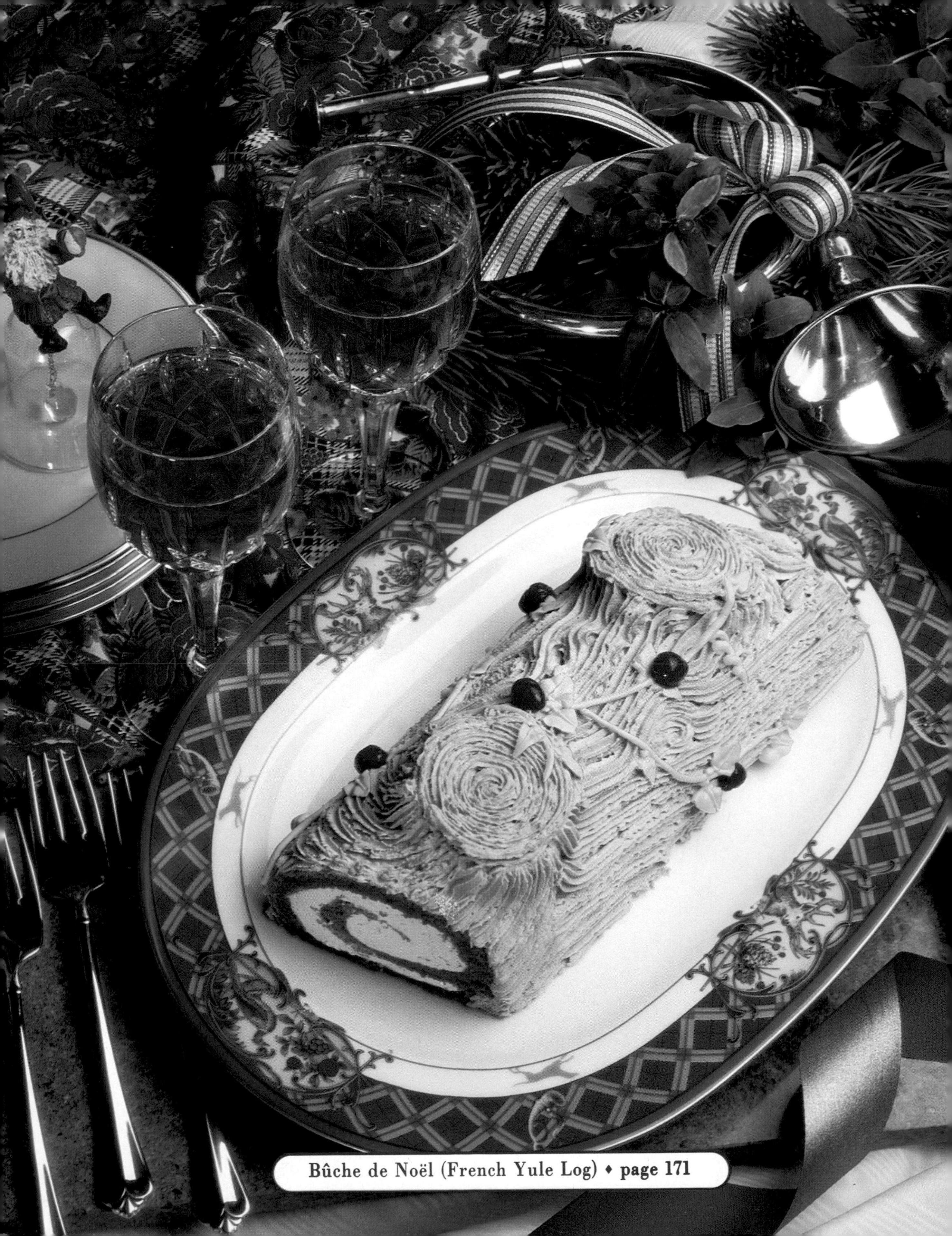

Bûche de Noël (French Yule Log) ♦ page 171

Pumpkin Pie

*

Yield:
9-inch pie
6 to 8 servings

This is my favorite pumpkin pie—perfectly spiced and wonderfully creamy. Pumpkin pie seems to be a true comfort food. Our customers agree, as they ask for it all year long.

As perfectly balanced spicing is so important to pumpkin pie, be sure that your spices are fresh before you begin. Because spices differ from one source to another and from one year to another, I've found it helpful to measure the spices and combine them together in a small bowl. Smell them. Do they conjure up the image of pumpkin pie? If not, adjust them by adding a little more cinnamon, or a bit of ginger or whatever is needed until the balance is just right. Then measure the amount of each spice called for in the recipe directly from this small bowl of spices.

Pumpkin Pie can be made dairy-free by substituting either almond milk (page 12) or soy milk (page 20) for cow's milk. Also, the recipe can be multiplied easily to make 2 to 20 or more pies.

Crust

Basic Pie Crust* (page 82): 9-inch bottom crust, partially baked

Filling

1⅔ cups canned pumpkin
½ teaspoon salt
1¼ teaspoons cinnamon
¼ teaspoon ginger
⅛ teaspoon nutmeg
⅛ teaspoon cloves
½ teaspoon vanilla extract
½ cup fruit sweetener
2 eggs
1⅔ cups milk* ***(use almond milk [4:1] or plain soy milk for dairy-free)***

Preheat the oven to 350° F. Prepare and partially bake the pie crust according to the directions on pages 77–79.

Meanwhile, prepare the pumpkin pie filling. In a medium-size bowl, whisk together the pumpkin, salt, spices, and vanilla. Stir in the sweetener and the eggs. When the mixture is smooth, stir in the milk. Pour the pumpkin pie mix into the partially baked crust.

Bake the pumpkin pie in the preheated oven for about 1 hour on a cookie sheet placed on either the floor of a gas oven or the lowest shelf in an electric oven. Pumpkin Pie is done when the center no longer wiggles when you shake the pan.

Pumpkin Pie is wonderful hot from the oven, at room temperature, or chilled. It is even more wonderful topped with Whipped Cream.

Baker's Tips

• Spices, especially once they have been ground, have a definite shelf life of about 1 year. Purchase only what you know you can use in a year and be willing to replace your spices when they're no longer what they used to be.

• The only time I haven't been disappointed substituting cooked and puréed pumpkin for canned pumpkin was when I used a kabocha squash (also known as hokaido pumpkin). Otherwise, the canned variety seems to have a much fuller taste and richer color (and there are no unknown ingredients on the label).

Pumpkin Mincemeat Pie

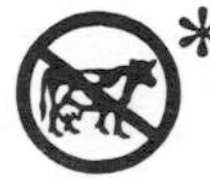

Yield:
9-inch pie
6 to 8 servings

This well-balanced Pumpkin Mincemeat pie is perfect for those who can never make up their mind whether to have Mince Pie or Pumpkin Pie—now they can have both, at once. The smooth and creamy pumpkin custard adds a wonderful texture and flavor contrast to the fruity and chunky mincemeat.

Mock Mincemeat (vegetarian mincemeat, made without meat) is more rounded in its flavor if it is prepared at least 1 to 2 days and up to a month in advance of preparing this pie. Refrigerated, Mock Mincemeat stores well for over a month.

Crust

Basic Pie Crust* (page 82): 9-inch bottom crust, preferably with a fluted edge, partially baked

Mock Mincemeat

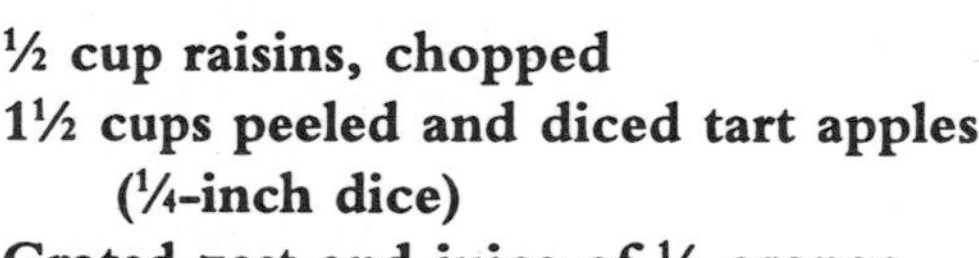

½ cup raisins, chopped
1½ cups peeled and diced tart apples (¼-inch dice)
Grated zest and juice of ⅓ orange
3 tablespoons unsweetened apple juice
2 tablespoons fruit sweetener
¼ teaspoon cinnamon
⅛ teaspoon nutmeg
Pinch cloves
½ cup walnuts

Pumpkin Custard

1 cup plus 2 tablespoons canned pumpkin
⅓ teaspoon salt
1 teaspoon cinnamon
Scant ¼ teaspoon ginger
Pinch cloves
Pinch nutmeg
½ teaspoon vanilla extract
⅓ cup fruit sweetener
1 egg plus 1 yolk
1 cup plus 2 tablespoons milk* *(use almond milk [4:1] or plain soy milk for dairy-free)*

Garnish

Whipped Cream* (page 181) *(optional)*
Toasted chopped walnuts

Preheat the oven to 350° F. Prepare and partially bake the pie crust according to the directions on pages 77–79.

To prepare the Mock Mincemeat filling, combine the raisins, apples, orange zest and juice, and the apple juice in a medium-size saucepan. Cover the pan and cook over medium heat until the apples are soft, 10 to 15 minutes. Remove the pan from the heat.

While the apple mixture is cooking, toast the walnuts in the preheated oven for 7 to 10 minutes, stirring occasionally. Allow the nuts to cool. Then medium-chop them with a knife or pulsing action in a food processor. When the apples are ready, stir in the sweetener, the spices, and the chopped walnuts. Refrigerate.

To prepare the pumpkin custard, whisk together the pumpkin, salt, spices, and vanilla in a medium-size bowl. Stir in the sweetener and the eggs. When the mixture is smooth, stir in the milk.

Spread the chilled mincemeat evenly in the bottom of the partially baked crust. Pour the pumpkin custard over the mincemeat to fill the crust.

To bake the pie, place it on a baking sheet in the preheated oven, directly on the oven floor of a gas oven or on the lowest shelf of an electric oven. Bake the pie for approximately 45 minutes, until the pumpkin custard no longer wiggles when you shake the pie.

When the pie is cool, garnish it with Whipped Cream and toasted chopped walnuts.

Maple Pecan Pie

*

Yield:
9-inch pie
6 to 8 servings

Traditional Pecan Pie is made even more irresistible with pure maple syrup used in combination with fruit sweetener. Maple syrup blends with and enhances the flavor of that most glorious of nuts, the pecan, and also keeps this American favorite from being too sweet.

Crust

Basic Pie Crust* (page 82): 9-inch bottom crust with a fluted edge, partially baked

Filling

1¾ cups pecans
1 teaspoon cinnamon
½ teaspoon salt
1 teaspoon vanilla extract
¾ cup pure maple syrup
¾ cup fruit sweetener
6 eggs

Garnish

Whipped Cream* (page 181) ***(optional)***
6 to 8 pecan halves

Preheat the oven to 350° F. Prepare and partially bake the pie crust according to the directions on pages 77–79.

Toast the pecans for filling and garnishing the pie in the preheated oven for 7 to 10 minutes, stirring occasionally. Reserve 6 to 8 perfect pecan halves for garnishing the finished pie. Put the remaining pecans in the partially baked pie crust.

In a medium-size bowl, combine the cinnamon, salt, vanilla, and ½ cup of the maple syrup. Use a whisk to evenly distribute the cinnamon. Then whisk in the remaining ¼ cup of maple syrup and all of the fruit sweetener. Whisk in the eggs, one at a time. Pour this filling into the crust over the pecans.

Bake the Maple Pecan Pie for approximately 45 minutes on a cookie sheet on either the floor of a gas oven or the lowest shelf in an electric oven. Maple Pecan Pie is done when it is golden brown, has puffed slightly, and does not shake in the middle when jiggled.

When the pie is cool, garnish it with Whipped Cream and toasted pecan halves.

Apple Custard Pie

Yield:
9-inch pie
6 to 8 servings

Apple Custard Pie is wonderfully refreshing, with its soft, comforting texture and healthy ingredients—apples and apple juice, spices, raw tahini, and kuzu. There are no eggs or dairy products, so it is very low in fat and free of cholesterol. So satisfying, delicious, and healthy—I could serve and probably eat Apple Custard Pie almost every day.

Crust

Nutty-Oat Crust (page 83), prebaked

Filling

2½ tart apples
2½ cups unsweetened apple juice
6 tablespoons apple juice concentrate
½ teaspoon cinnamon
⅛ teaspoon nutmeg
1 tablespoon fresh lemon juice
¼ teaspoon grated lemon zest
2½ tablespoons raw (untoasted) tahini
½ cup (2⅛ ounces) kuzu

Garnish

Tofu Cream (page 193) (optional)
¼ cup walnuts, toasted (optional)

Prepare and bake the Nutty-Oat Crust according to the directions.

Peel, core, and roughly chop the apples to equal 2½ cups. Blend the apples with 1 cup of the apple juice and the rest of the filling ingredients with a pulsing action in a food processor or blender just until the apples are rough and crunchy in texture. Do not blend them smooth.

Place the apple mixture, together with the remaining 1½ cups of the apple juice, in a medium-size saucepan. Bring to a boil over medium-high heat. Reduce the heat and simmer for 5 minutes to stabilize the kuzu, stirring continually.

Pour the hot custard into the prebaked Nutty-Oat Crust. Cover the surface of the pie entirely with plastic wrap. Chill the pie thoroughly before garnishing and serving.

Garnish the Apple Custard Pie with ground toasted walnuts and the Tofu Cream, if desired.

Variations

Molded Apple Custard. Instead of pouring Apple Custard into a Nutty-Oat Crust, divide the hot custard evenly between 5 or 6 ramekins or custard cups. Cover the cups with plastic wrap, and refrigerate the custard for 1 hour, until firm. Unmold the custard onto dessert plates and serve with hot Apple Currant Sauce (page 191) or Raspberry Purée (page 190). Garnish with chopped toasted walnuts.

Apple Custard Parfait. These parfaits have a softer texture than the molded Apple Custard, as they do not need to hold their shape outside of the parfait glasses. In preparing the Apple Custard, reduce the amount of kuzu to 3 tablespoons. Pour the hot custard into six 6-ounce parfait glasses.

Boysenberry Custard Pie

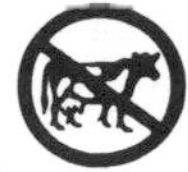  

Yield:
9-inch pie
6 to 8 servings

Such a beautiful royal color and comforting texture! Boysenberry Custard Pie is thickened with kuzu and not with eggs, so it is without cholesterol. If frozen boysenberries are difficult to find where you live, you can easily substitute frozen blackberries.

This custard also makes a wonderful parfait.

Crust

Nutty-Oat Crust (page 83), prebaked

Filling

3½ cups frozen boysenberries or blackberries
1¾ cups unsweetened apple juice
⅝ cup fruit sweetener
2½ tablespoons raw (untoasted) tahini
½ cup (2¼ ounces) kuzu
Pinch salt
1 tablespoon fresh lemon juice
1 tablespoon fresh orange juice

Garnish

Tofu Cream (page 193) (optional)

Prepare and bake the Nutty-Oat Crust according to the directions.

Measure the berries while they are frozen. As the berries defrost, purée them with the apple juice in a blender, then pour the purée through a medium strainer to remove the seeds. The purée should measure 3 cups. If not, add enough apple juice to make 3 cups.

In the blender, mix together all the ingredients except the fresh lemon and orange juices, and pour into a heavy-bottomed saucepan. Cook over medium heat until the mixture comes to the boil, whisking continuously. Reduce the heat and simmer for 5 minutes to stabilize the kuzu, continuing to stir to prevent the custard from burning and the kuzu from lumping. Remove from the heat and stir in the fresh citrus juices.

Pour the mixture into the prebaked Nutty-Oat Crust. Smooth the top of pie with a spatula and cover it closely with plastic wrap. Refrigerate the pie for 6 to 8 hours before garnishing with the Tofu Cream, if desired, and serving.

Variation

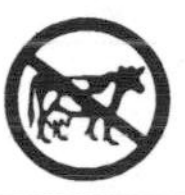  

Boysenberry Custard. Add 1 additional cup of apple juice, making 2¾ cups altogether. Continue with the recipe. Pour the hot custard into parfait glasses. Serve warm, at room temperature, or well chilled.

Banana Cream Pie

Yield:
9-inch pie
6 to 8 servings

Banana Cream Pie is a fabulous American classic. As bananas are available all year, this luscious treat can be made any time.

Be sure to prepare the Vanilla Custard at least 1 hour in advance, so that it is cold when you need it for the Banana Custard.

Crust

Basic Pie Crust (page 82): 9-inch bottom crust, prebaked

Banana Custard

2 cups Vanilla Custard (page 178)
¼ cup cool water
1⅓ tablespoons gelatin
¼ cup fruit sweetener
1½ teaspoons vanilla extract
2 medium-size ripe bananas

Whipped Cream Topping

2 tablespoons cool water
1 teaspoon gelatin
¼ cup fruit sweetener
2 teaspoons vanilla extract
1 cup heavy whipping cream

Prepare the Vanilla Custard according to the recipe directions.

Preheat the oven to 350° F. Prepare and bake the crust according to the recipe on pages 77–80.

To prepare the Banana Custard, place the cool water in a small bowl. Sprinkle on the gelatin and let it sit, undisturbed, for 5 minutes. Set the bowl into a small pan of simmering water for a couple of minutes until the gelatin is dissolved. Whisk the dissolved gelatin into the cold Vanilla Custard. Then stir in the sweetener and the vanilla extract. Stir the Banana Custard mixture until it begins to set. While the custard is setting, slice the bananas into ¼-inch slices, and fold them into the custard. Pour the Banana Custard into the prebaked crust. Refrigerate the filling for 30 minutes before topping with cream.

While the Banana Custard is chilling, prepare the Whipped Cream Topping. Place the cool water in a small bowl and sprinkle the gelatin on the water. Let it sit, undisturbed, for 5 minutes. Place the bowl into a small pan of simmering water until the gelatin is dissolved. Remove the bowl from the hot water and stir in the sweetener and the vanilla.

Whip the cream with an electric mixer on medium speed until the cream begins to thicken. While the cream is whipping, slowly pour in the gelatin mixture. Increase the mixer speed to high and continue to whip until the cream can stand in stiff peaks.

Top the chilled pie with the Whipped Cream Topping, leaving just enough topping to place in a pastry bag to decorate the edge of the pie. Refrigerate the completed Banana Cream Pie for 4 to 6 hours to set the filling thoroughly before cutting and serving.

Baker's Tip

• Gelatin must be completely dissolved before it is added it to other mixtures. A good method for dissolving it is to first "sponge" the gelatin: Sprinkle the gelatin over cool water in a small bowl and let it sit undisturbed for 5 minutes. ("Sponge" is an English term, referring to the way the gelatin crystals absorb all of the water.) Now place the bowl in a small pan of simmering water so that the heat can completely dissolve the sponge, producing clear, slightly amber-colored liquid gelatin.

Lemon Cream Pie

Yield:
9-inch pie
6 to 8 servings

Although fresh lemons are available year-round, sensational Lemon Cream Pie seems most appropriate during the hot summer months, when the crispness of the colors, the tartness of the lemon, and the softness of the cream seem to dispel the sometimes unbearable August heat. At the restaurant we usually begin making Lemon Cream Pies around the middle of June. That first pie with its yellow, white, and contrasting green mint leaves always brings oohs and aahs.

Be sure to prepare the Lemon Curd at least 1 hour in advance, so that it is cold when you need it for making the lemon filling.

Crust

Basic Pie Crust (page 82): 9-inch bottom crust, prebaked

Lemon Filling

2 cups Lemon Curd (page 177)
½ cup heavy whipping cream
1 cup fruit sweetener
3 tablespoons cool water
1½ teaspoons gelatin

Whipped Cream Topping

1 teaspoon gelatin
2 tablespoons cool water
¼ cup fruit sweetener
2 teaspoons vanilla extract
1 cup heavy whipping cream

Garnish

Lemon slices
Fresh mint sprigs

Prepare the Lemon Curd according to the recipe directions.

Preheat the oven to 350° F. Prepare and bake the crust according to the directions on pages 77–80.

To prepare the Lemon Filling, whip the cream with ½ cup of the sweetener to form soft peaks. Stir the remaining ½ cup of fruit sweetener into the Lemon Curd, and then fold the cold Lemon Curd into the softly whipped cream.

Place the cool water in a small bowl. Sprinkle on the gelatin, and let it sit undisturbed for 5 minutes. Set the bowl into a small pan of simmering water to dissolve the gelatin. Stir the dissolved gelatin into the lemon cream mixture, and pour it into the prebaked pie crust. Chill for 30 minutes to set the filling before topping with whipped cream.

While the Lemon Filling is chilling, prepare the Whipped Cream Topping. Place the cool water in a small bowl and sprinkle the gelatin on the water. Let it sit, undisturbed, for

5 minutes. Place the bowl into a small pan of simmering water until the gelatin is dissolved. Remove the bowl from the hot water and stir in the sweetener and the vanilla.

Whip the cream with an electric mixer on medium speed until the cream begins to thicken. While the cream is whipping, slowly pour in the gelatin mixture. Increase the mixer speed to high and continue to whip until the cream can stand in stiff peaks.

Top the chilled pie with the Whipped Cream Topping, leaving just enough topping to place in a pastry bag to decorate the edge of the pie. Refrigerate the completed Lemon Cream Pie from 4 to 6 hours to set the filling thoroughly before cutting and serving.

Garnish the chilled pie with thin slices of lemon and sprigs of fresh mint.

Mocha Mud Pie

Yield:
9-inch pie
6 to 8 servings

How can such a luscious pie have such an unusual name?

The "mud" refers to the richness of the mud at the bottom of the Mississippi River and is actually a compliment—you too will receive many compliments when you serve Mocha Mud Pie to your family and friends. We have customers at The Ranch Kitchen who come specifically for a piece of this rich and delicious cream pie.

It may be a bit fussy, putting all of the components together, but have patience and work one step at a time, and it will all be worth your effort.

Be sure to prepare the Vanilla Custard at least 1 hour in advance, so that it is cold when you need it for making the custard filling.

Custard

¾ cup Vanilla Custard (page 178)
1 teaspoon gelatin
2 tablespoons cool water

Crust

Basic Pie Crust (page 82): 9-inch bottom crust, prebaked

Sauce

⅔ cup Carob Fudge Sauce (page 192)

Mocha Cream

1 tablespoon cold water
½ teaspoon gelatin
1½ tablespoons instant coffee powder
1½ teaspoons sifted carob powder

2 tablespoons fruit sweetener
¾ cup heavy whipping cream

Whipped Cream Topping

1 tablespoon cool water
½ teaspoon gelatin
¼ cup fruit sweetener
¾ teaspoon vanilla extract
1 cup heavy whipping cream

Garnish

Carob powder or Pecan Praline (page 194) (optional)

Prepare the Vanilla Custard according to the recipe directions.

Preheat the oven to 350° F. Prepare and bake the crust according to the directions on pages 77–80.

Prepare the Carob Fudge Sauce and spread a thin layer of the sauce on the bottom of the prebaked crust. If the sauce is too thick to spread evenly, whisk in a few drops of water until it is of spreading consistency.

To prepare the Mocha Cream, place the cool water in a small metal bowl. Sprinkle the gelatin over the water and let sit undisturbed for 5 minutes. Place the bowl over simmering water to dissolve the gelatin. Remove the bowl from the water. Stir the instant coffee and carob powder into the 2 tablespoons of sweetener until blended, then stir into the dissolved gelatin.

Begin whipping the cream. When it is half-whipped, gradually add the gelatin mixture and continue to whip until the cream is stiff.

To prepare the Custard, dissolve the gelatin in the cool water as in making the Mocha Cream, and then stir the dissolved gelatin into the cold Vanilla Custard. Now fold the Mocha Cream into the custard and gelatin, and pour the filling into the prebaked pie shell. Smooth the top of the filling with a rubber spatula. Chill the pie for at least 30 minutes before topping with whipped cream.

While the Mocha Cream pie is chilling, prepare the Whipped Cream Topping. Place the cool water in a small bowl and sprinkle the gelatin on the water. Let it sit undisturbed for 5 minutes. Place the bowl into a small pan of simmering water to dissolve the gelatin. Remove the bowl from the hot water and stir in the sweetener and the vanilla.

Whip the cream with an electric mixer on medium speed until the cream begins to thicken. While the cream is whipping, slowly pour in the gelatin mixture. Increase the mixer speed to high and continue to whip until the cream can stand in stiff peaks.

Top the chilled pie with the Whipped Cream Topping, leaving just enough topping to place in a pastry bag to decorate the edge of the pie. Refrigerate the completed Mocha Mud Pie for 4 to 6 hours to set the filling thoroughly before cutting and serving.

Garnish the chilled pie with a light sifting of carob powder or a sprinkling of Pecan Praline.

Peach 'n' Berry Crisp

Yield:
9-inch by 13-inch pan
9 to 10 servings

Here is an embellishment on my mom's apple crisp recipe. I've been eating fruit crisps with different fruits for more than thirty years—and I still love them, especially when they're hot and bubbling from the oven. As a child I loved the "crisp" part the best. My mother still remembers the time she found her cooling apple crisp without any "crisp." For as soon as she left the room, I began to eat every delicious morsel of that topping . . . bit by bit by bit.

Fruit Filling

½ teaspoon cinnamon
¼ teaspoon nutmeg
2 tablespoons cornstarch
5 cups frozen blueberries
4 cups frozen sliced peaches
2½ cups frozen strawberries
1 tablespoon fresh lemon juice

Crisp Topping

½ cup walnuts
½ cup butter* *(substitute margarine or oil for dairy-free)*
6 tablespoons fruit sweetener
1½ cups rolled oats
¾ cup unbleached white flour* or whole wheat pastry flour or brown rice flour
1½ teaspoons cinnamon
½ teaspoon allspice

Preheat the oven to 350° F.

Toast the walnuts in the preheated oven for 7 to 10 minutes, stirring occasionally. Allow the nuts to cool. Then coarsely chop them with a knife or with a pulsing action in a food processor.

To prepare the Fruit Filling, combine the cinnamon, nutmeg, and cornstarch and toss with fruit in a medium-size bowl. Sprinkle the lemon juice over the fruit and toss again. Place the fruit in a lightly sprayed 9-inch by 13-inch pan. Cover with aluminum foil and bake at 350° F. for about 1 hour, until the fruit is very hot and the juices have begun to bubble.

Meanwhile, prepare the Crisp Topping:

If you are using cold butter or margarine, cut it into ½-inch pieces and set aside. Combine the rest of the topping ingredients and mix until crumbly. Mix in the butter or margarine until it is well distributed, though the mixture should remain crumbly.

If you are using oil, combine all of the topping ingredients (including the oil) and mix until the spices are well distributed and the mixture is crumbly.

Remove the pan of fruit from the oven. Remove the aluminum foil and crumble the crisp topping evenly over the fruit. Return the pan to the oven.

Bake, uncovered, for another 30 minutes, until the topping is crisp and golden brown and the filling is bubbly.

Serve right from the oven or at room temperature. The filling will become thicker as the crisp cools.

Baker's Tip

• For convenience, at The Ranch Kitchen we make this Peach 'n' Berry Crisp using frozen fruit. A variety of fresh fruit in season, combining both hard fruits, such as apples, with juicy fruits, such as peaches and berries, is equally delicious.

European Fruit Tarts and Tartlets

Fresh Plum Tart

Yield:
10-inch tart
7 to 10 servings

Each year when plum season comes around and I have my first bite of a Fresh Plum Tart, I am immediately reminded of European pastries and of picnics in the French countryside. It must be the inviting arrangement of the plums with their glistening caramelized edges, in combination with their irresistible flavor and the texture of the tart as a whole which inspires me. It is this same combination of natural flavors with little added sweetener that also makes this tart a delightful breakfast pastry.

A few years ago our summer organic fruit purveyor sold us tart, red-skinned plums with deep-red, sweet meat. Those special plums made the most sublime tart you can imagine. Not always having such extra-special plums, we will use almost-as-delicious, firm, ripe Santa Rosa plums or Italian prune plums instead.

Crust

Basic Pie Crust (page 82): 10-inch tart shell, partially baked

Nut Crumb Filling

¾ cup walnuts or pecans
3 to 4 slices day-old French or egg bread* ***(recipe contains egg whites only, if French bread is used)***
2 teaspoons cinnamon
½ teaspoon nutmeg
¼ cup fruit sweetener
2 tablespoons butter, melted

Plum Topping

3 to 4 pounds plums
1½ tablespoons fruit sweetener
1 tablespoon butter
Red Glaze (page 180)

Preheat the oven to 350° F. Prepare and partially bake the crust according to the directions on pages 77–79.

To prepare the Nut Crumb Filling, begin by toasting the nuts in the preheated oven for 7 to 10 minutes, stirring occasionally. Put aside. Use the food processor to process the sliced bread into very coarse crumbs. Add the nuts and spices, and continue to process until the nuts are coarsely chopped. With the motor running, drizzle in the fruit sweetener and melted butter until the mixture is evenly moistened. Place the filling in the bottom of a partially baked tart shell.

Cut the plums in quarters and remove their pits. Stand the quartered plums on end, skin side down, in closely touching circles starting at the edge and working to the center. Use as many plum quarters as necessary to completely cover the filling. (See illustration on next page.)

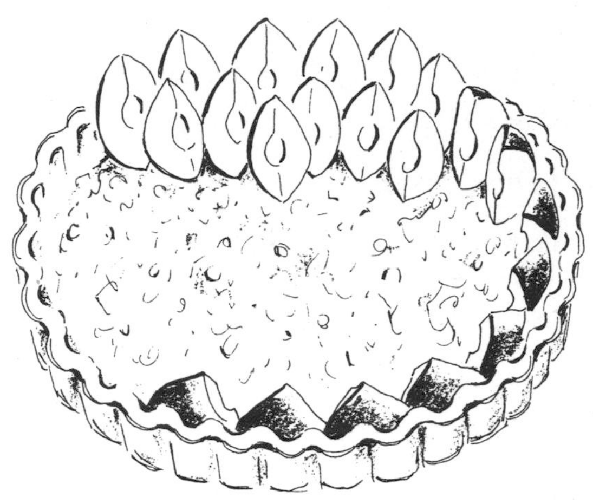

Drizzle the tart with 1½ tablespoons fruit sweetener and dot with 1 tablespoon of butter.

Place the completed tart on a baking sheet in the preheated oven on the lowest shelf of an electric oven or directly on the floor of a gas oven. Bake the tart for 45 to 60 minutes, until the edges of plums have begun to darken in color.

Place the Red Glaze in a small sauté pan and bring it to a boil. Remove the pan from the heat and cool the glaze for 1 minute. Brush the tart with the hot glaze.

Fresh Plum Tart can be served hot from the oven, but it has its best flavor when served at room temperature.

Baker's Tip

- The small amount of fruit sweetener drizzled on the fruit before baking aids in slightly caramelizing the fruit, giving it a richer taste and a European appearance to the finished tart.

Fresh Apricot Tart

Yield:
10-inch tart
7 to 10 servings

This fabulous, golden-domed tart is a wonderful way to enjoy ripe apricots during the few short weeks of their availability each summer. When apricot season has ended, you can prepare an equally wonderful Fresh Peach Tart in its stead.

Crust

Basic Pie Crust (page 82): 10-inch tart shell, partially baked

Nut Crumb Filling

¾ cup walnuts or pecans
3 to 4 slices day-old French or egg bread* ***(recipe contains egg whites only, if French bread is used)***
2 teaspoons cinnamon
½ teaspoon nutmeg
¼ cup fruit sweetener
2 tablespoons butter, melted

Apricot Topping

3 to 4 pounds apricots
1½ tablespoons fruit sweetener
1 tablespoon butter
Yellow Glaze (page 181)

Preheat the oven to 350° F. Prepare and partially bake the crust according to the directions on pages 77–79.

To prepare the Nut Crumb Filling, begin by toasting the nuts in the preheated oven for

7 to 10 minutes, stirring occasionally. Put aside. Use the food processor to process the sliced bread into very coarse crumbs. Add the nuts and spices, and continue to process until the nuts are coarsely chopped. With the motor running, drizzle in the fruit sweetener and melted butter until the mixture is evenly moistened. Place the filling in the bottom of a partially baked tart shell.

To peel the apricots, dip them in boiling water for 5 to 10 seconds to loosen their skin. Use the point of a small knife to peel them, cut them in halves, and remove their pits.

Arrange the apricot halves dome-side-up over the nut crumb filling into closely touching circles, beginning around the inside edge and working towards the center of the tart.

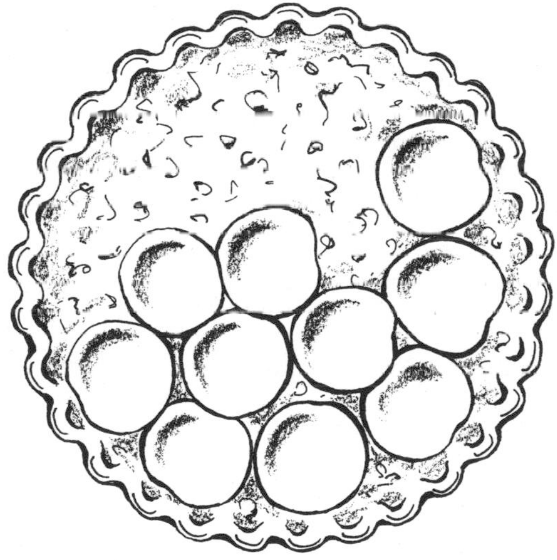

Drizzle the tart with the 1½ tablespoons of fruit sweetener and dot with 1 tablespoon of butter.

Place the completed tart on a baking sheet in the preheated oven on the lowest shelf of an electric oven or directly on the floor of a gas oven. Bake the tart for 45 to 60 minutes, until the fruit is soft and its edges have begun to darken in color.

Bring the Yellow Glaze to a boil in a small pan. Remove the pan from the heat and cool the glaze for 1 minute. Brush the tart with the hot glaze.

Serve Fresh Apricot Tart hot from the oven or at room temperature.

Variation

Fresh Peach Tart. Substitute fresh peaches for the apricots. Peel and pit the peaches and slice them ⅓ inch thick. Arrange two overlapping circles of sliced peaches, one around the inside edge, and the other in the center of the tart.

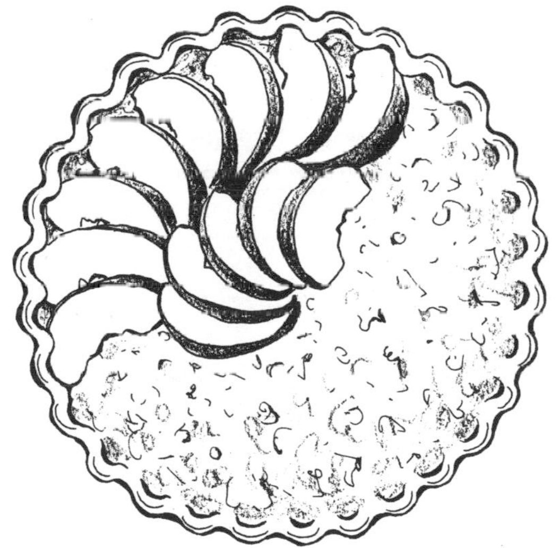

Fresh Strawberry Tart

Yield:
10-inch tart
7 to 10 servings

The promise offered by the many gleaming red peaks of strawberries is more than fulfilled in the satisfying taste of a Fresh Strawberry Tart. Because the strawberries are basically the whole show in this tart, it is best to use only fully ripe berries that are at their tastiest in flavor and their prettiest in appearance.

Crust

Basic Pie Crust (page 82): 10-inch tart shell, prebaked

Filling

¾ cup Vanilla Custard (page 178)
2 pint baskets strawberries

Garnish

1 cup Red Glaze (page 180)

Prepare the Vanilla Custard at least 1 hour in advance of preparing the Strawberry Tart, so that it is cold when you are ready to use it.

Preheat the oven to 350° F. Prepare and bake the crust according to the directions on pages 77–80.

Quickly wash the strawberries by dipping them in cool water and removing them immediately. Dry the berries in a single layer on a clean kitchen towel. Use the tip of a vegetable peeler to remove the hulls from the berries.

Bring the Red Glaze to a boil in a small pan. Remove the pan from the heat and cool the glaze for 1 minute. Brush the glaze thinly

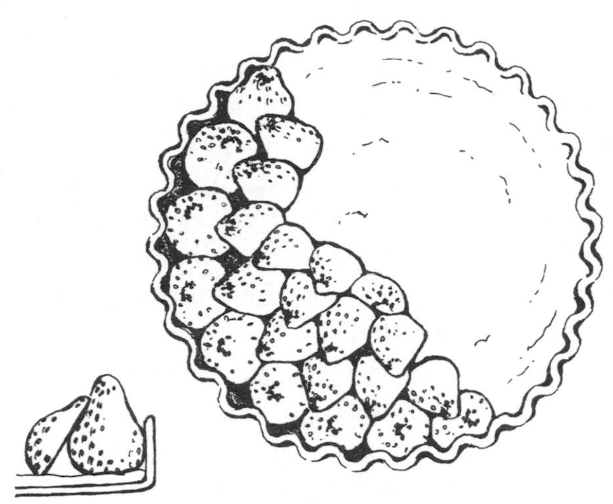

onto the bottom and inside edge of the prebaked tart shell.

Spread a thin layer of chilled Vanilla Custard on the bottom of the tart shell. Place a ring of whole strawberries around the outer edge of the tart with their peaks up. Slice the remaining berries in half lengthwise. Make a ring of the halved berries, closely touching one another and resting on the circle of whole berries. Continue with the remaining berry halves, placing them in concentric circles working from the outside in towards the center, closely overlapping the previous circle, so that none of the custard shows through the berries. Reheat the Red Glaze and brush it over all the berries.

For the tidiest cutting and serving of Fresh Strawberry Tart, it is best to refrigerate it for at least 30 minutes after assembling.

French Pear Tart

Yield:
10-inch tart
7 to 8 servings

French Pear Tart is another personal favorite. With its delectable chunky pear/applesauce filling, it gives all-American apple pie strong competition. I have adapted this recipe from a classic French Apple Tart made by Julia Child—surely one of America's best-loved chefs.

Some of my favorite types of pears to use in preparing French Pear Tart are Bartletts, Anjous, and Winter Nells. The best widely available apples, for both taste and texture, are tart ones, such as Pippins, Gravensteins, and Granny Smiths.

Crust

Basic Pie Crust (page 82): 10-inch tart shell, partially baked

Filling

3 pounds pears
1 pound tart green apples
⅓ cup fruit-sweetened apricot jam
1 tablespoon vanilla extract
2 tablespoons butter

Garnish

Yellow Glaze (page 181)
Sliced toasted almonds (optional)

Preheat the oven to 350° F. Prepare and bake the crust according to the directions on pages 77–80.

Peel, core, and roughly chop 2 pounds of the pears and all of the apples. Place the chopped pears and apples in a heavy-bottomed saucepan. Cover the pot tightly and cook the fruit over very low heat for about 20 minutes, stirring occasionally, until the fruit is tender but still chunky. The fruit will release its own juices as it cooks. Remove the pot from the heat and stir in the jam, vanilla, and butter. Set the chunky pear/applesauce aside to cool.

Peel, core, halve, and slice the remaining pears into ⅛-inch slices. Spread a thick layer of the cooled pear/applesauce over the bottom of the partially baked tart shell. Neatly fan the pear slices on top of the pear/applesauce, very

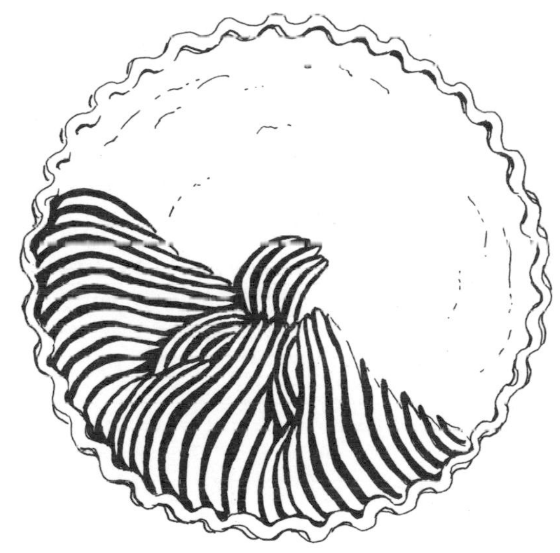

closely overlapping them, forming an outside circle and an inside circle.

Place the completed tart on a baking sheet in the preheated oven. Place the baking sheet on the lowest shelf of an electric oven or directly on the floor of a gas oven. Bake the tart for 35 to 45 minutes, until the pears are tender and lightly browned on their edges. Remove the tart from the oven.

Bring the Yellow Glaze to a boil in a small

pan. Remove from the heat and cool for 1 minute. Brush the tart with hot glaze and press toasted sliced almonds around the edge of the tart so that they stick to the glaze.

Serve hot or at room temperature.

Variations

French Apple Tart. Replace all the pears with apples. Fan the apple slices in closely overlapping circles on top of the chunky applesauce.

Crustless French Pear or Apple Tarts. A quick, crustless variation can be made using heat-proof glass or ceramic ramekins. Lightly spray the ramekins with lecithin spray. Then place the chunky filling directly into them. Cover each with half of a sliced pear or apple. Bake and glaze according to the recipe.

Linzertorte

Yield:
10-inch tart
7 to 10 servings

Linzertorte is one of the world's great desserts, with perfectly balanced spices, textures, and flavors. Here is a delicious fruit-sweetened alternative for this classic Austrian recipe. And, even though the name says it is a torte, it does seem to be a tart.

Linzertorte is best served at room temperature, where, if well-wrapped in plastic, it will keep well for about 2 weeks. Because of its good keeping qualities and sturdy nature, Linzertorte can be mailed to family and friends for holiday gift-giving.

Linzer Crust

1¼ cups almonds
14 tablespoons butter
½ cup fruit sweetener
3 egg yolks
½ teaspoon cinnamon
Pinch cloves
Pinch salt
1 teaspoon grated lemon zest
1 teaspoon fresh lemon juice
1 cup finely ground cookie crumbs
¾ cup whole wheat pastry flour
¾ cup white cake flour

Filling

1 cup fruit-sweetened seedless raspberry jam

Garnish

Egg Wash for Pies and Tarts (page 84)
1 cup sliced almonds
Coconut powder (page 194)

Preheat the oven to 350° F.

To prepare the linzer crust, toast the almonds in the preheated oven for 7 to 10 minutes. Allow the nuts to cool. Then process in a food processor, using a pulsing action, until they are finely chopped.

Use an electric mixer on medium-high speed to cream together the butter and sweetener until light and fluffy. Add the egg yolks one at a time, mixing well after each addition.

Reduce the speed to low and stir in the spices, lemon zest and juice, the finely ground almonds, cookie crumbs, and the flours. Chill the dough for at least 1 hour.

Spray the tart pan lightly with lecithin spray. Roll ⅔ of the chilled dough into a 12-inch circle on a lightly floured surface. Fit the circle of dough into the prepared tart pan, doubling the excess dough to the inside to form a double thickness around the sides of the tart. Spread the raspberry jam evenly on the bottom of the crust. Roll the remaining dough into ⅓-inch-wide ropes. Cut the ropes to just fit the inside of the tart, and form them into a diamond-lattice design on top of the jam.

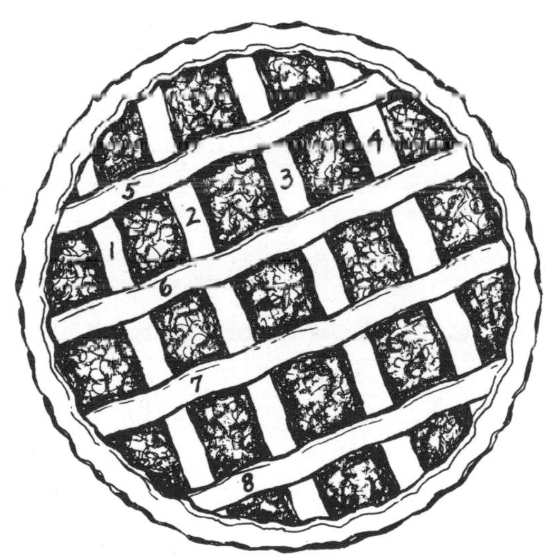

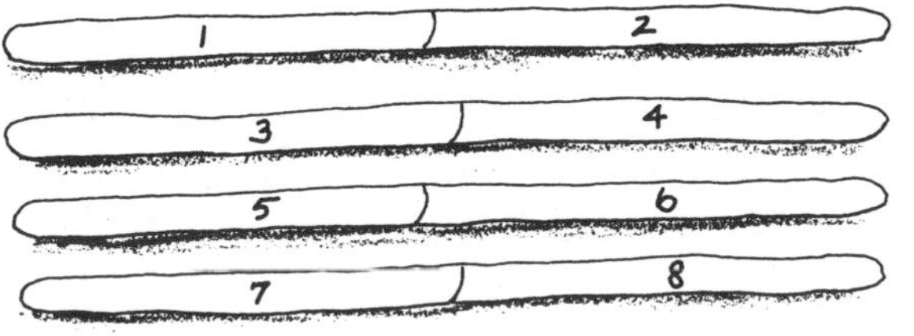

Prepare the Egg Wash and brush it onto the edge of the tart. Press the sliced almonds onto the edge.

Place the completed tart on a baking sheet in the preheated oven on the lowest shelf of an electric oven or directly on the floor of a gas oven. Bake the tart for 35 to 40 minutes, until the crust is lightly browned.

Cool the Linzertorte before removing it from the tart pan. When cool, sift Coconut Powder through a fine sieve evenly over the tart.

Serve and store Linzertorte at room temperature.

Baker's Tip

• Crumbs from any kind of cookie will do when making a Linzertorte. I've used everything from fruit-sweetened carob chip cookies to oatmeal cookies to spice cookies. Other times I have even substituted fruit-sweetened granola, after first removing the hard raisins.

Blueberry Lemon Tartlets

Yield:
6 tartlets

Blueberries and lemon are exceptionally complementary flavors, with the tartness of the Lemon Curd filling toned down just a bit by the sweet fruitiness of the Blueberry Sauce.

Basic Pie Crust (page 82): six 2½-inch to 3-inch tartlet shells, prebaked
¾ cup Lemon Curd (page 177)
¾ to 1 cup Blueberry Sauce (page 186)
½ cup Yellow Glaze (page 181)

Prepare both the Lemon Curd and Blueberry Sauce at least 1 hour in advance of assembling the tartlets, so that both mixtures are cold when you are ready to use them.

Preheat the oven to 350° F. Prepare and bake the tartlet shells according to the directions on pages 77–80.

In a small pan, heat the Yellow Glaze until it comes to the boil. Brush the hot glaze onto the inside of each tartlet shell.

Place 2 tablespoons of Lemon Curd on the bottom of each shell. Cover the Lemon Curd with a layer of Blueberry Sauce so that none of the Lemon Curd shows through.

Blueberry Lemon Tartlets are wonderful served at room temperature or lightly chilled. It is best to prepare and serve these tartlets on the same day; otherwise, the crust will become soggy and the Blueberry Sauce will begin to dry out and lose its sparkle.

Peach Roses

*

Yield:
6 tartlets

These exquisite Peach Roses are a delight to behold and a joy to prepare. I have been making Peach Rose tartlets for almost eighteen years, ever since I created my original one at my first restaurant bakery job. I still enjoy making them.

Do take the extra care necessary to slice the peaches thinly, in order to create the prettiest roses.

Basic Pie Crust* (page 82): six 2½-inch to 3-inch tartlet shells, prebaked
½ to ¾ cup Vanilla Custard (page 178)
6 to 8 ripe peaches
⅓ to ½ cup Yellow Glaze (page 181)
Finely chopped toasted almonds (optional)

Prepare the Vanilla Custard at least 1 hour in advance of preparing these tartlets, so that it is cold when you are ready to use it.

Preheat the oven to 350° F. Prepare and bake the tartlet shells according to the directions on pages 77–80.

Blanch the peaches in a pot of boiling water for 5 to 10 seconds to loosen their skins. Peel the peaches. Then slice them no more than ⅛ inch thick. To keep the slices from turning brown it is best to slice the peaches just before you plan to arrange them in the tartlet shells.

Heat the Yellow Glaze in a small pan until it comes to a boil. Brush the hot glaze on the inside of each tartlet shell. Place a ¼-inch layer of Vanilla Custard on the bottom of each shell.

Form the peach slices into a rose by standing one slice at a time on the custard, closely overlapping them in a circle. Begin just inside the crust and continue to overlap the peach slices as you fill in towards the center. For the very center of the rose, you will need a couple of very thin slices so that you can more easily shape them into a circle. Reheat the Yellow Glaze and brush it over each Peach Rose. An optional garnish would be to place finely chopped almonds around the edge of each tartlet.

Peach Roses are wonderful served at room temperature or slightly chilled. It is best to prepare and serve these tartlets on the same day, otherwise the crust will become soggy, and the peaches will lose their sparkle.

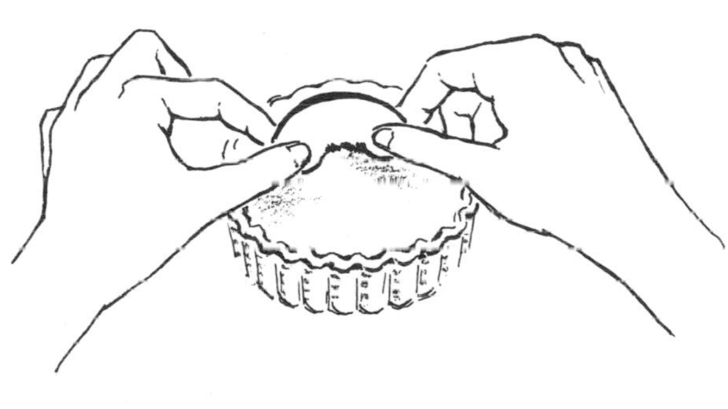

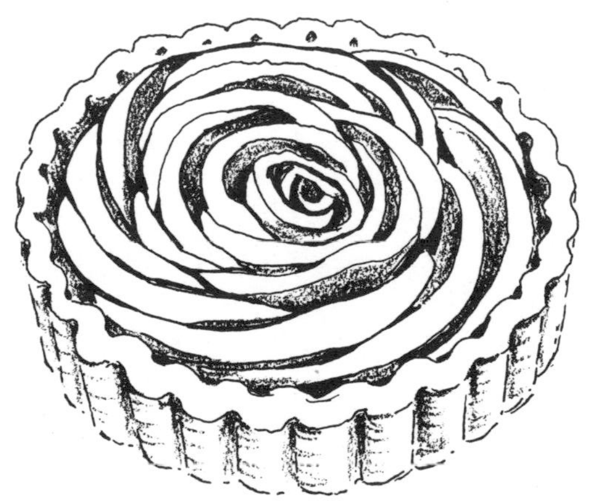

Strawberry Cream Tartlets

Yield:
6 tartlets

Individual tartlets featuring one large, magnificent, ripe, red strawberry are irresistible—especially so for children or for grown-ups who want only a taste of something sweet. Equally delicious are cream tartlets made from a luscious pyramid of raspberries or blackberries.

Basic Pie Crust* (page 82): Six 2½-inch to 3-inch tartlet shells, prebaked
⅓ to ½ cup Vanilla Custard (page 178)
1 to 2 pint baskets strawberries
½ to 1 cup Whipped Cream* (page 181)
(omit for dairy-free)
½ to ¾ cup Red Glaze (page 180)

Prepare the Vanilla Custard at least 1 hour in advance of preparing these tartlets, so that it is cold when you are ready to use it.

Preheat the oven to 350° F. Prepare and bake the tartlet shells according to the directions on pages 77–80.

The actual quantity of ingredients needed will depend upon the size of each tartlet shell.

Quickly wash the strawberries and place them in a single layer on a kitchen towel to dry. Choose 6 large strawberries, one for the center of each tartelet, and another 12 to 15 strawberries to surround them. Use the tip of a vegetable peeler to remove the hulls from all of the strawberries. Leave the 6 berries whole, and cut the others in half lengthwise.

In a small pan, bring the Red Glaze to the boil. Brush the hot glaze on the inside of each tartlet shell. Place a ¼-inch to ½-inch layer of custard on the bottom of each shell.

Place a large strawberry in the center of each tartlet with its peak up. Surround each whole berry with 3 to 5 strawberry halves (depending upon their size) leaning upon the

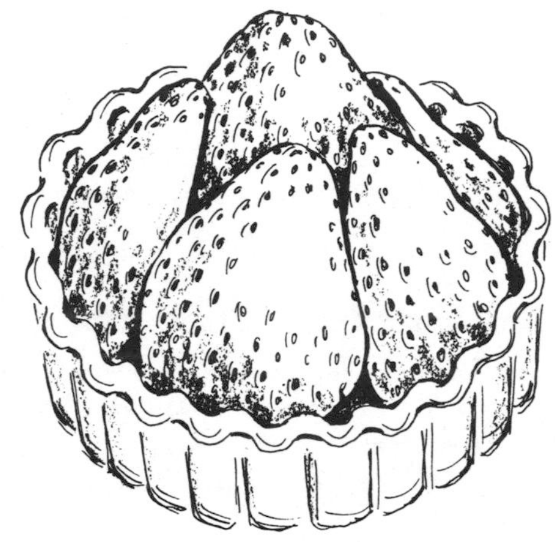

large strawberry. Place the strawberries so that they cover as much of the custard as possible.

Reheat the Red Glaze, and brush it over the fruit. When the glaze is dry, pipe a circle of whipped cream around the fruit.

Strawberry Cream Tartlets are wonderful served at room temperature or slightly chilled. It is best to prepare and serve these tartlets on the same day. Otherwise the crust will become soggy and the fruit will lose its sparkle.

Variations

Raspberry or Blackberry Cream Tartlets. Substitute 1 to 2 half-pints of fresh raspberries or blackberries for the strawberries. Do not wash the fresh berries; instead, roll them around on a baking pan lined with a clean kitchen

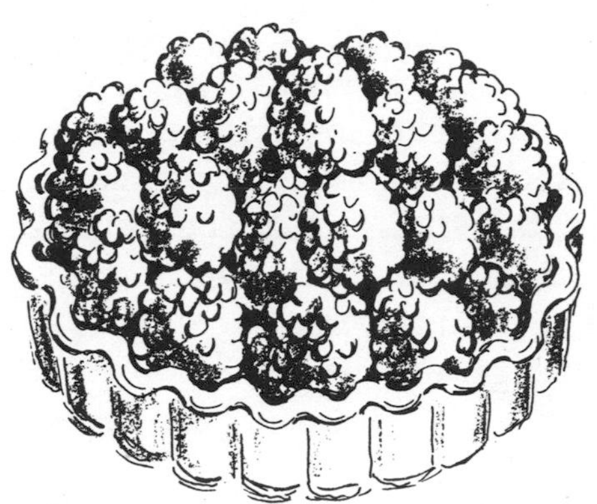

towel to remove any loose dirt or seeds. Arrange the berries in a pyramid on top of the custard, covering as much of the custard as possible. Pipe whipped cream stars to fill in the gaps between the berries.

Puff Pastry

Puff Pastry is by far the most delicate, challenging, and versatile of French pastries, and it is also the most time-consuming to prepare. It is worth searching specialty and gourmet stores for a good quality commercially made puff pastry that you can use instead of making your own; look for it in the freezer section. Ideally, puff pastry should consist of butter, flour, water, and salt, with very little else added. The puff pastry recipes included here are all made from frozen puff pastry sheets.

Puff pastry is made up of over a thousand layers of folded butter and flour. To prevent any of the layers of butter from prematurely melting, as well as for ease in handling, work quickly and always use puff pastry while it is still cold (but not frozen). When the cold pastry is put into a hot oven, it is the steam created by the melting thin layers of butter that makes the pastry rise 6 to 8 times in height and form its characteristic, almost miraculous, flakiness.

Frozen commercial puff pastry thaws sufficiently to use in about 10 to 15 minutes, depending upon the temperature of your kitchen. If the pastry is still partially frozen, you will not be able to unroll the sheet without breaking some of the layers of butter and flour. And, if the pastry is too defrosted, you will melt the layers of butter and flour. There seems to be a 10-minute to 15-minute period, again depending upon the temperature of your kitchen, when it is best to work with puff pastry. If at any time it softens, with the butter on the verge of melting, place the pastry in the refrigerator for a few minutes to firm it up again before continuing.

Very lightly flour your work table, your hands, and your rolling pin to keep the puff pastry from sticking when you roll it out to the desired size and thickness. When it is necessary to have a larger sheet of pastry than you have, you can slightly overlap two or more sheets of pastry. Attach the edge of one to the other with a small amount of water. Roll over this edge with a rolling pin, and proceed with it as 1 sheet of pastry. However, be extra careful in transferring the pastry to your baking pan, to keep the seam from coming apart.To avoid this problem, you can work with the pastry directly on the paper-lined baking sheet.

Puff pastry can be formed into many different size pastries. The unbaked, formed pastries can be frozen for 2 to 3 months, but for the highest-rising pastries, thaw them in the refrigerator before baking.

From my experience, puff pastry rises and browns the best in a constant, slightly hot oven at 375° F. All puff pastry is at its tastiest when baked and served on the same day.

Because of the flakiness and fragility of puff pastry, the neatest way to cut puff pastry creations is with either an electric knife or a very sharp serrated knife.

Making Tart Shells from Puff Pastry Sheets

Puff pastry can be used to form delicious, easy, and attractive tart shells in a variety of sizes and shapes.

Rectangular Tart Shells

Start with one 10-inch by 15-inch sheet of puff pastry. Cut out a 6-inch by 15-inch rectangle of puff pastry and place it on a paper-lined baking sheet. Cut four ½-inch-wide strips from the pastry trim: Two 15 inches long, and two strips 5 inches long. Brush the top edge of the large rectangle with cold water. Place the strips flat on the top edge of the rectangle to form a border. Prick the bottom of the pastry, inside the border, all over with the tines of a fork. Use the tip of a small, sharp knife to lightly score the pastry around the inside edge of the border. To seal the pastry strips to the bottom dough, press the top of the border with your little finger, and press the outside edge with the back of a knife held upright in your other hand, working all the way around the tart shell. Place the completed rectangular tart shell in the refrigerator for a minimum of 20 minutes before baking.

Preheat the oven to 375° F. Bake the pastry in the preheated oven for 25 to 35 minutes, until the tart shell is golden brown and well puffed. After the first 15 or 20 minutes of baking, re-prick the bottom of the tart shell with the tines of a fork in order to prevent it from puffing up too much.

Let the tart shell cool completely before filling. Run the point of a sharp knife along the scored border, and gently lift the inside pastry out. This piece can become a "cover," or it can be inverted and returned to the tart shell to form a crispier and thicker bottom.

Round Tart Shells

Start with one 10-inch by 11-inch sheet of puff pastry. Cut out a 10-inch circle of puff pastry and place it on a baking-paper-lined baking sheet. Cut a curved strip, ½ inch wide, from the remaining pastry, long enough to fit around the circle. Brush the top edge of the circle with cold water. Place the curved strip on the top edge of the pastry circle to form a border, cutting off any excess. Prick the bottom of the tart shell, inside the border, all over with the tines of a fork. Use the tip of a small,

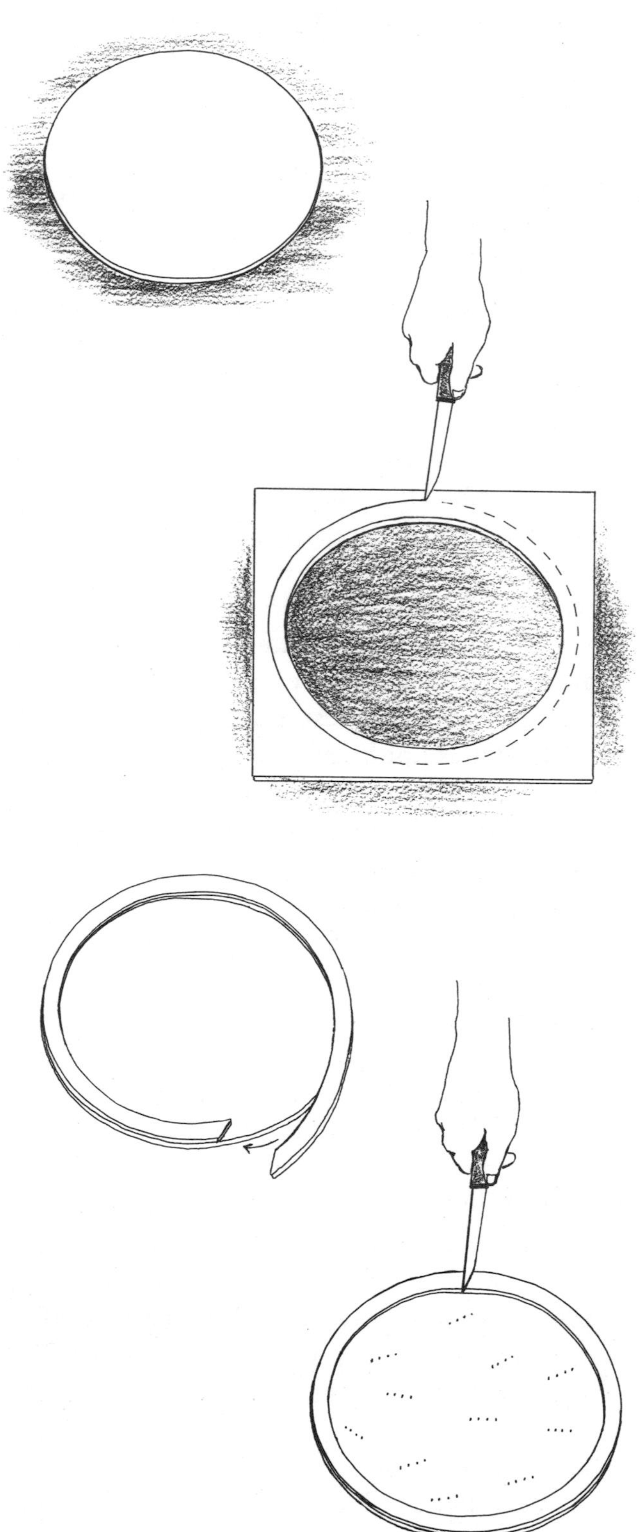

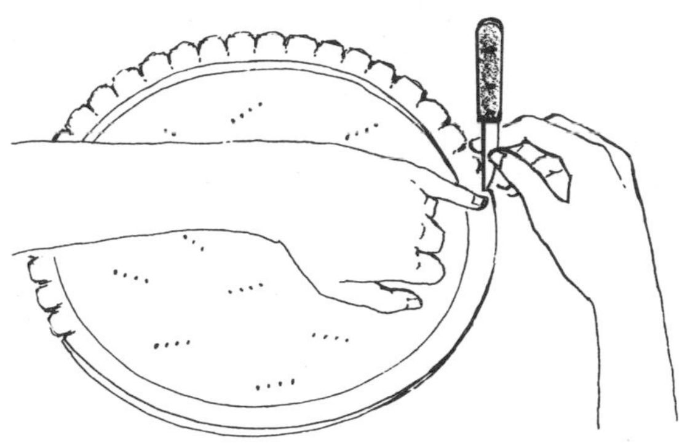

sharp knife to lightly score the pastry around the inside edge of the border. To seal the border to the bottom dough, press the top of the curved strip with your little finger, and press the outside edge with the back of a knife held upright in your other hand, working all the way around the tart shell. Chill the tart shell for a minimum of 20 minutes before baking.

Preheat the oven to 375° F. Bake the pastry in the preheated oven for 25 to 35 minutes, until the tart shell is golden brown and well puffed. After the first 15 or 20 minutes of baking, re-prick the bottom of the tart shell with the tines of a fork in order to prevent it from puffing up too much.

Let the tart shell cool completely before filling. Run the point of a sharp knife along the scored border, and gently lift the inside pastry out. This piece can become a "cover," or it can be inverted and returned to the tart shell to form a crispier and thicker bottom.

Small Tart Shells

Start with one 10-inch by 15-inch sheet of puff pastry. Use the point of a sharp knife to cut six 4½-inch circles from the sheet of puff pastry. Place the pastry circles on a paper-lined baking sheet. On each pastry circle use the point of a small knife to score a circle ½ inch in from the edge of the pastry to form a border. Use the tines of a fork to prick inside the scored circle. Chill the pastry circles for a minimum of 20 minutes before baking.

Preheat the oven to 375° F. Bake the pastry in the preheated oven for 25 to 35 minutes, until the tart shells are golden brown and well puffed. After the first 15 or 20 minutes of baking, re-prick the bottom of the tart shell with the tines of a fork in order to prevent it from puffing up too much.

Let the tart shell cool completely before

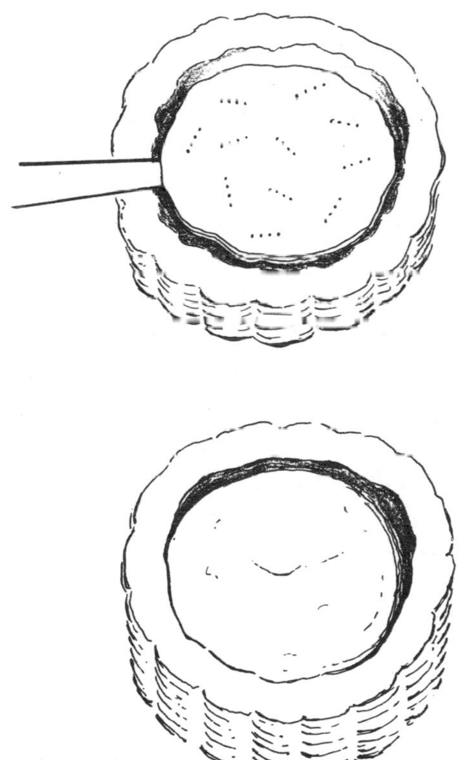

filling. Run the point of a sharp knife along the scored border, and gently lift the inside pastry out. These pieces can become "covers" or they can be inverted and returned to the tart shells to form crispier and thicker bottoms.

Tarte Tatin

Yield:
10-inch tart
7 to 10 servings

This is probably the world's only sugar-free Tarte Tatin. Tarte Tatin is a most wonderful caramelized, upside-down apple tart. Many people would agree that it is one of the world's greatest desserts, especially made this way by slowly cooking the apples and caramelizing them in their own juices. A few years ago in Los Angeles, many of the better restaurants were competing with each other for the best Tarte Tatin. I learned this technique from Jacques Auber, the pastry chef at Le Bel Age Hotel in West Hollywood, California. His Tarte Tatin was definitely one of the best. With a few adjustments, here is Jacques' Tarte Tatin made with fruit sweetener.

There is nothing like the texture of the apples when cooked this way. Because the apples are quartered, each quarter, though much reduced in size and shape, retains its integrity throughout. Thus, it is very important which apples you choose to make Tarte Tatin. Following in Jacques' footsteps, I choose very crisp and very fresh Red Delicious apples. They must be very crisp and fresh, for if they are not fresh, if even a bit mealy, they will make a disappointing tart. It is very important to make this tart in a heavy-bottomed pan. (At the hotel we used copper; at The Ranch Kitchen I use heavy stainless steel pans with an aluminum core.) Any size saucepan will do. (Once for a buffet I made a Tarte Tatin in an 18-inch diameter sauté pan—difficult to manage, but a spectacular centerpiece). Just adjust the quantity of ingredients proportionately. This recipe is for a 10-inch pan, which will need 20 apples; an 8-inch pan, having about ⅓ less volume, would need 13 to 14 apples; and a 12-inch pan with almost ⅓ more volume would need 26 to 27 apples. It is more delicious to err on the side of extra apples.

A note of caution: *Do not use a cast-iron skillet as there seems to be a reaction that takes place, making the entire tart very metallic tasting for some people.*

Because several hours of slow cooking, refrigerating, and freezing are required for the Tarte Tatin, it is necessary to begin preparing it the day before it is to be served.

20 Red Delicious apples
8 tablespoons (4 ounces) butter
¾ cup fruit sweetener
10-inch round of puff pastry
¼ cup Yellow Glaze (page 181)

Peel, core, and quarter the apples. Over very low heat, melt the butter in the bottom of the pan in which you are going to cook the Tarte Tatin, along with ¼ cup of the fruit sweetener. Keep the pan over the heat while you stand the quartered apples on end and pack them tightly in concentric circles in the pan.

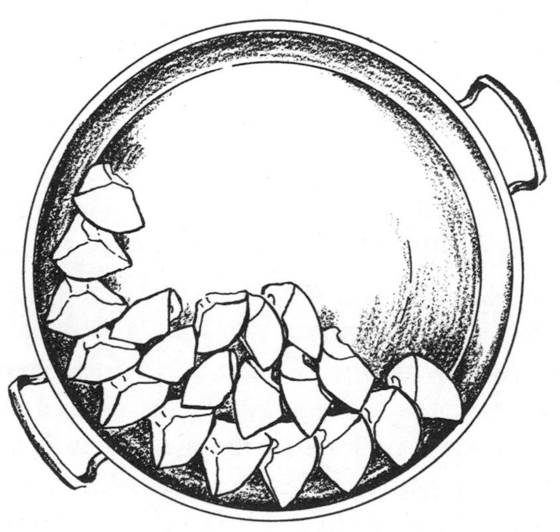

Alternate the direction of the apples from circle to circle. Drizzle the remaining fruit sweetener over the apples. Use a flat saucepan lid to gently weight the apples down. As you will notice, not all of the apple quarters will fit in the pan in the beginning. Add the remaining apple quarters during the first hour of cooking, as the apples in the pan soften and reduce in size. Check the cooking apples every 15 minutes during that first hour, in order to pack in the remaining apple quarters. Just push the apples in the pan together more tightly, and insert the uncooked quarters in between the cooking apples.

Continue to cook over very low heat for approximately 3 hours until the pan juices are a deep, golden brown. Adjust the heat so that the juices in the pan are just simmering. Shake the pan occasionally to make sure the apples are not sticking to the bottom of the pan. This is especially important during the last hour of cooking. Remove the pan from the heat. When the pan has cooled, refrigerate the cooked apples for at least 12 hours.

Preheat the oven to 375° F. Prepare a round of puff pastry to fit just inside your pan. Prick the pastry all over with the tines of a fork to keep it from puffing too much while baking. Place the pastry directly on the chilled apples in the pan. Bake the apples in the preheated oven for 30 to 40 minutes, until the pastry is golden and puffed. Remove the pan from the oven. Let the tart cool before placing it in the freezer for about 4 hours.

Place the pan on the stove over medium heat, just until you are able to use your hand to loosen the tart in the pan. When you are sure that the tart is not sticking to the bottom of the pan (you can swirl it in the pan using your full hand), invert the tart onto a serving platter.

Bring the Yellow Glaze to a boil in a small pan. Remove from the heat and cool for 1 minute. Brush the top of the tart with hot glaze.

To assure the fullest flavor, serve Tarte Tatin at room temperature and do not refrigerate.

Mixed Fruit Tarts

Yield:
10-inch tart
6 to 8 servings

The contrast of colors, textures, and flavors makes mixed fruit puff pastry tarts exquisite.

¾ to 1 cup Vanilla Custard (page 178)
10-inch round puff pastry tart shell (page 116)
2 to 4 cups fresh fruit of your choice
¾ to 1 cup Red or Yellow Glaze (page 180 or 181)

Prepare the Vanilla Custard at least 1 hour in advance, so that it is well chilled when you use it.

Preheat the oven to 350° F. Prepare and bake the puff pastry crust according to the recipe directions. If the bottom of the tart shell has puffed a lot, use a sharp knife to remove the top layers of the shell in one piece, and then invert them in the shell to become part of the bottom of the tart.

Bring the glaze to a boil in a small pan.

Remove the pan from the heat and brush the bottom of the tart with the hot glaze. Spread a ¼-inch-thick layer of chilled Vanilla Custard on top of the cooled glaze.

Arrange the fruit in concentric circles over the custard, working from the outside towards the center. Place the fruit either in overlapping layers or very closely touching, so that none of the custard shows through the fruit.

Reheat the glaze to boiling and let it cool for 1 minute. Brush it over the fruit. Chill fresh fruit tarts for 1 hour before serving.

Baker's Tips

• Remember that Yellow Glaze is used for yellow, green, or other light-colored fruits and that Red Glaze is used with red, purple, or other dark-colored fruits.

• For the prettiest Mixed Fruit Tarts, use ripe but not overripe fruit in a variety of shapes and color, for example:

Mango or papaya slices are a magnificent golden yellow.

Kiwis offer a unique touch of green.

Blueberries and blackberries are a great color contrast to other fruits.

Strawberries left whole or halved are a perfect choice with their red color and heart shape.

Bananas offer an ivory color and give an incomparable taste when used in small amounts.

Raspberries are delicious and beautiful.

• When arranging the fruit, remember that your creativity is the only limit. Almost any design can be beautiful just because fresh fruit is so beautiful. You can choose a design of concentric overlapping circles, or perhaps create a mixed fruit tart as the French do by having sections of only one kind of fruit. When glazing a tart of both light and dark-colored fruits, it is acceptable to use Yellow Glaze over all of the fruit. However, the red fruits will not be as rich and vibrant as if you had brushed them with Red Glaze.

Raspberry Treasure Chests

Yield:
6 pastries

Raspberries are so special and delicate in flavor that they are best served whole with the simplest of ingredients, so that their pure raspberry flavor comes through. Raspberry Treasure Chests are a perfect example of a simple raspberry dessert, with the shining raspberry jewels as the booty.

¾ to 1 cup Vanilla Custard (page 178)
Six 4-inch puff pastry tartlet shells, prebaked (page 117)
3 half-pint baskets fresh raspberries
1 cup Red Glaze (page 180)
6 fresh mint sprigs

Prepare the Vanilla Custard at least 1 hour in advance of preparing the Raspberry Treasure Chests, so that it is cold when you are ready to use it.

Preheat the oven to 350° F. Prepare and bake the puff pastry tartlets according to the recipe directions.

Use the tip of a small knife to remove the puffed centers of the small prebaked tartlet shells. Reserve the centers.

Sort through the raspberries and discard any moldy or mushy fruit. Roll the good berries around on a baking pan lined with a clean kitchen towel to remove any loose dirt or seeds.

Bring the Red Glaze to a boil in a small pan. Remove the pan from the heat and brush the bottom of the tartlet shells with the hot glaze. Spread a ¼-inch-thick layer of chilled Vanilla Custard on top of the cooled glaze.

Arrange the raspberries peak-side-up over the custard so that none of the custard shows through the fruit. Reheat the Red Glaze to boiling and let it cool for 1 minute. Brush it over the raspberries.

To serve the Treasure Chests, place each one on a small doily with its reserved pastry center angled at its side, partially covering the raspberries. Garnish each tartlet with a sprig of mint amidst the raspberries.

Peach-Raspberry Rectangle

Yield:
5-inch by 15-inch tart
6 to 8 servings

This is one of my favorite tarts—not just because of the mouth-watering and colorful combination of fresh peaches and raspberries but also because of its rectangular shape, perfect for summer dessert buffets.

¾ to 1 cup Vanilla Custard (page 178)
5-inch by 15-inch rectangular puff pastry tart shell, prebaked (page 115)
2 half-pint baskets fresh raspberries
3 to 4 medium-size peaches, peeled and sliced ¼ inch thick
½ cup Red Glaze (page 180)
1 cup Yellow Glaze (page 181)
Fresh mint sprigs

Prepare the Vanilla Custard at least 1 hour in advance of preparing the tart, so that it is cold when you are ready to use it.

Preheat the oven to 350° F. Prepare and bake the puff pastry crust according to the recipe directions.

Sort through the raspberries and discard any moldy or mushy fruit. Roll the good berries around on a baking pan lined with a clean kitchen towel to remove any loose dirt or seeds.

Place the peaches in a pot of boiling water for 5 to 10 seconds to loosen their skins. Peel the peaches. Then slice them no more than ¼ inch thick. To keep the slices from turning brown it is best to slice the peaches just before you are going to arrange them in the tart shell.

If the bottom of the tart shell has puffed a lot, use a sharp knife to remove the top layers of the shell in one piece, and then invert them in the shell to become part of the bottom of the tart.

Bring the Yellow Glaze to a boil in a small pan. Remove the pan from the heat and brush the bottom of the tartelet shell with the hot glaze. Spread a ¼-inch-thick layer of chilled Vanilla Custard on top of the cooled glaze.

Arrange the sliced peaches in 3 diagonal fans across the width of the tart, leaving space between the fans. Fill in the spaces around the sliced peaches with fresh raspberries. Place the raspberries so that none of the custard shows through the fruit.

In separate pans, heat the Red and Yellow Glazes until they boil. Let the glazes cool for 1 minute. Brush the Yellow Glaze onto the peach slices and brush the Red Glaze onto the whole raspberries. Garnish the finished tart with fresh sprigs of mint.

Chill the Peach-Raspberry tart for 1 hour before cutting. Rectangular tarts can be cut in wedges or in rectangles. Be sure to cut the tart so that there will be both peaches and raspberries in each portion.

Fresh Banana Tart

Yield:
10-inch tart
6 to 8 servings

Bananas, carob, and Vanilla Custard with a flaky puff pastry crust—a delicious combination of flavors and textures.

10-inch round puff pastry tart shell, prebaked (page 116)
½ to ¾ cup Vanilla Custard (page 178)
¼ to ⅓ cup walnuts
¾ to 1 cup Yellow Glaze (page 181)
⅓ cup Carob Glaze (page 192)
2 to 3 ripe bananas

Prepare the Vanilla Custard at least 1 hour in advance of preparing the Banana Tart, so that it is cold when you are ready to use it.

Preheat the oven to 350° F. Prepare and bake the puff pastry crust according to the recipe directions.

Toast the walnuts in the preheated oven for 7 to 10 minutes, stirring occasionally. Allow the nuts to cool. Then finely chop them with a knife or with a pulsing action in a food processor, and set them aside.

If the bottom of the prebaked tart shell has puffed a lot, use a sharp knife to remove the top layers of the shell in one piece, and then invert them in the shell to become part of the bottom of the tart.

Bring the Yellow Glaze to a boil in a small pan. Remove the pan from the heat and bush the bottom of the tart with the hot glaze.

Heat the Carob Glaze in a small bowl placed over a pan of boiling water. Spread a thin layer of the Carob Glaze on the bottom of the tart shell, over the cooled Yellow Glaze. Spread a

¼-inch-thick layer of chilled Vanilla Custard on top of the cool Carob Glaze.

Slice the bananas into ⅛-inch-thick slices. Arrange the sliced bananas in overlapping concentric circles on top of the custard, working from the outside of the tart in towards the middle. Reheat the Yellow Glaze to boiling and let it cool for 1 minute. Brush the glaze over the sliced bananas and the edge of the tart. Press the finely chopped walnuts around the edge of the tart so that they stick to the glaze. Chill the Fresh Banana Tart for 1 hour before serving.

Apple Turnovers

Yield:
6 pastries

Small triangles of puff pastry enfolding a delicious apple filling make these Apple Turnovers a most special treat. You can adjust the amount of sweetening based on whether you serve these turnovers at breakfast, as an afternoon snack, or for dessert.

2 teaspoons walnuts
1½ tablespoons raisins
⅔ cup peeled, diced tart apples
¼ teaspoon cinnamon
Pinch nutmeg
Pinch salt
⅔ teaspoon unbleached white flour
1 to 3 teaspoons fruit sweetener
10-inch by 15-inch sheet puff pastry
Egg Wash for Pies and Tarts* (page 84)
(omit for egg-free)

Preheat the oven to 375° F.

Toast the walnuts in the preheated oven for 7 to 10 minutes, stirring occasionally. Allow the nuts to cool. Then process them in a food processor, using a pulsing action, until they are finely chopped.

Plump the raisins by bringing ½ cup of water to a boil and adding the raisins. When the water returns to the boil, turn off the heat. Let the raisins plump in the water for at least 10 minutes. Drain the raisins, saving any raisin water for another use. Set the raisins aside.

Place the diced apples in a small bowl and stir in the cinnamon, nutmeg, salt, flour, fruit sweetener, walnuts, and raisins.

Cut the puff pastry sheet into six 5-inch squares. Prepare the Egg Wash.

Make one turnover at a time. Place 2 tablespoons of the apple filling in the center of each square. Brush the Egg Wash on the edges of the square. Fold the dough over the filling to form a triangle and seal the edges with light pressure from the tines of a fork. Place the completed turnovers on baking paper-lined pans. Brush the tops with Egg Wash. With a sharp knife make 3 small slits on top of each turnover to release steam while baking.

Bake the turnovers in the preheated oven for 35 to 45 minutes, until the pastry is well puffed and golden brown.

Bake only the number of Apple Turnovers you can enjoy in one day. The others can be frozen unbaked for 2 to 3 months, defrosted in the refrigerator, and then baked as needed.

Nut Strudel

Yield:
5 to 6 servings

Nut Strudel, with its golden puff pastry enclosing a richly flavored nut filling, is a delight at breakfast or at tea. At the restaurant, we regularly feature a flaky puff pastry strudel on our Sunday brunch buffets.

One Christmas we gave Nut Strudels as thank-you gifts to our purveyors and neighbors. The following Christmas, one of the neighbors phoned to ask if we would be giving gifts again, and could she please receive another Nut Strudel just like the one she received last year!

⅓ cup raisins
1¾ cups nuts (walnuts, pecans, almonds, hazelnuts, or any combination)
1 egg
¼ cup fruit sweetener
1 cup butter, melted
½ teaspoon cinnamon
½ teaspoon grated lemon zest
¼ cup fruit-sweetened orange marmalade
¾ cup finely ground cookie crumbs
1 sheet of frozen 10-inch by 15-inch by ⅛-inch puff pastry
Egg Wash for Pies and Tarts (page 84)

Preheat the oven to 350° F.

Bring ½ cup of water to a boil and add the raisins. When the water returns to the boil, turn off the heat. Let the raisins plump in the water for at least 10 minutes. Drain the raisins, saving any raisin water for another use.

Toast the nuts in the preheated oven for 7 to 10 minutes. Allow the nuts to cool. Then process them in a food processor, using a pulsing action, until finely chopped.

Increase the oven temperature to 375° F.

Using an electric mixer, beat the egg with the fruit sweetener until thick and creamy. Stir in the melted butter, cinnamon, lemon zest, orange marmalade, cookie crumbs, nuts, and plumped raisins.

On your work surface, lay out the frozen puff pastry sheet. Cut it to form a rectangle 8½

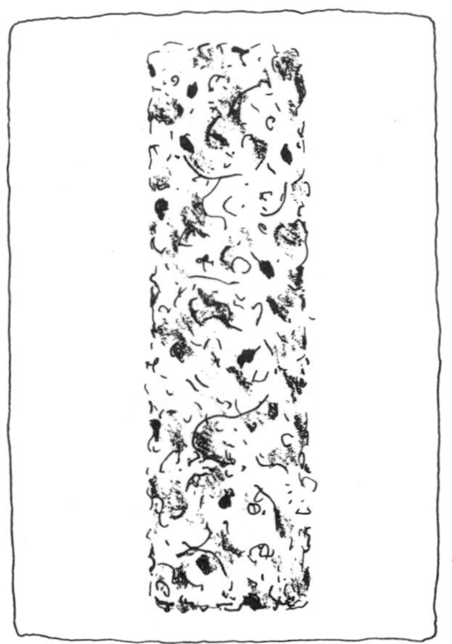

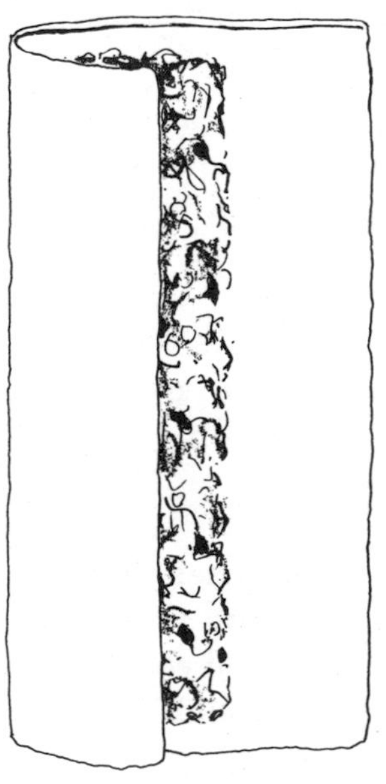

inches by 15 inches. Cut the pastry trim into about 20 strips measuring 5 inches by ¼ inch. Place the nut filling down the center of the puff pastry rectangle.

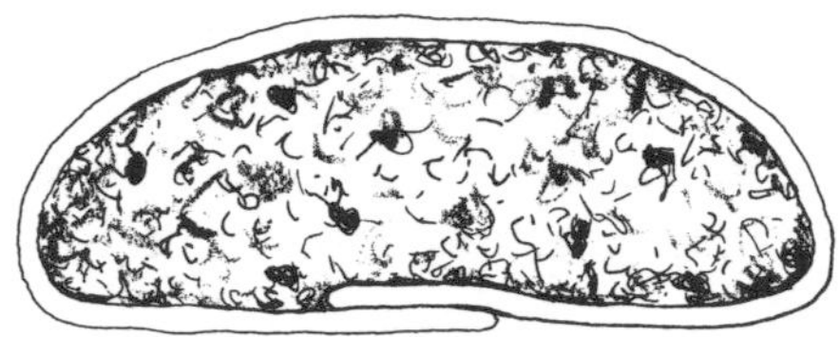

Prepare the Egg Wash, and use a soft brush to brush it on the edges of the pastry. When the pastry has defrosted, fold the lengthwise sides of the pastry over the filling. Place the filled pastry seam-side down on a baking-paper-lined baking sheet. Seal the short edges together by pressing lightly with the tines of a fork. Brush the top of the strudel with Egg Wash. Arrange the thin strips from the pastry trim in a diamond-lattice pattern on top of the strudel. Refrigerate the strudel for at least 20 minutes before baking.

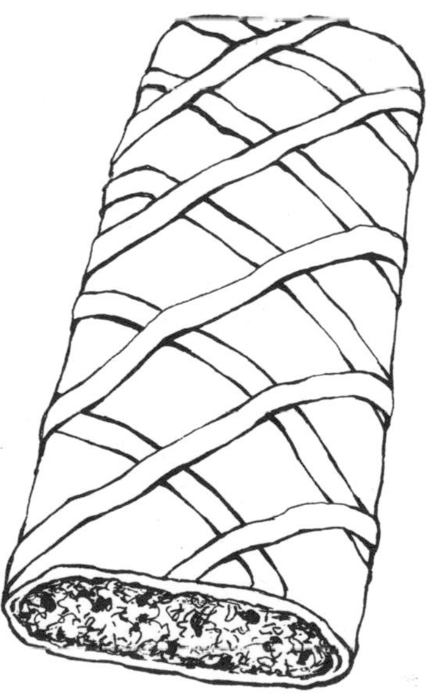

Bake the pastry in the preheated oven for 35 to 45 minutes, until it is well puffed and golden brown.

Serve Nut Strudel hot from the oven. As with all puff pastries, Nut Strudel is best when baked and served on the same day.

Variation

Apple Nut Strudel. Place an overlapping layer of two peeled and cored tart cooking apples sliced ⅛ inch thick down the center of the puff pastry. Top the apples with the nut filling. Roll and bake as above.

Baker's Tip

- As these strudels freeze well, they can be always available. Let the pastries freeze solid after preparing them. Then wrap them tightly in plastic wrap and aluminum foil and return them to the freezer.

To use them, unwrap them and place them seam-side down on a paper-lined baking sheet, lightly covered with plastic wrap, in the refrigerator overnight to thaw. The next day bake them in a preheated 375° F. oven for 35 to 45 minutes, until golden brown.

Peach Strudel

Yield:
5-inch by 15-inch strudel
5 to 6 servings

Use fresh or frozen peaches for a golden pastry delicious inside and out.

2 tablespoons walnuts
3 cups frozen unsweetened sliced peaches or 3 to 4 medium-size peaches
3 tablespoons fruit sweetener
1 tablespoon flour
1 teaspoon cinnamon
¼ teaspoon nutmeg
Pinch salt
¼ cup date pieces
1 cup bread and/or cake crumbs
1 tablespoon butter, melted
10-inch by 15-inch sheet puff pastry
Egg Wash for Pies and Tarts* (page 84) ***(omit for egg-free)***

Garnish

Coconut Powder (page 194) (optional)

Preheat the oven to 350° F.

Toast the walnuts in the preheated oven for 7 to 10 minutes, stirring occasionally. Allow the nuts to cool. Then chop them coarsely with a knife. Increase the oven temperature to 375° F.

If you are using fresh peaches, peel them by placing them in a pot of boiling water for 5 to 10 seconds to loosen their skins. Peel the peaches. Then slice them no more than ¼ inch thick. You should have 3 cups of fruit. To keep the slices from turning brown, slice the peaches just before combining them with the rest of the filling ingredients.

In a medium-size bowl, toss the fresh or defrosted frozen sliced peaches with the fruit sweetener. In a small bowl, combine the cinnamon, nutmeg, flour, and salt. Toss it with the sweetened peaches, along with the date pieces and toasted walnuts.

In another small bowl, combine the bread and/or cake crumbs with the melted butter.

On your work surface, lay out the frozen puff pastry sheet. Place the peach filling lengthwise down the center of the pastry. Cover the filling evenly with the crumbs.

Prepare the Egg Wash, and use a soft brush to brush it on the edges of the pastry. Fold the lengthwise sides of the pastry over the filling. Place the filled pastry seam-side down on a baking-paper-lined baking sheet. Seal the short edges together by pressing lightly with the tines of a fork. Brush the top of the strudel with Egg Wash. Use a sharp knife to make three diagonal slashes across the top of the strudel to release steam while baking.

Bake in the preheated oven for 40 to 45 minutes, until the strudel is well puffed and golden brown.

Let the pastry cool to room temperature before dusting it with Coconut Powder passed through a fine strainer. Bake and serve Peach Strudel on the same day.

Variation

Apple Strudel. Substitute peeled apples, sliced ⅛ inch thick, for the peaches, and ⅓ cup plumped golden raisins for the date pieces.

Almond Blossoms

Yield:
18 pastries

These make a wonderful sweet mouthful: a bit sweet, a bit crisp and flaky, and a bit creamy.

I used a scalloped-edged cookie cutter the first time I made these pastries for a Sunday brunch. The completed pastries looked just like flowers and thus their name.

The puff pastry can be formed in advance and then defrosted in the refrigerator as needed. The filling can be prepared and refrigerated for up to 3 days before filling and baking the pastries.

10-inch by 15-inch sheet puff pastry
2¼ cups almonds
⅓ cup fruit sweetener
1 egg
1 egg yolk
Grated zest of 1 lemon
1 teaspoon vanilla extract

Use a 2½-inch scalloped-edge or plain round biscuit cutter to cut rounds of puff pastry to fit mini muffin cups. Gently ease each round in place. Use the tines of a fork to prick the bottom of each pastry round. Refrigerate the pastry while preparing the filling.

Preheat the oven to 375° F.

Toast the almonds in the preheated oven for 7 to 10 minutes, stirring occasionally. Allow the nuts to cool. Then process them in a food processor, using a pulsing action, until they are finely chopped. Add the remaining ingredients in the order given and process until well blended. Spoon the filling into the pastry-lined muffin cups.

Bake the pastries in the preheated oven for about 20 minutes, until the pastries are golden brown.

Cool the Almond Blossoms for a few minutes in their pan before removing them. Serve at room temperature.

Almond Straws

Yield:
15 pastries

Almond straws are crunchy, flaky, and fun to eat as an accompaniment to a creamy custard or with a cup of tea.

10-inch by 15-inch sheet puff pastry
3 to 4 tablespoons sliced almonds
2 tablespoons fruit sweetener
1½ teaspoons cinnamon

Preheat the oven to 350° F.

Toast the sliced almonds in the preheated oven for 7 to 10 minutes, stirring occasionally.

Roll the puff pastry sheet into an 11¼-inch by 17-inch rectangle.

In a small bowl, combine the fruit sweetener and the cinnamon. Brush the cinnamon mixture over the bottom half of the puff pastry rectangle. Sprinkle the sliced, toasted almonds over the cinnamon mixture. Fold the unbrushed half of dough over the brushed half and gently press both halves together with a rolling pin.

With a sharp knife, cut ¾-inch strips from the double-layered rectangle. Twist each strip 5 or 6 times until it appears as a solid spiral. Place the twisted strips on a paper-lined baking pan, pressing the edges down. Retwist each strip as necessary to help them retain their shape. Refrigerate for 20 minutes.

Increase the oven temperature to 375° F. Bake the Almond Straws for about 20 minutes, until they are well puffed and golden brown.

Bake only the number of Almond Straws you can enjoy in one day. The others can be frozen unbaked for 2 to 3 months, defrosted in the refrigerator, and then baked as needed.

Cream Puff Pastry

This basic pastry is unexpectedly easy to make. It is such an essential part of the baking repertoire that from one cook to another, or from one book to another, the recipe proportions and techniques are usually the same. It is the chemistry of the ingredients and their preparation that brings forth the miracle of the pastry's tripling or quadrupling in size in the hot oven, with the expanding flour and eggs forming a structure that enfolds the steam created by the heat.

Here are some basic points to remember when preparing cream puff pastry:

- The butter must be completely melted and the water must have come to a full boil before you add the flour. You must add the flour all at once and beat vigorously with a wooden spoon until you have a solid mass of dough that pulls away from the sides and bottom of the pan. Reduce the heat and continue to cook the dough for another 2 to 3 minutes to evaporate the excess liquid.

- Add the eggs one at a time, beating well after each addition until the dough is well blended and smooth. The dough should be just stiff enough to stand in a peak. If not, beat in a portion of another beaten egg, a little at a time, until the dough is the right consistency. The dough should be soft and yet retain its shape when piped or dropped from a spoon onto a paper-lined baking pan.

- Place the formed pastries into a hot, preheated 375° F. oven, and bake the pastry until it is puffed, golden brown, and crisp to the touch. If the puffs are removed from the oven too soon, they will collapse as they cool. Use the tip of a knife or a toothpick to put a small hole in each puff, then return the pastries to a turned-off oven to completely dry for another 20 minutes.

• To retain the crispness of the puffs, fill them the same day, preferably within an hour of serving.

• Freezing is the best method for storing extra unfilled puffs. Heat them, direct from the freezer, in a 350° F. oven for a couple of minutes to restore their crispness.

Cream Puff Pastry

Yield:
1½ cups pastry dough
6 medium-size to large pastries

Cream puff pastry can be piped from a pastry bag or dropped from a spoon. However, for the most elegant eclairs and swans, it is preferable to use a pastry bag. Simpler puffs may be filled with sweet or savory fillings, from ice cream, whipped cream, or vanilla custard to herbed cheese, crab salad, or creamed chicken.

4 tablespoons butter
½ cup water
½ cup unbleached white flour
Pinch salt
2 eggs

Preheat the oven to 375° F and line a baking pan with baking paper.

Cut the butter into ½-inch pieces. In a small saucepan bring the butter and the water to a rolling boil over medium heat. When the butter is completely melted, turn the heat down very low and pour in the flour and salt all at once. With a wooden spoon, beat the mixture vigorously until it pulls away from the sides of the pan and forms a solid mass, 1 to 2 minutes.

Remove the saucepan from the heat and transfer the dough to a mixing bowl. Using a wire whisk or an electric mixer on medium speed, beat in the eggs one at a time. Make sure each egg is fully incorporated before adding the next egg. The pastry dough must be stiff enough to just stand in a peak. If it is too stiff, add a small portion of a beaten egg. The dough should be soft and yet firm enough to retain its shape when dropped or piped. Transfer the dough to a pastry bag. Pipe or spoon desired shapes onto the prepared pan, placing them 1 to 2 inches apart.

Bake the pastry on the middle shelf of the preheated oven for 25 to 30 minutes. Pastries should be well puffed and a rich golden brown. Use a toothpick to make a small hole in each pastry to allow the trapped steam to escape. Return the pastries to the oven with the heat turned off for another 20 minutes, so the pastries can thoroughly dry.

Let the pastries cool completely before filling them.

Carob Cream Eclairs

Yield:
6 pastries

Eclairs are such a luscious combination of soft cream and crisp pastry and rich carob that there is just one word to describe them . . . delicious. They are surprisingly easy and fast to prepare. If time is short and you have no Vanilla Custard on hand, fill the eclairs with whipped cream.

1 recipe Cream Puff Pastry (page 129)
½ cup Red Glaze (page 180)
1 cup Carob Glaze (page 192)
½ cup heavy whipping cream
1 tablespoon fruit sweetener
½ teaspoon vanilla extract
½ cup Vanilla Custard (page 178)

Preheat the oven to 375° F. Line a baking pan with baking paper.

Make the Cream Puff Pastry according to the recipe directions. Pipe the pastry through a pastry bag or use a spoon to form six 3-inch to 4-inch eclair shells. Bake the pastries in the preheated oven until they are puffed and a rich golden brown, about 30 minutes. Use a toothpick to make a small hole in each pastry to allow the trapped steam to escape. Return the pastries to the turned-off oven for another 20 minutes, to thoroughly dry them.

While the eclair shells are still warm, cut off the top fourth of each shell. Use your fingers to remove any damp dough filaments inside.

Heat the Red Glaze in a small pan. Dip the top of the tops in the hot Red Glaze.

Heat the Carob Glaze in a small bowl over a pan of hot water. When the Red Glaze is dry, dip the top of the tops into the warmed Carob Glaze. Set tops aside to dry.

About an hour before serving the eclairs, whip the cream with 1 tablespoon fruit sweetener and ½ teaspoon vanilla until it forms stiff peaks. Stir the cream into the custard. Use a pastry bag or a spoon to fill the eclairs with the custard and cream mixture.

Cover each bottom with its carob-dipped top.

Variation

Carob Strawberry Eclairs. A colorful and elegant springtime eclair. Slice a cup of strawberries and place the strawberries in the bottoms of the eclairs, standing them up so they'll show. Fill with custard and cream filling and top with carob-dipped tops.

Cream Puff Swans

Yield:
6 pastries

As dramatic as Cream Puff Swans are, as with all cream puff pastry desserts, you will be surprised at how easy they are to make.

For a reception a few years ago, I made 150 Cream Puff Swans. They were spectacular—they looked almost alive: each swan sitting in its own pool of ruby red Raspberry Sauce, and each with its own personality.

1 recipe Cream Puff Pastry (page 129)
½ cup whipping cream
1 tablespoon fruit sweetener
½ teaspoon vanilla extract
½ cup Vanilla Custard (page 178)
⅓ cup Coconut Powder (page 194)
¾ cup Raspberry Sauce (page 175)

Preheat the oven to 375° F. Line a baking pan with baking paper.

Make the Cream Puff Pastry according to the recipe directions. Pipe the pastry through a pastry bag or use a spoon to form six 3-inch ovals for the swans' bodies on the baking pan. Use a round tip with a ¼-inch opening in a pastry bag to form the heads and necks in one piece, piping a shape similar to a question mark. Pipe directly onto the same pan as the bodies.

Bake the pastries in the preheated oven until they are puffed and a rich golden brown, 20 to 30 minutes. The heads will be baked in about 20 minutes and they should be removed from the oven at that time. Use a toothpick to make a small hole in each pastry body to allow the trapped steam to escape. Return the pastry bodies to the turned-off oven for another 20 minutes to thoroughly dry them.

About an hour before serving the swans, use a serrated knife to cut off the top third of each swan body. Cut this piece lengthwise into two pieces, which will be used to form the wings. Use your fingers to remove any damp dough filaments inside the swan body.

Whip the cream with 1 tablespoon fruit sweetener and ½ teaspoon vanilla until it forms stiff peaks. Stir the cream into the custard. Use a pastry bag or a spoon to fill each body with the custard and cream mixture.

Position the head and neck in the cream at one end of the body. Position the wings at a 45° angle to the body, with the cut side in the cream.

Sift Coconut Powder onto each swan.

To serve, place a pool of Raspberry Sauce in the center of each dessert plate. Place a swan in each pool. Serve at once.

5

Specialty Cakes for Every Occasion

In all of life's special celebrations and memorable occasions, simple and elegant cakes take stage center as few other confections can. Cakes seem to give more pleasure in the present and bring back more memories from the past than any other bakery treat. In this chapter you will find recipes translating many of the classic European and American cakes into healthier, sugar-free favorites—from a traditional Bavarian Black Forest Torte to a French Christmas Yule Log, a layered Strawberry and Cream Cake to a relaxed Sunday morning Coffeecake, a Celebration Carrot Cake with Cream Cheese Frosting to a tea-time Poppy Seed Cake with Lemon Sauce, and many more.

The cakes are arranged in two groups. The first group includes recipes for the basic cakes themselves—everything from an exquisitely textured Vanilla Sponge Cake to a carrot, walnut, pineapple, and coconut-rich Carrot Cake, to a soufflé-light Carob Cake Roll, to an unbelievable egg-free and dairy-free Toasted Hazelnut Torte. These basic cakes can be served simply at tea with a friend or at a picnic for twenty, with a sauce of fresh or frozen fruit or a dusting of powdered coconut.

The second part of the chapter gives the recipes for assembling masterpieces from the basic cakes by combining them with custard or curd, fresh fruit, creams and frostings, sauces and fillings, and toppings and glazes. I believe the building of cake masterpieces is the most creative aspect of baking, for it is here that all of your hard-won skills become reality.

Expectations are always high around cakes, and there is always someone who will love everything you do. But sometimes you will know that next time you could do it a little differently—that you could be a little gentler in folding the batter, or more patient in the trimming of the layers, or more artistic in decorating the cake.

When assembling your masterpieces, be aware of the time involved, as many of these cakes take extra time for cooking and cooling the fillings and for refrigerating the cakes (from a few hours to overnight) before their final decorating.

Skill and accuracy seem to be much more important in preparing cakes than in any other aspect of baking. Improper measuring, heavy-handed folding, and inaccurate oven temperatures are only a few of the factors that can affect the taste, appearance, and texture of finished cakes. As your techniques improve, so will your cakes and so will your pleasure in preparing them.

Let's begin with a few tips on preparing the basic cakes themselves. Familiarize yourself with each recipe before you begin, as different cakes—even with similar ingredients—are handled in different ways. Sometimes the butter is creamed with the sweetener and sometimes the eggs are whipped with the sweetener. It is helpful not to assume that because you made a cake one way, every cake should be made the same way.

Measuring and Folding

Accurate measurements are essential in preparing cakes. This is not the place to guess on the amount of flour—measure. For dry measurements, these recipes presuppose that you dip a cup into the flour and use a knife to cut off the excess without shaking or settling the flour in the cup.

Liquids should be measured in liquid measuring cups, as there is a difference in volume between liquid and dry measuring cups.

Folding is a very important technique to master, especially when making cakes which rely upon the air whipped into eggs for their lightness and volume.

The folding process is best done with your hand, fingers together like a spatula. Always use a bowl larger than the amount of your ingredients, so as to have plenty of room to work.

Hold the mixing bowl with your left hand. Your right hand enters at about 4:30 o'clock, palm facing up and away from you. Move your hand to the bottom of the bowl and bring it

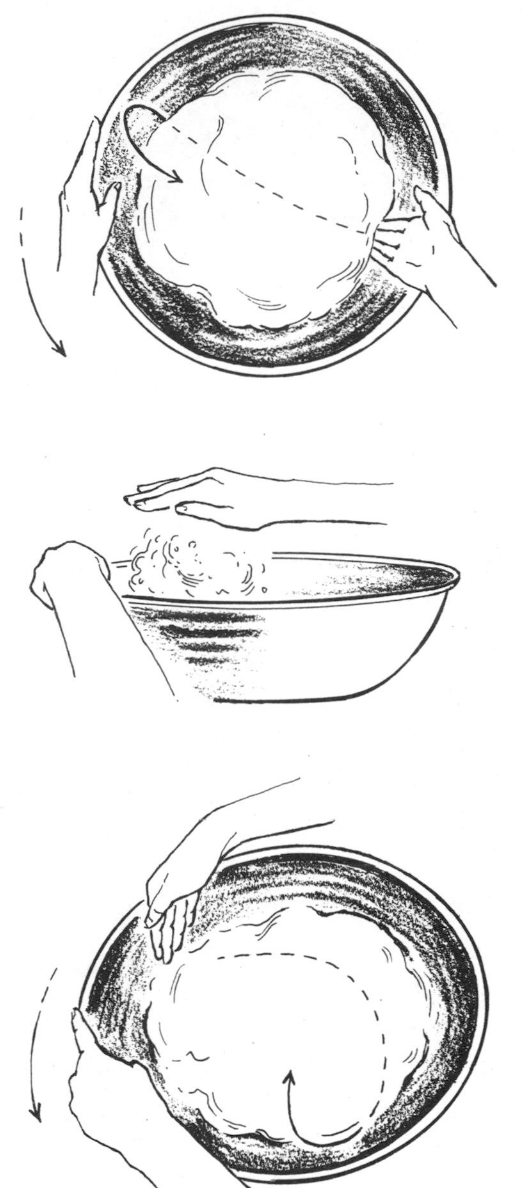

out at the far side, folding its contents on top of the other ingredients. At the same time, your left hand gives the bowl a quarter turn counter-clockwise.

The right hand now re-enters at the far side of the bowl at about 11:30, and follows along the side of the bowl, working its way to the bottom by the time it is closest to you at 6:00. The right hand comes out of the bowl, palm facing away from you, and folds its contents on top of the other ingredients as the left hand gives the bowl another quarter turn counter-clockwise.

These steps are repeated, using quick, gentle, and thorough movements. Fold just enough to incorporate the ingredients, being careful not to overmix and deflate the batter. The advantage of using your hand for folding is that you can feel where there is a lump of flour or a piece of egg shell. Then you can break up the flour and distribute it or remove the broken shell.

When folding *egg whites* into another mixture, first add ⅓ of the stiffly whipped whites to the other mixture and use your hand with your fingers spread apart to gently stir in the whites. This will lighten the mixture so it can combine more easily with the remaining whites without deflating them.

The remaining whites are then folded in, in two parts, alternating with the flour. When the first half of the whites is two-thirds incorporated, then the second half of the whites and the flour are folded in.

REMOVING CAKES FROM THE PANS

When the cakes have cooled, run a small knife along the inside edge of the cake pan to loosen the cake, being sure to hold the knife against the pan so as not to cut into the cake.

For ease in handling cakes while filling and frosting them, place them on cardboard cake circles. These can be purchased from cake-decorating stores and some kitchenware stores, or even from local bakeries. If the cake layers are to be frozen, it is a good idea to place the layers on the cake boards so that the layers remain flat while in the freezer.

Place a cardboard round on top of the cake and invert the cake onto it. Remove the cake pan, leaving the baking paper in place. Reinvert the cake onto another cardboard round so that the top of the cake is up and the bottom of the cake is down.

Cutting and Trimming Layer Cakes

Cakes that are to be layered with filling and frosting need to be thoroughly cooled before they are cut and trimmed. For the prettiest cakes, each of the layers should be level and equal in size.

The bottom crust of each cake is the sturdiest part of the cake. As often as possible, use a bottom crust for the bottom of the cake and another bottom crust for the top of the cake. For ease of handling, when you trim the layers, leave the baking paper in place. Remove the paper just before putting the layer in place if it is the bottom of the cake, and just after putting the layer in place if it is for the top of the cake. If it is necessary to use a bottom as a middle layer, then trim off the thin, darker layer of the bottom crust before proceeding with the filling of the cake.

Place each cake bottom (paper side down) on a cardboard circle. Use a long serrated knife to trim off the thin top crust of the cake, leaving the top of the cake level. Then cut the cake into the number of layers required.

With your right hand, hold the long serrated knife horizontally. Begin cutting with a gentle sawing motion. With the palm of your

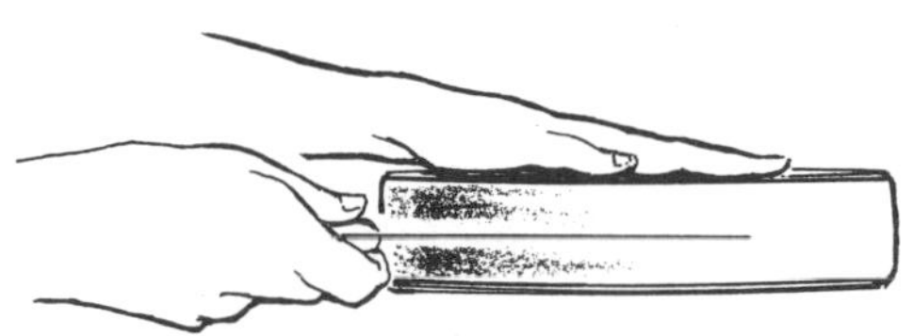

left hand, give the cake about one-eighth of a turn at a time. Keep your eyes and your attention focused on holding the knife straight. Do not attempt to cut deeply into the cake at any one spot. As you turn the cake, you will naturally move toward the center and eventually cut all the way through. For ease in handling, slide a cardboard circle under each layer.

Filling and Frosting Layer Cakes

Because many cream-based frosting and fillings deflate if not used shortly after preparing them, and many fruits begin to lose their bright color when exposed to the air, it is wise to trim and cut the cake layers before preparing such frostings, fillings, and fruits.

When filling cakes, the axiom "More is better" does not hold true. Too much fruit or filling will encourage the layers to slide about, making the finished "leaning tower" most difficult to cut and serve. For similar reasons, do not use a runny or very soft filling—it will spill out the sides, causing the layers to slip about and making the cake difficult to serve. A too-soft filling will also make the cake too moist and soggy to eat.

When fresh fruit is placed between the layers, cut the fruit into uniform slices so that the cake layers will remain level. By placing a thin amount of filling both under and on top of the fruit, you stabilize the fruit and even out the natural ridges and valleys created by its shape.

Once the cake is filled, glaze it entirely with a thin layer of room-temperature jam glaze. This layer of glaze is a flavor-enhancer and acts as a "crumb-coat," keeping the crumbs in place on the cake when you frost it. Closely cover the cake with a large piece of plastic wrap. As time allows, refrigerate the cake for at least a couple of hours to overnight before the final frosting and decorating. This rest in the refrigerator not only sets the filling but also allows the flavors to marry.

Before removing the plastic wrap from the chilled cake, use your hands to smooth and straighten the sides and top of the cake. Remove the plastic and frost and decorate the cake. It is important that the cake be even before you frost it, as frosting should be used to mask only minor flaws. If the construction flaws are acute, it is better not to frost the cake smoothly, but rather to use your decorating spatula to form luxurious circles and swirls. Encrusting the frosting with nuts is another way to hide minor flaws.

However, when your cakes are perfectly level and straight, any sort of frosting or embellishment will only add to the appearance.

As the cake is on a cardboard round, it is very stable and easy to work with. If you do not have a cake turntable, place the cake directly on your work surface, or if you have a strong left arm and hand, hold the cake in the palm of your hand.

Covering cakes with cream-based frostings requires large movements done quickly and confidently. A lot of slow, small movements will cause the frosting to break down (lose its texture), which will then require a thorough encrusting with nuts. A good way to practice frosting a cake is to cover the cake with jam glaze. A number of extra strokes (as long as they are not done with too heavy a hand) won't show and will give you some practice. (If you really want to practice, prepare a batch of instant mashed potatoes to frosting consistency, and frost and refrost an inverted cake pan to your heart's content.)

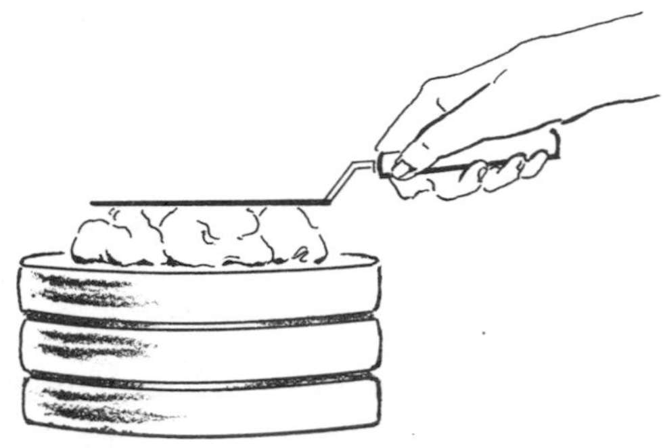

I like to frost a cake beginning at the top. Always put on a great glob of frosting to begin with, smoothing it to cover the top of the cake using a back and forth movement. Work the frosting out to the sides holding the decorating spatula at a 25° to 35° angle and using large movements. Then add more frosting to the sides. Holding the spatula parallel with the cake and with the spatula angled slightly outward, smooth the frosting on the sides, working around the cake and turning the cake as you work. If you have done all this quickly, you

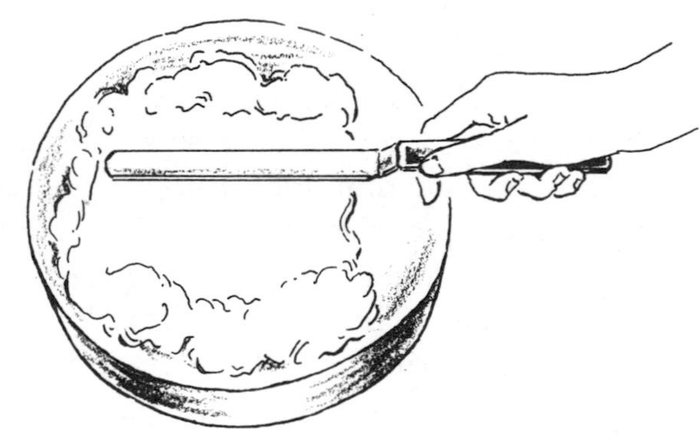

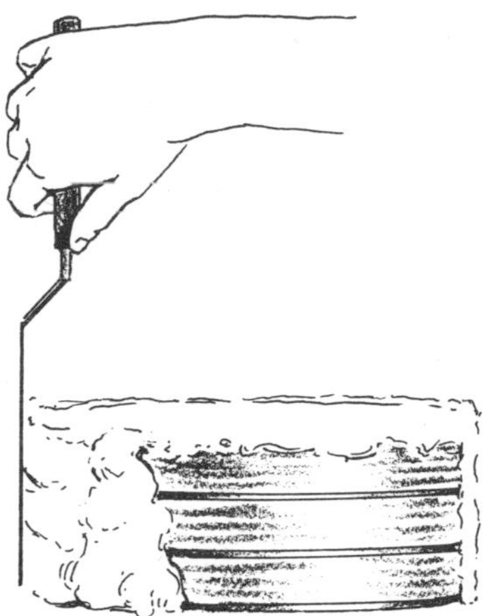

can then use a hot, dry knife (dipped in hot water and dried thoroughly with a clean kitchen towel) to perfectly smooth the frosting.

Once the cake is frosted and/or decorated with nuts, put it onto a serving platter.

Decorating with Nuts

Toasted and thinly sliced, chopped, or ground walnuts, almonds, hazelnuts, and pecans are all wonderfully delicious textural additions to finished cakes. Pressed onto the sides of a glazed cake they cover the sides sufficiently so that no other, richer frosting is needed. Nuts can be sprinkled all over a cake to mask minor construction or frosting flaws. And, of course, nuts can be used as an aspect of the design.

To press nuts onto a cake, put more nuts than you will need into a plate or pie tin. Place the cake (it should be on a cardboard round) on the palm of your left hand. Hold the cake at a 45° angle a few inches above the plate of nuts. Pick up a handful of nuts with your right hand and press them onto the sides of the cake, letting the excess fall back into the plate. Continue rotating the cake in the palm of your left hand and pressing on the nuts with your right hand until the sides are covered evenly all around. If the top of the cake is to be covered also, sprinkle the nuts evenly over the top.

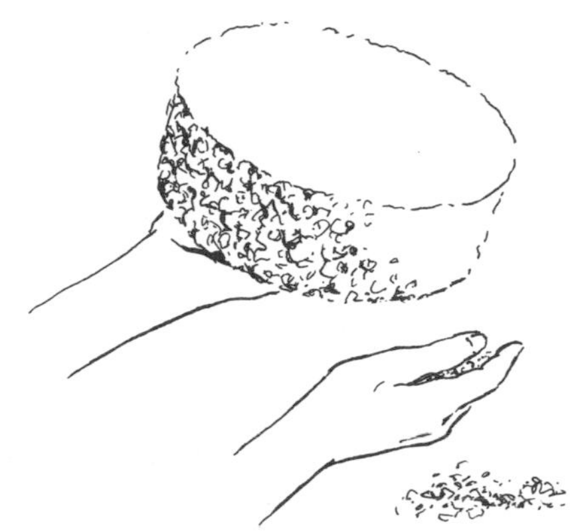

Decorating with Fruit

When decorating with fresh fruit, choose the most perfect fruit for the top of the cake: the biggest and reddest strawberries with the prettiest green leaves, or the biggest raspberries or blackberries, or the greenest, most evenly sliced kiwis. Whole fruits or those cut in half such as strawberries and cherries, can be dipped in hot jam glaze, set aside to dry for a moment, and then set in place. When using sliced fruit or whole fruits such as raspberries or blackberries, it is best to set them in place before brushing them with hot glaze.

Use Red Glaze for red, purple, blue, or other dark-colored fruits; and use Yellow Glaze for yellow, green, gold, or other light-colored fruits. For the prettiest finish, jam glazes should first be strained free of any fruit or cake crumbs before using.

If you are decorating with fruit sauces such as blueberry, strawberry, and cranberry, the sauces must be drained of excess liquid before the fruit is spooned or hand-placed on the top of a cake.

DECORATING WITH A PASTRY BAG

The most beautiful cakes are finished with a decorative edge of frosting. Even the most basic skill in using a pastry bag is a skill worth acquiring, for not only can cakes and pies be made more lovely, but using a pastry bag is a quick and efficient method of forming and filling cream puff pastries and some drop cookies, such as macaroons and soft butter cookies.

Control in the use of a pastry bag takes practice and patience. Rather than practice with a pastry bag directly on your cakes, make up a batch of instant mashed potatoes and reuse them over and over again, piping designs on the back and sides of an inverted cake pan.

Polyester 8-inch and 10-inch pastry bags are probably the most practical for the home baker. They can be used many times over but must be washed inside and out in soap and water after each use and dried thoroughly. Be sure to remove and wash the plastic coupler each time the pastry bag is washed.

It is necessary to cut the opening in a new pastry bag a bit larger, in order to accommodate a plastic coupler or one of the larger metal tips. Place the coupler at the very bottom of the bag with the desired tip, or fit the bag with a large metal tip. Plastic couplers are very handy for using more than one tip with the same frosting without having to empty or change bags; however, the large metal tips have larger openings than the tips used with couplers. The larger-size tips are more appropriate for piping larger and more luxurious designs.

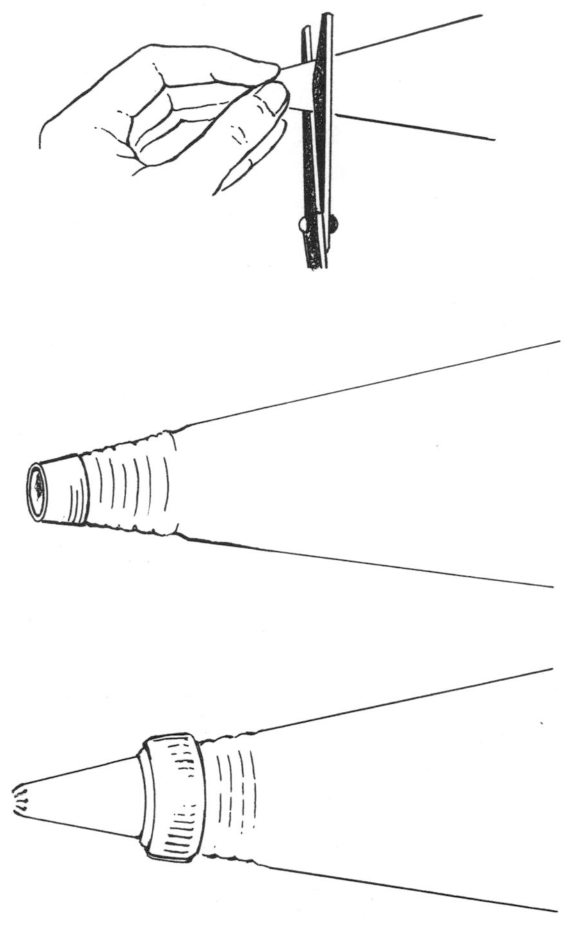

To fill the pastry bag, fold down the top third of the bag to form a large collar. Hold the bag on the outside beneath the collar, and fill the inside of the bag to the top of the collar. Unfold the collar and use your thumb and first two fingers to push all the frosting towards the tip. Twist the bag closed just above the frosting, so that the bag is taut in your hand, held in the space between your thumb and forefinger.

The right hand is responsible for placing even pressure on the bag and for moving it. Use the fingers of the right hand and the thumb to do the squeezing. The left hand is used for steadying and guiding the pastry bag. It should not do the squeezing. (In the beginning when I did use my left hand for squeezing, the extra pressure would push the frosting up and out the top end of the bag—and always onto my shoes.) As the icing is piped out of the bag continue to retwist the top of the bag, so that

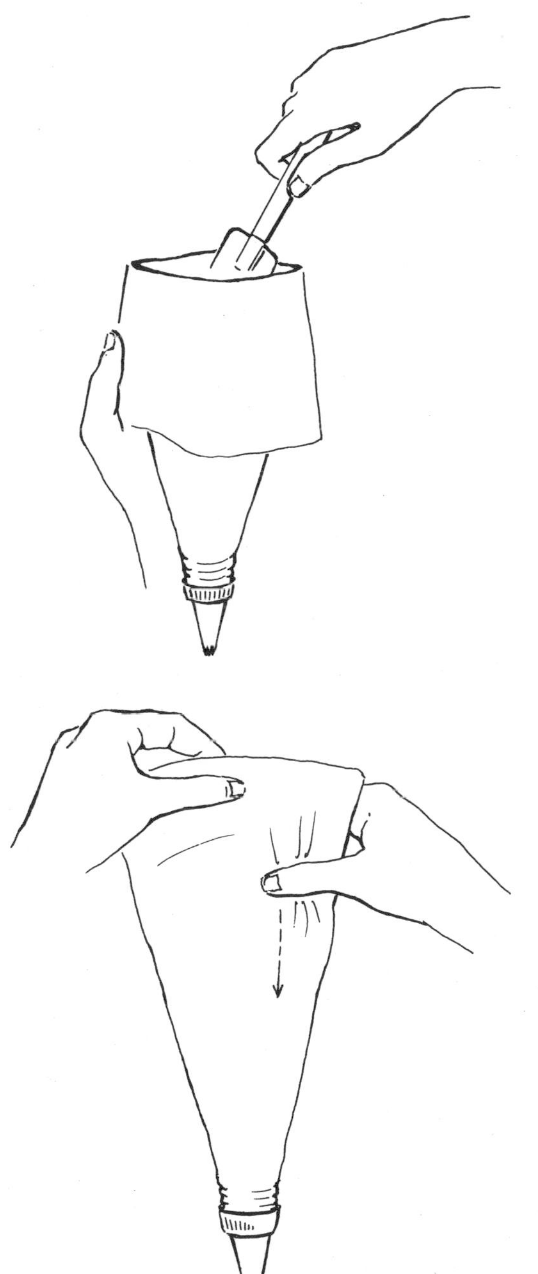

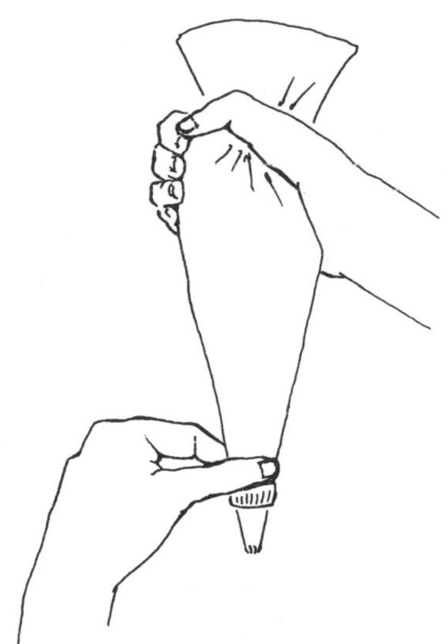

the bag is always taut in your hand, allowing for maximum control.

The two basic designs to master first are the extremely versatile and graceful rosette and shell. With a flourish, the rosette tops individual desserts, such as a strawberry shortcake or an ice cream sundae, or it can be used to mark individual portions on the top of pies or cakes. The shell design, whether straight, curved, or reversed, is the most often used design in cake decorating.

Both of these basic designs require a star tip, of any size. As you increase the size of the tip, the design becomes larger and more luxurious.

For a *rosette,* hold the pastry bag at a 90° angle, ¼ to ½ inch from the surface. With even

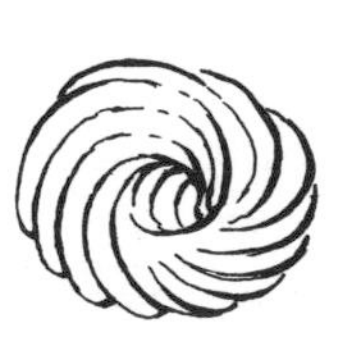

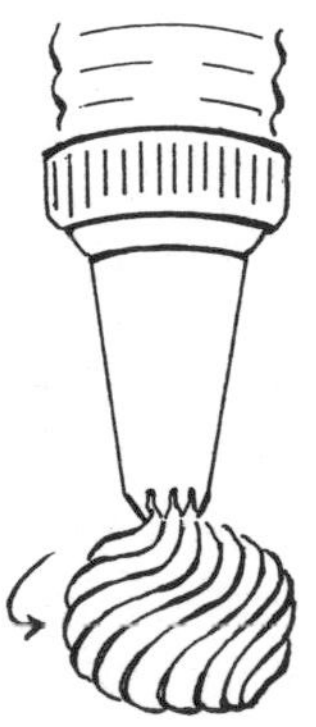

pressure, pipe a circle of frosting, not lifting the pastry bag until you have stopped pressing in order to avoid making a "tail" on the rosettes.

For the *shell* design, hold the pastry bag at a 75° angle, ¼ to ½ inch from the surface. Apply pressure so that the frosting fans out. Then lessen the pressure as you draw the bag away from the fan, lowering the tube to the surface to form the frosting into a point. Do not lift the bag until you have stopped pressing.

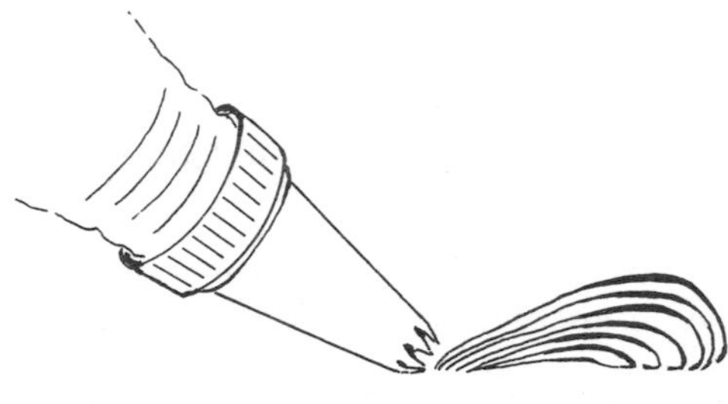

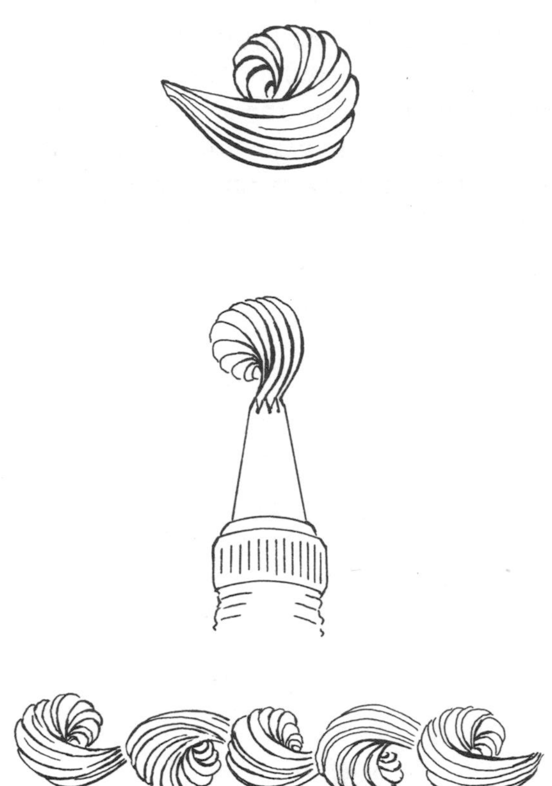

To have a *continuous shell* pattern, one shell after another, pipe the next shell at the point of the preceding shell. In the beginning, it is helpful to pipe one shell at a time, taking a breath between shells. When you feel competent, go ahead and pipe a few in a row, remembering to breathe as you go. I have noticed that when people hold on to their breath, forgetting to breathe, their designs get smaller and tighter and less uniform until they are hardly even recognizable at all . . . (breathe!).

For *curved shells,* the fan part of the design is curved slightly like a question mark, with the point of the shell still in the center as with the regular shell. A *reverse shell* pattern uses curved shells, alternating the direction of the curve with each shell.

There are many other piped decorations that can be accomplished using the basic tips: Round tips for dots, writing, and vines; leaf tips for leaves; rose tips for roses and rosebuds, ruffles, and sweet peas; and the drop flower tips for dainty little flowers. Perfecting your skill with decorating is much fun. Each design takes a bit of experimenting, but with practice the improvement is quick and steady.

The Basic Cakes . . .

Gingerbread

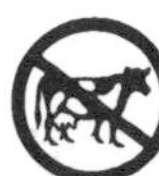

Yield:
9-inch by 9-inch square
9 servings

This sensational Gingerbread was developed just a few months ago for a nearby university kitchen. I had been asked to suggest a number of fruit-sweetened, nondairy desserts. When they chose gingerbread, I discovered that I no longer had a recipe. So a quick browse through a number of books, pulling the combination of spices from one, the quantity of spices from another, the proportion of dry to wet ingredients from still another; then putting it all together my way (e.g., replacing the dairy products with applesauce, part of the flour with ground nuts, and the sugar with fruit sweetener), created this recipe for Gingerbread. It is so wonderful that we now serve it at The Ranch Kitchen as well.

When still slightly warm from the oven, Gingerbread's texture is at its most tender. And for an even more delectable treat, serve Gingerbread with hot Lemon Sauce (page 189).

Wet Ingredients

½ cup fruit sweetener
¼ cup oil
2 eggs
1 teaspoon vanilla extract
1 cup unsweetened applesauce

Dry Ingredients

¼ cup walnuts
1½ cups whole wheat pastry flour
½ teaspoon salt
1½ teaspoons baking soda
2 teaspoons ginger
1 teaspoon cinnamon
⅛ teaspoon nutmeg
⅛ teaspoon cloves

Preheat the oven to 350° F. Lightly spray a 9-inch square pan with lecithin spray.

Toast the walnuts in the oven for 7 to 10 minutes, stirring occasionally. Allow the nuts to cool. Then process them in a food processor, using a pulsing action, until finely ground. Be careful not to overprocess or you will end up with a paste.

Use an electric mixer on medium-high speed to whisk the sweetener and oil together until thickened. Continuing on medium-high speed, add the eggs one at a time, beating well after each addition. Reduce the speed and stir in the vanilla extract.

Sift together the dry ingredients and stir in the ground toasted walnuts.

With the mixer on its lowest speed, add the dry ingredients in 2 parts, alternating with the applesauce. Mix just until the flour is incorporated.

Pour the batter into the prepared pan. Place the pan on the middle shelf in the preheated oven and bake for 25 to 35 minutes, until the Gingerbread springs back when touched lightly in its center.

Cool the Gingerbread in its pan on a wire rack. Store Gingerbread well wrapped in plastic at room temperature.

Toasted Almond Torte

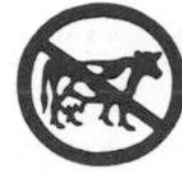 

Yield:
Two 10-inch layers
One 9-inch by 13-inch rectangle
12 to 16 servings

Toasted Almond Torte is an exceptional cake! It is hard to believe it is made without eggs or dairy products. Toasted Almond Torte has a wonderful European quality about it, with rich and complex flavors and textures. This is an excellent cake to make to introduce you and your family to the world of healthier baking.

Toasted Almond Torte can be baked in a rectangle and served simply with a fruit sauce, or baked in rounds and split into layers to form the basis of an elegant Strawberry or Raspberry Toasted Almond Torte (page 158).

Dry Ingredients

2 cups almonds
2 cups whole wheat pastry flour
2 cups unbleached white flour
3 tablespoons baking powder
½ teaspoon salt

Wet Ingredients

1 cup unsweetened applesauce
1¼ cups plain soy milk or almond milk (4:1)
¾ cup oil
¾ cup fruit sweetener
1½ cups unsweetened apple juice
1 teaspoon vanilla extract
1 teaspoon almond extract

Preheat the oven to 350° F. Line the bottoms of two 10-inch cake pans or one 9-inch by 13-inch rectangular pan with baking paper.

Toast the almonds in the preheated oven for 7 to 10 minutes, stirring occasionally. Let the nuts cool. Then process in a food processor, using the pulsing action, until they are finely ground. Do not overprocess or you will end up with an oily paste.

Sift the flours, baking powder, and salt into a large bowl; stir in the ground almonds. Make a well in the center. Combine the wet ingredients in the order given, and stir them into the dry ingredients just until combined. Pour the batter into the prepared pans.

Bake the cakes in the preheated oven for 45 to 60 minutes for the rounds, or 50 to 60 minutes for the rectangle, until they are golden brown and spring back lightly when touched in the middle.

Place the pans on a wire rack to cool before removing the cakes onto cardboard rounds. The cakes must be completely cool before you cut and layer them.

Serve the cake simply with Red Raspberry Sauce (page 175), Blueberry Sauce (page 186), or Strawberry Sauce (pages 188 and 189) or as an elegant Strawberry or Raspberry Toasted Almond Torte (page 158).

Variation

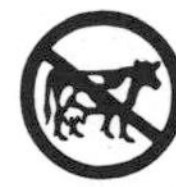 

Toasted Hazelnut Torte. Substitute 2 cups of toasted finely ground hazelnuts for the almonds.

Baker's Tip

• Although "torte" often refers to a multi-layered confection, it actually means a cake in which up to half of the flour has been replaced with finely ground nuts or crumbs.

Coffee Cake

Yield:
9-inch by 13-inch pan
10 to 12 servings

This is the perfect Sunday morning cake. Lots of crunchy crumb topping (everybody's favorite part) covers this rich, moist, and not-too-sweet breakfast favorite. Coffee Cake had become so popular at The Ranch Kitchen that a few years ago when there was some major construction in the area, we would sell it by the pan to the local construction crews.

As might be expected, Coffee Cake is most tender when served hot from the oven.

Crumb Topping

1⅓ cups walnuts
1⅛ cups unbleached white flour
⅓ cup fruit sweetener
2 teaspoons cinnamon
Pinch salt
4 tablespoons cold butter

Batter

4½ cups unbleached white flour
1⅓ cups fruit sweetener
2¼ teaspoons cinnamon
½ teaspoon salt
1½ cups butter, melted
2 teaspoons baking powder
2 teaspoons baking soda
2 eggs
2 cups buttermilk
1 teaspoon vanilla extract

Preheat the oven to 350° F. Lightly spray a 9-inch by 13-inch pan with lecithin spray.

To prepare the Crumb Topping, toast the walnuts in the preheated oven for 7 to 10 minutes, stirring occasionally. Let the nuts cool. Then process in a food processor, using the pulsing action, until they are coarsely chopped. Use an electric mixer on low speed to mix the flour, fruit sweetener, cinnamon, and salt just until crumbly. Then stir in the toasted walnuts. Cut the butter into ½-inch pieces and add it to the nut mixture, keeping the mixture crumbly. Set aside.

To prepare the Coffee Cake batter, use an electric mixer on low speed to combine the flour, sweetener, cinnamon, and salt just until they resemble coarse cornmeal. With the mixer running, pour in the melted butter. Mix until a smooth batter is created. It is important to stop the mixer occasionally and scrape the bottom and sides of the mixing bowl to ensure even mixing and a lump-free batter. Remove 1 cup of this batter and add it to the Crumb Topping above, mixing with your fingers until it is evenly dispersed, though the mixture must remain crumbly.

Stir the baking powder and the baking soda into the rest of the batter. Add the eggs one at a time, beating well after each addition. Add the buttermilk gradually, then the vanilla, again scraping the bowl with a rubber spatula to ensure even mixing. Spread the Coffee Cake evenly in the prepared pan. Use your hands to evenly distribute the Crumb Topping over the top of the cake.

Bake the cake in the preheated oven for 45 to 50 minutes until it is golden brown and springs back when touched lightly in the center. Serve Coffee Cake hot from the oven.

Variation

Dairy-Free Coffee Cake. Substitute margarine for the butter and either almond milk (4:1) or soy milk for the buttermilk.

Basic Carrot Cake

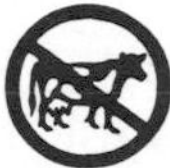

Yield:
Three 8-inch layers for one cake
8 to 10 servings

This is Carrot Cake at its best—the reason Carrot Cake earned such a good reputation in the first place. It is moist and deliciously abundant with grated carrots, shredded coconut, ground walnuts, and crushed pineapple.

For less trimming and handling of the layers, bake your Carrot Cake as we do, in two layers, one twice as large as the other. Then, you'll need to cut the larger of the two layers in half to yield three layers altogether.

For a luscious dessert, see Celebration Carrot Cake (page 158), which is filled and frosted with Cream Cheese Frosting with Raisins and Nuts.

Wet Ingredients

¾ cup walnuts
3 to 4 medium-size carrots
¾ cup drained, crushed, unsweetened pineapple
¾ cup shredded unsweetened coconut
¾ cup oil
1 cup fruit sweetener
2 eggs
1½ teaspoons vanilla extract

Dry Ingredients

1½ cups cake flour
1½ teaspoons cinnamon
1½ teaspoons baking soda
¾ teaspoon nutmeg

Preheat the oven to 350° F. Line the bottom of two 8-inch round cake pans with parchment paper.

Toast the walnuts in the preheated oven for 7 to 10 minutes, stirring occasionally. Let the nuts cool. Then process in a food processor, using the pulsing action, until they are finely ground. Do not overprocess or you will end up with an oily paste.

Peel the carrots and medium-grate them to equal 1½ cups. Drain the canned pineapple, reserving the juice for another use. Combine the grated carrots, drained pineapple, coconut, and ground walnuts. Set aside.

With an electric mixer on medium-high speed, whisk the oil and sweetener until thickened.

Sift the dry ingredients together 3 times.

When the oil and sweetener are thick, add the eggs one at a time, waiting until one is incorporated before adding the next. Stir in the vanilla. On the lowest speed, stir in the sifted dry ingredients and the carrot mixture.

Pour the batter into the prepared pans, putting two-thirds of the batter in one pan and one-third of the batter in the other pan.

Bake the cakes in the preheated oven for 30 to 35 minutes for the smaller layer, and for 35 to 40 minutes for the larger layer. The cakes are done if they bounce back when touched lightly in their center.

Place the pans on a wire rack to cool before removing the cakes onto cardboard rounds. The cakes must be completely cool before you cut and layer them.

Serve Carrot Cake simply with whipped cream or hot Lemon Sauce (page 189).

Banana Walnut Cake

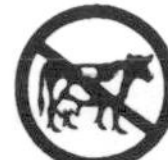

Yield:
10-inch cake
12 to 16 servings

This is a moist, light, and well-flavored cake from The Ranch Kitchen's first summer. Its rich banana taste earned its role in our first most popular cake, the "Carobou." The Carobou was layered with Creamy Carob Frosting (page 183) and sliced bananas, then covered with a rich Carob Glaze (page 192), and garnished with toasted, chopped walnuts. The cake received its name the very first day when I put it into the freezer for a few moments to firm up—and then promptly forgot about it. As a pun on its now frozen state, it was dubbed the "Carobou." The name stayed and so did its popularity. Our Carobou Cake received the 1984 Grand Prize at the Montana State Fair.

Banana Walnut Cake can be more simply frosted with Cream Cheese Frosting with Raisins and Nuts (page 185). Or perhaps you might prefer to keep it nondairy, by layering it with Yellow Glaze (page 181), topping it with a design of glazed fresh bananas, and pressing toasted, finely chopped walnuts onto its sides.

Dry Ingredients

¾ cup walnuts
2 cups cake flour
2 teaspoons baking soda
½ teaspoon baking powder
½ teaspoon cinnamon
¼ teaspoon salt

Wet Ingredients

½ cup oil
¾ cup fruit sweetener
3 eggs
1 teaspoon vanilla extract
¾ cup mashed bananas (1 to 2 medium-size bananas)

Preheat the oven to 350° F. Line one 10-inch cake pan with baking paper.

Toast the walnuts in the preheated oven for 7 to 10 minutes, stirring occasionally. Let the nuts cool. Then process in a food processor, using the pulsing action, until they are finely ground. Do not overprocess or you will end up with a paste.

Sift the remaining dry ingredients together and stir in the ground walnuts.

Using an electric mixer on medium-high speed, whisk the oil and the sweetener together until thickened, about 5 minutes. Add the eggs one at a time, beating well after each addition. Stir in the vanilla and the mashed bananas.

On the lowest speed, add the sifted dry ingredients and mix together for 1 minute. Pour the batter into the prepared 10-inch round pan.

Bake the cake in the preheated oven for 35 to 40 minutes, until it is golden brown and springs back when touched lightly in the center.

Place the pan on a wire rack to cool before removing the cake onto a cardboard round. The cake must be completely cool before you cut and layer it.

Serve Banana Walnut Cake simply with whipped cream or Cream Cheese Frosting with Raisins and Nuts.

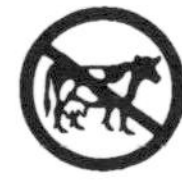

Variation

Applesauce Almond Cake. Substitute unsweetened applesauce for the mashed bananas and toasted, finely ground almonds for the walnuts.

Vanilla Sponge Cake

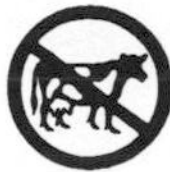 *

Yield:
Two 8-inch or 10-inch cakes
10 to 16 servings

This exceptional cake is my favorite. It is an exquisitely textured, perfectly flavored, light, and moist cake with almost no equal for versatility. I doubt there is any flavor, fruit, sauce, filling, or frosting that would not be complemented by its presence. And, the recipe enlarges so well that we've successfully made large 24-inch by 16-inch sheet cakes, or 18-inch round cakes for the bottom tier of large wedding cakes. (To so enlarge this recipe, you must have at least a 20-quart-capacity mixer in order to properly whip the egg whites.)

With a few substitutions, this is also the basic formula for an "unchocolate (carob) cake." I believe you will find its flavor unique in its own right—dark, rich, and full-flavored. Visually it is a delight to substitute a layer of carob cake in between two of vanilla. Carob cake is a bit more fragile than its vanilla sister, so treat it especially gently.

You can play with the basic flavor of this sponge cake in other ways as well—with the addition of lemon or orange zest, or the adjustment in the quantity and flavor of the extract from vanilla to peach to almond to your choice.

If you are allergic to wheat flour, you can substitute brown rice flour for the cake flour.

Once baked, Vanilla Sponge Cake can be filled with any fruit in season and frosted with any frosting—almost like having a clean white canvas with which to create your masterpiece.

There are many basic techniques given in this recipe for working with egg whites and yolks. Once you have mastered these techniques you will be able to make a number of different cakes perfectly every time.

A stationary electric mixer is recommended for

	Quantities		Ingredients
	8-inch cakes	**10-inch cakes**	
Wet Ingredients			
	4	**6**	**egg yolks**
	⅔ cup	**1 cup**	**fruit sweetener**
	7 tablespoons	**10 tablespoons**	**oil**
	⅔ cup	**1 cup**	**unsweetened applesauce**
	2 teaspoons	**1 tablespoon**	**vanilla extract**
	2 teaspoons	**1 tablespoon**	**peach extract†**
Dry Ingredients			
	1⅞ cups	**2¾ cups**	**cake flour*** ***(substitute brown rice flour for wheat-free)***
	1½ teaspoons	**2 teaspoons**	**baking powder**
	½ teaspoon	**¾ teaspoon**	**baking soda**
	¾ teaspoon	**1¼ teaspoons**	**salt**
Egg White Mixture			
	8	**10**	**egg whites**
	¼ cup	**⅓ cup**	**fruit sweetener**

† Peach extract is optional, though delicious. Replace it with 1 teaspoon additional vanilla extract, or 1½ teaspoons almond extract.

preparing this cake and a second mixing bowl and whip (or beaters) makes the mixing of this cake more convenient. Vanilla Sponge Cake takes approximately 30 minutes to prepare for baking and another 45 minutes to bake.

Preheat the oven to 350° F. Line the bottoms of two 8-inch or 10-inch round cake pans with baking paper.

Whip the yolks and sweetener on medium-high speed for 7 to 10 minutes until very light and fluffy. (This may take a few minutes longer with a hand-held electric mixer.)

Sift the dry ingredients together 3 times into a large bowl.

Increase the mixer speed to high and slowly drizzle the oil into the egg yolk mixture. Reduce the speed to low and stir in the applesauce and extracts. Transfer the egg yolk mixture to a large bowl.

Once the yolk mixture is ready, you will need to proceed very quickly until the cakes are in the oven.

If you have only one whip and one mixing bowl for your mixer, wash and dry them quickly and thoroughly before proceeding.

Whip the egg whites and sweetener together on high speed until they form stiff peaks. Alternately fold the stiffly beaten whites and the sifted dry ingredients into the yolk mixture, one-third of each at a time. It is important that you fold both gently and thoroughly, without deflating either the yolks or the whites. Distribute the batter between the prepared 8-inch or 10-inch pans. Tap the pans once or twice on the table to bring any air bubbles to the surface.

Bake the cakes in the preheated oven for approximately 45 minutes, until they are golden brown and spring back when touched lightly in the middle.

Place the pans on a wire rack to cool before removing the cakes onto cardboard rounds. The cakes must be completely cool before you cut and layer them.

Variations

Carob Sponge Cake. Use the Vanilla Sponge Cake recipe, substituting as follows:

For 8-inch cakes: ⅔ cup carob powder and 1¼ cups cake flour for the flour. Almond extract for the peach extract. Increase the oil by 1 tablespoon to ½ cup.

For 10-inch cakes: ¾ cup carob powder and 2 cups cake flour for the flour. Almond extract for the peach extract. Increase the oil by 2 tablespoons to equal ¾ cup.

Baker's Tip

- Both the Vanilla and Carob Sponge Cakes freeze beautifully for up to 2 months if they are well wrapped. Be sure to protect them from heavier items until they are solidly frozen.

Applesauce Spice Cake

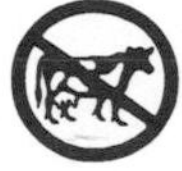 

Yield:
Two 10-inch cake layers
12 to 16 servings

Applesauce lends a wonderful moistness to this cake, and the fragrant cinnamon, cloves, and nutmeg give it a rich, perfectly balanced flavor. Its light and fluffy texture is in no way altered even when it is made with brown rice flour. Applesauce Spice Cake can, of course, be made with unbleached white flour, white cake flour, or whole wheat pastry flour, with equally delicious results.

Because of the preparation technique, which requires the extended beating of both the egg yolks and egg whites, a stationary electric mixer is recommended. An additional mixing bowl and whip (or beaters) is also convenient.

Serve Applesauce Spice Cake simply with Apple Currant Sauce (page 191) and/or lightly whipped cream. For a more special presentation, prepare the Gâteau Normandy (page 160), layering the cake with a tempting combination of Apple Butter and Vanilla Custard.

Wet Ingredients

7 egg yolks
½ cup fruit sweetener
10 tablespoons oil
¾ cup unsweetened applesauce
6 tablespoons Apple Butter (page 193)
Grated zest of 1 lemon
1¼ teaspoons fresh lemon juice
2½ teaspoons vanilla extract

Dry Ingredients

2½ cups brown rice flour
1¾ teaspoons baking powder
½ teaspoon baking soda
½ teaspoon salt
2½ teaspoons cinnamon
1 teaspoon cloves
1 teaspoon nutmeg

Egg White Mixture

7 egg whites
2 tablespoons fruit sweetener

Preheat the oven to 350° F. Line two 10-inch cake pans with baking paper.

Use an electric mixer on medium-high speed to whip the yolks and the sweetener until very light and fluffy, about 7 to 10 minutes.

Meanwhile, sift the dry ingredients 3 times into a medium-size bowl.

Increase the mixer speed to high and drizzle the oil into the yolk mixture. Reduce the mixer speed and gently stir in the applesauce, apple butter, lemon zest and juice, and vanilla. Transfer the mixture to a large bowl.

Once the yolk mixture is ready, you will need to work very fast to prepare this cake for the oven.

If you have only one whip and one mixing bowl for your mixer, wash and dry them quickly and thoroughly before proceeding.

Whip the egg whites and 2 tablespoons sweetener together on high speed until they form stiff peaks. Alternately fold the whites and the sifted dry ingredients into the yolk mixture, one-third of each at a time. It is important that you fold both gently and thoroughly without deflating either the yolks or the whites. Distribute the batter between the prepared 10-inch round pans. Tap the pans once or twice on the table to bring any air bubbles to the surface.

Bake the cakes in the preheated oven for 35 to 40 minutes, until they are golden brown and spring back when touched lightly on the surface.

Place the pans on a wire rack to cool before removing the cakes onto cardboard rounds. The cakes must be completely cool before you cut and layer them.

Serve Applesauce Spice Cake simply with whipped cream, or prepare a more elaborate Gâteau Normandy.

Poppy Seed Cake

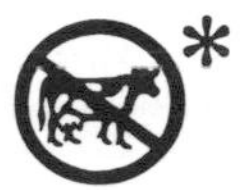

*

Yield:
10-inch tube pan
10 to 12 servings

Many people consider Poppy Seed Cake to be their favorite of all cakes. I understand their choice, especially when the cake is paired with a sublime Lemon Sauce (page 189).

Instead of storing it in the refrigerator, store Poppy Seed cake well wrapped at room temperature, where it will keep for about 3 days.

Wet Ingredients

¾ cup poppy seeds
¾ cup milk* *(use plain soy milk or almond milk [4:1] for dairy-free)*
1 cup butter* *(substitute margarine for dairy-free)*
⅔ cup fruit sweetener
4 egg yolks
2 teaspoons vanilla extract

Dry Ingredients

2 cups cake flour
2 teaspoons baking powder
½ teaspoon baking soda
¼ teaspoon salt

Egg White Mixture

4 egg whites
⅓ cup fruit sweetener

Preheat the oven to 350° F. Lightly spray a 10-inch tube pan with lecithin spray.

Grind the poppy seeds in a coffee grinder

and place them in a small pan with the milk. Bring the mixture to a boil and remove from the heat.

Sift the dry ingredients together 3 times. Cream the butter or margarine and the ⅔ cup of fruit sweetener until light and fluffy. Add the egg yolks one at a time, beating well after each addition. Stir in the vanilla and the cooled poppy seed mixture. Transfer the mixture to a medium-size bowl.

Use an electric mixer on high speed to whip the egg whites with the ⅓ cup of sweetener until they form stiff peaks. Alternately fold the stiffly beaten whites and the sifted dry ingredients into the poppy-seed mixture, one-third of each at a time. It is important that you fold both gently and thoroughly without deflating either the yolks or the whites. Pour the batter into the prepared 10-inch tube pan, smoothing the top.

Bake the cake in the preheated oven for 35 to 45 minutes, until it is golden and springs back when touched lightly in the center.

Place the pan on a wire rack to cool before removing the cake onto a cardboard round.

Serve Poppy Seed Cake at room temperature with Lemon Sauce (page 189).

Carob Cake Roll

Yield:
10-inch by 15-inch or
12-inch by 17-inch jelly roll pan
5 to 6 servings or 7 to 8 servings

Feather-light and deliciously moist, elegant Carob Cake Roll is quick and easy to prepare—and wonderful. As the cake roll is made with a minimum of flour, the structure of the cake comes from perfectly whipped egg yolks and egg whites. It is very important that you fold the ingredients together quickly and lightly, to maintain their structure. For ease in rolling, fill your Carob Cake Roll within 15 minutes of removing it from the oven.

This recipe has been adapted from a chocolate cake recipe of Rose Levy Beranbaum, author of The Cake Bible. *Equally versatile and delicious, Carob Cake Roll is the basis of both a Raspberry Cream Roll (page 170) and a festive Bûche de Noël (page 171).*

The amounts of the ingredients for 2 different sizes of cake roll are included below: The first amounts are for the home-size jelly roll pan, 10 inches by 15 inches; and the second amounts are for the larger, professional-size jelly roll pan, 12 inches by 17 inches. This larger pan can be purchased at restaurant supply stores as well as at some kitchenware shops.

Quantities		Ingredients
10" x 15" pan	12" x 17" pan	
¼ cup	⅓ cup	carob powder
1⅓ tablespoons	2 tablespoons	butter, softened
3 tablespoons	4 tablespoons	boiling water
1 teaspoon	1 teaspoon	vanilla extract
3 tablespoons	4 tablespoons	fruit sweetener
4	6	egg yolks
4	6	egg whites
4 teaspoons	2 tablespoons	fruit sweetener
3 tablespoons	4 tablespoons	cake flour

Preheat the oven to 350° F. Line either a 10-inch by 15-inch or a 12-inch by 17-inch jelly roll pan with baking paper.

Place the carob powder and softened butter into a small bowl. Pour in the boiling water and mix with a fork until smooth. Stir in the vanilla.

Use an electric mixer to whip the egg yolks and sweetener until very light and fluffy, 7 to 10 minutes. Stir in the carob mixture and transfer the new mixture to a medium-size mixing bowl.

If you have only one whip and one mixing bowl for your mixer, wash and dry them quickly and thoroughly before proceeding.

Whip the egg whites and sweetener until stiff peaks are formed. Alternately fold the whites and the cake flour into the carob/egg yolk mixture. It is important that you fold both gently and thoroughly without deflating either the yolks or the whites. Spread the cake batter evenly into the prepared jelly roll pan.

Bake the cake in the preheated oven until it springs back when touched lightly in the center, 15 minutes for the smaller pan, or 18 minutes for the larger pan.

Remove the cake from the oven and immediately cover it with a damp cloth to keep the cake moist. Let the cake cool for about 10 minutes before removing it from the pan. Place a sheet of baking paper on your work surface. Remove the dampened towel and loosen the edges of the cake with a sharp knife. Invert the cake onto the baking paper. Gently peel away the baking paper from the bottom of the cake (now the top of the cake).

Immediately spread on a very thin layer of jam glaze and 1⅓ cups of filling for the smaller cake, 2 cups of filling for the larger cake. With the point of a sharp knife, lightly score the cake ½ inch in from the edge closest to you. Then with the support of the baking paper, roll the cake up and place it seam-side down, either on a rectangular piece of cardboard or directly on a serving platter.

Baker's Tips

• Carob Cake Roll is moist enough to roll up easily without cracking. To assist in the rolling, use the point of a very sharp knife to lightly score the cake ½ inch in from the long edge closest to you. This will make the cake roll more easily and will make the first roll a little bit tighter.

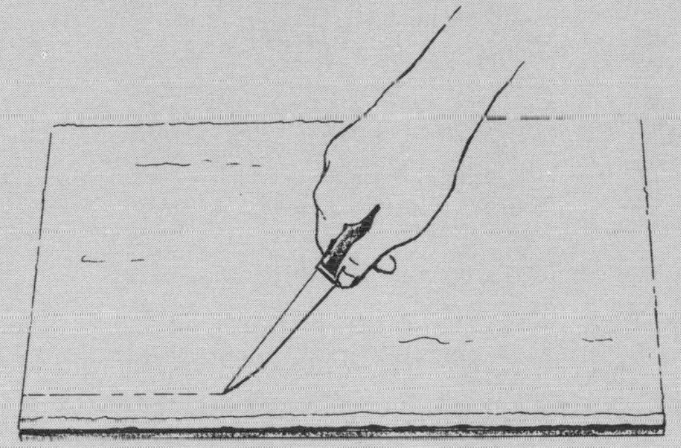

• I have never found it necessary to prepare the cake for rolling by first rolling it up in a clean kitchen towel until cool, then gently unrolling it, spreading it with filling, and rerolling it. If this method does work for you, please continue to use it.

Cheesecake with Blueberry Sauce

Yield:
10-inch cheesecake
12 to 16 servings

Richly flavored with a hint of fresh lemon, and perfectly moist and creamy textured from the combination of cream cheese, sour cream, and whipped cream, this cheesecake is sublime.

I have adapted this recipe from one given to me by Jacques Auber, a French pastry chef extraordinaire, who in his first job in America quickly learned to satisfy his American patrons' love for cheesecake.

Jacques' cheesecake was beautiful to behold, as it was luxuriously masked with whipped cream. Here is a lighter version, sauced with blueberries. Or you may choose any of the other sauces in Chapter 6 to serve with it. At The Ranch Kitchen, we serve cheesecake with Cranberry Raspberry Topping (page 187) in November and December, Strawberry Sauce (pages 188 and 189) or Raspberry Sauce (page 175) during the summer, and Blueberry Sauce (page 186) almost all of the time.

Prepare this cheesecake the day before you serve it, as it requires at least 12 hours in the freezer for the best texture.

Crust

10-inch Granola Crust (page 83)

Cheesecake

2 pounds cream cheese, at room temperature
2 tablespoons plus 1 teaspoon cornstarch
¾ cup fruit sweetener
Grated zest and juice of 1 lemon
1½ teaspoons vanilla extract
⅔ cup sour cream
½ cup whipping cream
3 eggs

Topping

1 recipe Blueberry Sauce (page 186)

Preheat the oven to 350° F. Line the bottom of a 10-inch cake pan with baking paper. Do *not* use a springform pan with this cheesecake recipe.

Prepare the Granola Crust according to the recipe directions, pressing it evenly into the bottom of the pan. Bake the crust in the preheated oven for 10 minutes. Let the crust cool while you prepare the cheesecake filling.

Using an electric mixer, mix the cream cheese until it is very smooth. Add the rest of the cheesecake ingredients in the order listed, mixing well after each addition. Frequently, scrape the bottom and sides of the mixing bowl with a rubber spatula to ensure that the mixture remains free of lumps. Pour the batter over the prebaked crust. Set the cheesecake into a larger pan, and fill the larger pan with 1 inch of hot water. Place both pans (one inside the other) on the middle shelf of the preheated oven.

Reduce the oven temperature to 325° F and bake the cheesecake for 1 hour. Without opening the oven door, turn off the heat and leave the cheesecake in the oven for another hour. Remove the cheesecake from the oven and let it cool to room temperature, about 1 hour. Freeze the cheesecake for at least 12 hours before unmolding.

To unmold the cheesecake, rotate it in the cake pan over a low flame on a gas burner or on an electric stove burner preheated on medium, to release the sides and bottom of the cheesecake. Run a thin knife between the edge of the cake and the inside edge of the pan. Place a cardboard circle on the top of the pan and invert it. Remove the pan and the baking paper from the bottom of the crust. Place another cardboard circle on the bottom of the crust and reinvert the cheesecake. Refrigerate the cheesecake until 1 hour before serving.

Prepare the Blueberry Sauce according to the recipe directions; it can be served either warm or cold. Cover the entire top of the cheesecake with Blueberry Sauce, or pass the sauce separately and have your guests help themselves.

Baker's Tips

• Cheesecake tastes the best and has the best texture when it is eaten at room temperature, although it cuts the easiest and cleanest when it is still partially frozen. Use a hot, dry knife when cutting cheesecake.

• Cheesecake can be prepared in advance and stored in the freezer for up to 3 months before serving. After inverting the cheesecake onto a cardboard round, wrap it well in plastic wrap and aluminum foil. Then freeze.

Holiday Cake

Yield:
10-inch tube pan
10 to 16 servings

A lovely, spicy, fruity cake, perfect for gift-giving during the holidays. Holiday Cake has less fruit than a traditional fruit cake, so there is more light and fluffy cake to enjoy.

One transplanted Australian friend asked for this cake, with a variety of additional fruits added, to be her wedding cake. She was following the Australian tradition of celebrating weddings with fruit cakes. Her husband-to-be, himself a transplant from Hawaii, had beautiful dendrobrium orchids sent from Hawaii to Montana for his bride's bouquet and for decorating the cake. From the orchids on the outside to the cake on the inside, it was beautiful, delicious, and unique.

Holiday Cake really doesn't need any frosting. It can be most tastily combined with Raspberry Sauce (page 175), Lemon Sauce (page 189), or light and spicy Apple Currant Sauce (page 191).

Wet Ingredients

1⅓ cups pecans or walnuts
1 cup raisins
1 cup currants and/or yellow raisins
1 cup date pieces
¼ cup fruit-sweetened orange marmalade
⅔ cup butter
⅔ cup fruit sweetener
2 eggs
2⅓ cups unsweetened applesauce

Dry Ingredients

2⅔ cups unbleached white flour
1½ teaspoons cinnamon
1½ teaspoons allspice
¾ teaspoon cloves
¼ teaspoon nutmeg
1 tablespoon baking powder
¾ teaspoon baking soda
¾ teaspoon salt

Preheat the oven to 350° F. Lightly spray a 10-inch tube pan with lecithin spray.

Toast the pecans or walnuts in the preheated oven for 7 to 10 minutes, stirring occasionally. Allow the nuts to cool. Then process in a food processor, using the pulsing action, until coarsely chopped.

Bring 2½ cups of water to a boil and add the raisins and currants and/or yellow raisins. When the water returns to the boil, turn off the heat. Let the raisins plump in the water for 10 minutes. Drain the raisins, saving any raisin water for another use.

Sift the dry ingredients together 3 times.

Combine the date pieces, coarsely chopped nuts, and well-drained plumped raisins and/or currants with the orange marmalade.

With an electric mixer on medium-high speed, cream together the butter and sweetener in a large bowl. When light and fluffy, add the eggs one at a time, beating well after each addition. (If the mixture begins to curdle, add a tablespoon of flour.) Stir in half of the dry mix, then the applesauce, then the remaining dry mix. Fold in the fruit and nut mixture. Spoon the batter into the prepared 10-inch tube pan.

Bake the cake for approximately 1¾ hours, until a toothpick inserted in the center comes out clean.

Place the pan on a wire rack to cool before removing the cake onto a cardboard round.

Serve Holiday Cake warm or at room temperature with a light sauce. Store the cake well wrapped in plastic wrap at room temperature, where it will stay moist for a week or longer.

The Ranch Kitchen Fruitcake

Yield:
10-inch tube pan
20 to 24 thin servings

Capture the richness of holiday traditions with our excellent fruitcake. The Ranch Kitchen Fruitcake is prepared from a variety of delicious dried fruits—dates, pineapples, peaches, figs, raisins, and prunes. The richly spiced cake is a wonderful blend of tastes, textures, and colors. And since no alcohol is used, the marvelous flavors of the cake and the fruit prevail.

Once you have aged the cake in the fruit syrup for a couple of weeks, it is ready to be served. Freezing is recommended for long-term storage. I had one cake in the freezer for more than 2 years. With a bit of trepidation I removed it from the freezer. Once defrosted, it was every bit as wonderful as it was in the beginning.

You can substitute any combination of dried fruit that appeals to you. I can't think of any fruit that won't work. The purpose of letting the fruit sit overnight in the orange marmalade is not only to soften it, but also to enhance its flavor.

Fruitcake bakes well in a medium-slow oven for a long time. Be sure to cover the top of your fruitcake with foil if it seems to be getting too dark before it has finished baking.

Fruit and Nut Mixture

¾ cup chopped dried pineapple
½ cup chopped dried peaches
½ cup chopped dried figs
½ cup chopped dried prunes
½ cup golden raisins
½ cup raisins
½ cup date pieces
1 cup fruit-sweetened orange marmalade
2 teaspoons vanilla extract
2 teaspoons almond extract
¾ cup pecans
3 to 4 medium-size carrots

Wet Ingredients

1 cup butter
¾ cup fruit sweetener
3 eggs

Dry Ingredients

1¾ cups unbleached white flour
2 teaspoons baking powder
½ teaspoon baking soda
2 teaspoons cinnamon
½ teaspoon salt
¼ teaspoon nutmeg
¼ teaspoon allspice

Lacing Juice

1 cup unsweetened apple juice
¼ cup unsweetened orange juice

Garnish

½ cup Yellow Glaze (page 181)
12 pecan halves, toasted

Cut the pineapple, peaches, figs, and prunes into ½-inch dices. While preparing these fruits, plump the raisins. Bring 1¼ cups of water to a boil and add the raisins. When the water returns to the boil, turn off the heat and let the raisins plump in the water for at least 10 minutes. Drain the raisins, saving any raisin water for another use.

In a medium-size bowl, toss together the diced fruit, date pieces, and the drained, plumped raisins with the orange marmalade and extracts. Cover the bowl with plastic wrap and let the fruit mixture sit out overnight at room temperature.

The next day, preheat the oven to 325° F. Lightly spray a tube pan with lecithin spray.

Toast the pecans in the preheated oven for 7 to 10 minutes, stirring occasionally. Allow the nuts to cool. Then process in a food processor, using the pulsing action, until coarsely chopped. Peel the carrots and finely grate them to make 1½ cups.

With an electric mixer, cream the butter and ¾ cup sweetener. When light and fluffy, add the eggs one at a time, beating well after each addition.

Sift the dry ingredients together 3 times.

Stir the coarsely chopped pecans and finely grated carrots into the fruit mixture.

Stir the sifted dry ingredients into the butter mixture. Then stir in the fruit and nut mixture. Spoon the batter into the prepared tube pan and smooth the top.

Bake the cake in the preheated oven for 1½ to 2 hours, until it springs back when touched lightly in the center. Cool the cake in the pan on a wire rack before removing it.

Combine the lacing juices in a small bowl while the cake is cooling. Spoon half of the Lacing Juice over the fruitcake. Soak a piece of cheesecloth in the remaining juice and wrap the fruitcake in this juice-soaked cheesecloth. Wrap the entire cake in plastic wrap.

Age the well-wrapped fruitcake in a cool place for 1 week. After this week, prepare a ½ recipe of fresh Lacing Juice. Remove the plastic wrap and re-lace the fruitcake through the cheesecloth. Rewrap in plastic.

Let the fruitcake continue to age for at least another week before serving. When the fruitcake is ready to serve, toast the pecan halves in a preheated 350° F. oven for 7 to 10 minutes, stirring occasionally. Heat the Yellow Glaze in a small pan and brush the glaze onto the top of the fruitcake. Garnish the top of the cake with the toasted pecan halves. Use a very sharp serrated knife or an electric knife to thinly slice the cake for serving.

Baker's Tips

- As this fruitcake is not preserved in brandy or other alcohol, the fruitcake *must* be kept in the freezer for long-term storage.

- Lacing is an English term I learned at London's Cordon Bleu School. It means to sprinkle or brush a cake with syrup so that the cake absorbs both moisture and flavor.

. . . Made Into Masterpieces

Strawberry Shortcake

Yield:
9 shortcakes

An old-fashioned all-American favorite and a recent Ranch Kitchen favorite, Strawberry Shortcakes, filled with bright red strawberries, are a beautiful reminder that spring is indeed "busting out all over." We first served Strawberry Shortcake at the restaurant a few years ago on Mother's Day. They were an absolute hit; we could barely keep up with the demand. That same year we had a special order for more than 2,000 Strawberry Shortcakes! It was almost a 3-day operation and required many extra helping hands. It is amazing how much fun it was to prepare shortcakes in quantity and see tray after tray, cart after cart of assembled shortcakes awaiting their moment of glory . . . and the smiles on all the faces of those who received them.

These shortcakes use a flaky biscuit as their base, and a combination of both fresh and frozen strawberries for beautiful color and to ensure sufficient sauce to last through the very last delicious mouthful.

Shortcakes

9 Buttermilk Biscuits (page 60)

Strawberry Mixture

4 to 5 cups fresh strawberries
2 cups frozen strawberries, defrosted
3 to 4 tablespoons fruit sweetener

Whipped Cream

2 cups heavy cream
¼ cup fruit sweetener
2 teaspoons vanilla extract

Prepare and bake the Buttermilk Biscuits according to the recipe directions.

Wash the fresh strawberries by quickly dipping them in water and immediately drying them on kitchen towels. Use the tip of a vegetable peeler to hull all the berries, except for 9 perfect ones to garnish the tops of the shortcakes. Slice 2 cups of the hulled berries and put them into a small bowl. Stir the fruit sweetener into the sliced strawberries, and macerate them for 30 minutes at room temperature.

Meanwhile, coarsely mash the remaining 1 cup of hulled fresh berries with the defrosted frozen berries. Stir the macerated sliced strawberries with their juices into the mashed berries.

Whip the cream with the fruit sweetener until thick and light. Place the whipped cream into a pastry bag fitted with a large star tip.

Divide each biscuit in half horizontally. Place the bottom half of each biscuit on an individual serving dish. Cover each biscuit half with ⅓ cup of the strawberry mixture. Pipe a ½-inch high round of cream to cover the strawberries. Place the top half of each biscuit on top of the cream. Spoon ¼ cup strawberry mixture over each shortcake. Top each shortcake with a large rosette of cream and a perfect whole strawberry.

Strawberry Shortcake is at its best when served within an hour of being assembled.

Baker's Tip

• *Macerate* is a French word referring to the process of combining fruit with a liqueur or syrup until the fruit becomes softer and more flavorful.

Peach Hazelnut Torte

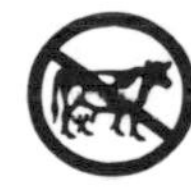 

Yield:
10-inch cake
12 to 16 servings

Toasted hazelnuts and peach jam combine to make this a most delicious and elegant cake with a decidedly European flavor. As the torte is made without eggs or dairy products—which help keep baked goods moist—plan to serve it within one day of preparation for the best flavor and most tender texture.

Two 10-inch Toasted Hazelnut Torte layers (page 142)
2 to 3 cups hazelnuts
10-ounce jar fruit-sweetened peach jam
1 cup Yellow Glaze (page 181)

Prepare the torte according to the recipe directions on page 142.

Preheat the oven to 350° F. Toast the hazelnuts for 7 to 10 minutes, stirring occasionally. If the hazelnuts still have their skins on, rub the nuts, a few at a time, in a clean kitchen towel to remove them. Process the nuts in a food processor, using the pulsing action, until they are finely ground.

Trim the tops of all cake layers to make them level. Then divide each layer in half, making 4 layers altogether. Reserve the bottom of one of the layers for the top of the cake. Place the other bottom layer of cake, bottom-side down, on a cardboard circle. Spread on ⅓ of the peach jam. Sandwich the remaining layers together, dividing the remaining jam between them, ending with a layer of cake on top.

Cover the entire cake with a thin layer of room-temperature Yellow Glaze. Press the finely ground hazelnuts onto the sides and top of the cake.

Serve Peach Hazelnut Torte at room temperature.

Variations

Raspberry Toasted Almond Torte. Substitute Toasted Almond Torte (page 142) for the Hazelnut Torte, unsweetened raspberry jam for the peach jam, Red Glaze (page 180) for the Yellow Glaze, and toasted ground almonds for the ground hazelnuts. An optional garnish would be lightly glazed whole fresh raspberries and fresh sprigs of mint around the top of the cake.

Strawberry Toasted Almond Torte. Substitute Toasted Almond Torte (page 142) for the Hazelnut Torte, unsweetened strawberry jam for the peach jam and add a layer of thinly sliced strawberries between each layer of cake. Garnish the top of the cake with glazed sliced or whole strawberries.

Raspberry Custard Torte. Divide 2 cups of Vanilla Custard (page 178) and 2 cups of Red Raspberry Filling (page 175) between the layers of a Toasted Almond or Hazelnut Torte (page 142). Cover the entire cake with a thin layer of Red Glaze (page 180). Press the finely ground almonds or hazelnuts onto the sides and top of the cake.

Celebration Carrot Cake

Yield:
8-inch cake
10 to 12 servings

At The Ranch Kitchen, we fill and frost our Carrot Cake with delectable Cream Cheese Frosting with Raisins and Nuts. To bring out the very best flavor and texture of both the cake and the frosting, serve your Celebration Carrot Cake at room temperature.

1 recipe Carrot Cake (page 144)
1 recipe Cream Cheese Frosting with Raisins and Nuts (page 185)
Few drops *each* yellow, red, and green food coloring

Prepare and bake the Carrot Cake according to the recipe directions. When the cakes are thoroughly cool, use a serrated knife or an electric knife to cut the larger layer in half, making 3 layers altogether. Trim all 3 layers so that they are level and of equal size.

Prepare the Cream Cheese Frosting according to the recipe directions. Just before adding the raisins and nuts, remove a very small amount of the frosting to each of 2 small bowls to be colored for decorative carrots and leaves. Color the frosting in 1 bowl orange for the carrots, and color the frosting in the other bowl green for the carrot tops. (Use a light touch with the food coloring as it will continue to darken as it sits.) Now stir the chopped raisins and nuts into the Cream Cheese Frosting.

Place one layer of cake, preferably one with the bottom still intact, on a cardboard circle, with its bottom side down. Spread on a ¼-inch-thick layer of frosting. Top with a second layer of cake and spread on a ¼-inch layer of frosting. Top with the last layer of cake. Use the remaining frosting to generously frost the top and sides of the cake. Use the decorating spatula to gently swirl the frosting.

Place the 2 colored frostings into 2 different pastry bags. Fit the pastry bag with the orange frosting for the carrots with a #9 plain round tip. Fit the pastry bag with the green frosting for the leaves with a #233 multi-opening tip. Pipe the carrots and their leaves decoratively around the cake. At the The Ranch Kitchen we score the cake into portions and pipe one carrot on each portion.

To set the frosting, refrigerate the completed Carrot Cake for at least 1 hour. However, as both the Carrot Cake and the Cream Cheese Frosting taste best when served at room temperature, remove the cake from the refrigerator at least 30 minutes before serving.

Kiwi Lemon Cake

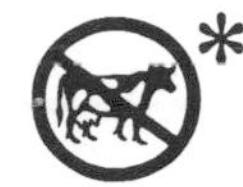

Yield:
10-inch cake
12 to 16 servings

A luscious tart and sweet cake that can be made all through the year, as kiwis seem to be always available. Be sure to use kiwis when they are ripe, when they give to slight pressure, or they will be too tart to enjoy. Combined with the gentle sharpness of lemon curd and the tart sweetness of the orange marmalade, the flavor of kiwis is well complemented. Don't strain the orange marmalade. Those chunky shreds of orange rind add interest and flavor.

This is a wonderful cake to serve on dessert buffets because of its unique and attractive green color and tart flavor. Also, it can become a dairy-free cake when margarine is used in preparing the Lemon Curd. Be sure to prepare the Lemon Curd at least an hour in advance of assembling the cake.

To firm up the filling and blend the flavors, Kiwi Lemon Cake benefits from an overnight stay in the refrigerator before the final decorating.

2 ten-inch Vanilla Sponge Cake layers (page 146)
2 cups Lemon Curd* (page 177) *(prepare with margarine for dairy-free)*
¾ to 1 cup Yellow Glaze (page 181)
1½ cups sliced almonds
7 to 8 ripe kiwis
1½ cups fruit-sweetened orange marmalade

Prepare and bake the Vanilla Sponge Cakes according to the recipe directions, placing two-thirds of the batter in one pan, and one-third of the batter in the other pan, so that you can slice the larger cake layer in half to make two layers.

Prepare the Lemon Curd and refrigerate it until well chilled, for about 1 to 2 hours. Prepare the Yellow Glaze and let it come to room temperature.

Toast the sliced almonds in a preheated 350° F. oven for 7 to 10 minutes, stirring occasionally.

Peel and slice 5 of the kiwis into ¼-inch slices.

Trim the cake layers so that you have 3 equal-size and level cake layers.

Place one layer of cake, preferably one with the bottom still intact, on a cardboard circle, with its bottom side down. With a cake spatula, spread a thin layer of orange marmalade on the cake. Next spread on a thin layer of chilled Lemon Curd. Then place a closely touching layer of sliced kiwis on top of the lemon curd. Now spread another thin layer of lemon curd over the sliced kiwis. Top with the next layer of cake and repeat the process from the orange marmalade through to the second layer of lemon curd. Top with the last layer of cake.

Cover the entire cake with a thin coat of orange marmalade. Closely wrap the cake with plastic wrap and refrigerate it overnight if possible.

When ready for the final decoration, peel and slice the remaining kiwis.

Remove the plastic wrap from the cake and cover the top with perfect slices of kiwi. Place them very close together, covering as much of the top surface of the cake as possible. In a small pan, bring the Yellow Glaze to a boil and cool for 1 minute before brushing it over the kiwis and onto the sides of the cake.

Press the toasted sliced almonds onto the glazed sides.

Refrigerate Kiwi Lemon Cake for 1 hour before serving.

Baker's Tips

- If you have the time for the filled cake to be refrigerated overnight before its final decoration, it will be a more flavorful cake and easier to cut.
- Once peeled and sliced, kiwis bruise easily and quickly lose their clear color. Don't peel or slice the kiwis for the top of the cake until you are ready to put them in place.

Gâteau Normandy

 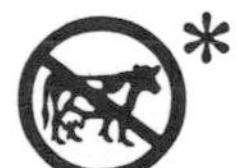*

Yield:
10-inch cake
12 to 16 servings

A sophisticated name for a comforting and delicious cake. Normandy is the region in France known for its wonderful apples, sweet butter, and cream, and gâteau *is French for a fancy cake. Placed together they have become the name for a fancy, old-fashioned cake layered with homemade Apple Butter (page 193) and Vanilla Custard (page 178), and frosted with cream or studded with chopped walnuts.*

If you are assembling Gâteau Normandy using homemade apple butter, remember that apple butter takes 5 to 6 hours to prepare, and at least another hour or two to chill. Vanilla Custard also must have at least 1 hour to chill before using.

2 ten-inch Applesauce Spice Cake layers (page 148)
2¼ cups Apple Butter (page 193)
¾ cup Vanilla Custard (page 178)
¾ to 1 cup Yellow Glaze (page 181)
2 cups walnuts, toasted and finely chopped, or ½ recipe Whipped Cream* (page 181) *(optional)*

Prepare and bake the Applesauce Spice Cake layers according to the recipe directions.

In a small bowl, combine 1½ cups of well-chilled Apple Butter with the Vanilla Custard. Prepare 1 recipe Yellow Glaze and let it come to room temperature.

Cut each cake layer in half, and trim the layers so that they are level and of equal size. Place one of the bottom cake layers on a cardboard circle, with its bottom side down. Spread on a thin coat of Yellow Glaze. Spread on ¾ cup of the custard and apple butter mixture. Sandwich the remaining layers of cake in the same manner, ending with a layer of cake on top. Cover the entire cake with a thin coat of Yellow Glaze.

Spread the remaining ¾ cup apple butter on the top of the cake.

To finish the cake, either press finely chopped and toasted walnuts onto its sides or frost with Whipped Cream, reserving 1 cup of cream to pipe decoratively around the top edge of the cake.

Refrigerate Gâteau Normandy for at least 1 hour before serving.

Strawberry Custard Cake

Yield:
10-inch cake
12 to 16 servings

This is a very elegant affair, with beautiful red ripe strawberries, soft and creamy Vanilla Custard, toasted chopped almonds, and light and fluffy Vanilla Sponge Cake. It is rather unbelievable that Strawberry Custard Cake is made without dairy products or refined white sugar. You will find it the perfect ending for many meals.

This cake is made visually even more appealing when it is made with two layers of Carob Sponge Cake sandwiched around one layer of Vanilla Sponge Cake. In this case, bake one-half recipe of the Carob Sponge Cake and one-half recipe of the Vanilla Sponge Cake.

Strawberry Custard Cake can be baked and assembled in as little as 3 hours, or if you have the time, it can be done over a 2-day period. Be sure to prepare the Vanilla Custard at least 1 hour before it is needed so it will be well chilled and thickened before using.

2 ten-inch Vanilla Sponge Cake layers (page 146) or 1 ten-inch Vanilla Sponge Cake layer and 1 ten-inch Carob Sponge Cake layer (page 147)
2 cups Vanilla Custard (page 178)
1 to 1½ cups Red Glaze (page 180)
2 to 2½ cups sliced almonds
2 pint baskets strawberries

Prepare and bake the Vanilla Sponge Cake (and Carob Sponge Cake) according to the recipe directions. If you are making the cake completely from the Vanilla Sponge Cake, bake the cake with two-thirds of the batter in one pan and one-third of the batter in the other pan. If you are using both carob and vanilla cakes, you will end up with an extra layer of vanilla cake. This layer can be wrapped in plastic and frozen for up to 2 months.

Prepare the Vanilla Custard and refrigerate it until well chilled, about 1 to 2 hours. Prepare the Red Glaze and let it come to room temperature.

Toast the sliced almonds in a preheated 350° F oven for 7 to 10 minutes, stirring occasionally.

Quickly wash the strawberries by dipping them in cool water and removing them immediately. Dry the berries in a single layer on a clean kitchen towel. Use the tip of a vegetable peeler to remove the hulls from the berries.

Trim the cake layers so that you have 3 level and equal-size layers of cake.

Place one layer of cake, preferably one with the bottom still intact, on a cardboard circle, with its bottom side down. With a cake spatula, spread a thin layer of Red Glaze on the cake. Next spread on a thin layer of chilled Vanilla Custard. Then place a closely touching layer of thinly sliced strawberries on top of the custard. Now spread another thin layer of custard over the sliced strawberries. Top with the next layer of cake and repeat the process from the Red Glaze through to the second layer of custard. Top with the last layer of cake.

Spread the Red Glaze thinly over the top and sides of cake. Cover the cake closely with plastic wrap and refrigerate it for at least a couple of hours to overnight.

After the cake has chilled and you are ready to decorate it, slice the remaining strawberries in half lengthwise. Place the strawberries closely touching in a circle around the top edge of the cake with their points facing the center. Overlap the remaining berries with their points facing outward in closely touching concentric circles, filling in towards the center.

Place the Red Glaze in a small pot and bring to a boil. Let the glaze cool for 1 minute. Then brush it on the strawberries and the sides of the cake. Press the toasted almonds onto the glazed sides of the cake.

Refrigerate the Strawberry Custard Cake for at least 1 hour before serving.

Baker's Tips

- Delicious variations can be created substituting fresh peaches, nectarines, blackberries, raspberries, or kiwis for the fresh strawberries.

- If you have the time to refrigerate the cake once it is assembled and before it is decorated, it will hold its shape better when it is cut and served. After the cake has chilled, and with the plastic still in place, use your hands to smooth and shape the cake.

Strawberry Cream Cake

Yield:
8-inch cake
10 to 12 servings

The perfect cake, luscious in taste and beautiful to behold. Strawberry and Raspberry Cream Cakes are the choice of many brides during the summer months when strawberries and raspberries are at their reddest and ripest. These cakes are deliciously simple with the clear flavors of berries and cream and are artfully elegant with the contrasting colors and textures.

Strawberry Cream Cake can be quickly baked and assembled in less than 2 hours, although it does benefit from a thorough chilling in the refrigerator if you have the time.

One birthday party I catered in Malibu, California, featured a Strawberry Cream Cake as the birthday cake for the guest of honor. As I wanted to impress the guests with a sugar-free confection, I decided to wait until the morning of the party to bake it, so the cake would be at its very freshest. When I arrived at the home for the party, the first thing I did was to prepare the cake. While it was baking and cooling, I prepared the luncheon. While the guests were enjoying their luncheon by the ocean, I assembled and decorated the cake. The cake was indeed a success, receiving many raves over its freshness, coupled with expressions of disbelief that it could really have been so delicious and yet made without refined sugar.

It is also possible to assemble Strawberry Cream Cake up to a day in advance of frosting and garnishing.

2 eight-inch Vanilla Sponge Cake layers (page 146)
1 to 1½ cups Red Glaze (page 180)
2 pint baskets strawberries
1 recipe Whipped Cream/Cream Cheese Frosting (page 182)

Prepare and bake the Vanilla Sponge Cake according to the recipe directions, placing two-thirds of the batter in one pan, and one-third of the batter in the other pan, so that you can slice the larger cake layer in half to make two layers.

Prepare the Red Glaze and let it come to room temperature.

Quickly wash the strawberries by dipping them in cool water and removing them immediately. Dry the berries in a single layer on a clean kitchen towel. Keep the leaves on 5 to 6 perfect strawberries to use for garnishing the top of the cake. Use the tip of a vegetable peeler to remove the hulls from the rest of the berries.

Trim the cake layers so that you have 3 level and equal-size layers of cake.

Prepare the Whipped Cream/Cream Cheese Frosting.

Place one layer of cake, preferably one with the bottom still intact, on a cardboard circle, with its bottom side down. With a cake spatula, spread a thin layer of Red Glaze on the cake. Next spread on a ⅛-inch thick layer of Whipped Cream/Cream Cheese Frosting. Then place a closely touching layer of sliced strawberries on top of the frosting, and then cover them with another thin layer of frosting. Top with the next layer of cake and repeat the process from the Red Glaze through to the second layer of frosting. Top with the last layer of cake.

Spread Red Glaze thinly over the top and sides of the cake. Cover the cake tightly with plastic wrap and refrigerate it for at least a couple of hours to overnight.

After the cake has chilled, smoothly frost the top and sides of the cake with the rewhipped Whipped Cream/Cream Cheese Frosting, reserving 1 cup for piping the garnish. Place the reserved frosting in a pastry bag and decoratively pipe frosting around top edge of cake. Pipe the cream into 10 to 12 rosettes or shells on the top of the cake.

Slice the reserved 5 to 6 whole strawberries in half lengthwise through their leaves, leaving them intact. Heat the Red Glaze in a small pan. Holding the strawberries by their leaves, dip them one at a time into the hot glaze and put them on a plate to dry for a moment.

Place one glazed strawberry half on each rosette or shell of cream.

Refrigerate the cake for at least 1 hour before serving.

Variation

Raspberry Cream Cake. Substitute 3 small baskets of raspberries for the strawberries. Do not wash the raspberries, but sort through them for moldy or mushy ones. Roll the good ones around on a baking pan lined with a clean kitchen towel to remove any loose dirt or seeds. Put aside 10 to 12 perfect raspberries to use for garnish. Arrange the remaining raspberries between the cake layers. Place the raspberries on their sides to keep the finished cake from being too tall. Garnish the top of the cake with the reserved raspberries and sprigs of fresh mint.

Peaches 'n' Cream Cake

Yield:
10-inch cake
12 to 16 servings

Peaches 'n' Cream Cake was created the year the bakery received a wooden crate full of organic peaches from Washington. Those juicy peaches were a beautiful deep, rosy peach color with an equally rosy flavor that would penetrate throughout every cake, pie, or tart in which they were used. May you be so fortunate as to find such perfect peaches. When you need a beautiful and delicious cake in a hurry, you can prepare your Peaches 'n' Cream Cake—including time for baking and cooling—in about 3 hours, if you don't refrigerate the cake before frosting and decorating it.

2 ten-inch Vanilla Sponge Cake layers (page 146)
2 to 3 cups walnuts
1 to ½ cups Yellow Glaze (page 181)
4 to 6 fresh, ripe peaches
1 recipe Peaches 'n' Cream Frosting (page 177)

Prepare and bake the Vanilla Sponge Cake according to the recipe directions, placing two-thirds of the batter in one pan and one-third of the batter in the other pan, so that you can slice the larger cake layer in half to make 2 layers.

Toast the walnuts in a preheated 350° F oven for 7 to 10 minutes, stirring occasionally. Let the nuts cool. Then process in a food processor using the pulsing action until they are finely chopped.

Prepare the Yellow Glaze and let it come to room temperature.

Trim the cake layers so that you have 3 level and equal-size layers of cake.

Place the peaches in a pot of boiling water for 10 seconds to loosen their skins. Peel the peaches. Then slice them into ⅛-inch-thick slices.

Prepare the Peaches 'n' Cream Frosting according to the recipe directions.

Place one layer of cake, preferably one with the bottom still intact, on a cardboard circle, with its bottom side down. With a cake spatula, spread a thin layer of Yellow Glaze on the cake. Next spread on a thin layer of Peaches 'n' Cream Frosting. Then place a closely touching layer of sliced peaches on top of the frosting. Now spread another thin layer of frosting over the sliced peaches. Top with the next layer of cake and repeat the process from the Yellow Glaze through to the second layer of frosting. Top with the last layer of cake.

Cover the entire cake with a thin coat of Yellow Glaze. Cover the cake closely with plastic wrap and refrigerate it at least a couple of hours to overnight. After the cake has chilled, smoothly frost the top and sides of the cake with Peaches 'n' Cream Frosting, reserving 1 cup for piping the garnish.

On the top of the cake, place a circle of overlapping peach slices ¾ inch in from the outside edge. In a small pan, bring the Yellow Glaze to a boil. Let the glaze cool for 1 minute. Then brush it on the circle of peach slices. Avoid dripping the glaze on the frosting. Place a 2-inch to 3-inch circle of ground walnuts in the center of the cake inside the circle of peaches. Press the remaining ground walnuts onto the sides of the cake.

Put the reserved frosting in a pastry bag and decoratively pipe it around the top edge of cake to the edge of the peaches, and again on the inside edge of peaches around the outer edge of the ground walnuts.

Refrigerate the Peaches 'n' Cream Cake for at least 1 hour before serving.

Baker's Tip

• To stabilize fresh fruit in between layers of cake, place thin layers of frosting or custard on either side of the fruit. When the frosting or the custard chill, they will help hold the fruit in place. When serving the cake, to help hold the fruit layers in place, use a very sharp serrated-edge knife or an electric knife to cut the cake.

July Fourth Cake

Yield:
8-inch cake
10 to 12 servings

What would a Fourth of July celebration be without a red, white, and blue cake? Here is The Ranch Kitchen's sumptuous July Fourth Cake, with fresh strawberries, whipped cream, and glistening blueberries. And, of course, if you would like, you can bake the cake into a rectangle, and then form the fruit on top into Old Glory, with piped stars of whipped cream to represent as many states as you have room for.

2 eight-inch Vanilla Sponge Cake layers (page 146)
1 recipe Blueberry Sauce (page 186)
¾ to 1 cup Red Glaze (page 180)
1 pint basket fresh strawberries
1 recipe Whipped Cream/Cream Cheese Frosting (page 182)

Prepare and bake the Vanilla Sponge Cake layers according to the recipe directions, placing two-thirds of the batter in one pan and one-third of the batter in the other pan, so that you can slice the larger cake layer in half to make 2 layers.

Prepare the Blueberry Sauce at least 1 hour in advance so that it will be well chilled when needed. Prepare the Red Glaze and let it come to room temperature.

Quickly wash the strawberries by dipping them in cool water and removing them immediately. Dry the berries in a single layer on a clean kitchen towel. Keep the leaves on 5 to 6 perfect strawberries to use for garnishing the top of the cake. Use the tip of a vegetable peeler to remove the hulls from the rest of the berries.

Trim the cake layers so that you have 3 level and equal-size layers of cake.

Place the Blueberry Sauce in a strainer to drain the liquid from the berries, saving it for another use. Prepare the Whipped Cream/Cream Cheese Frosting.

Place one layer of cake, preferably one with the bottom still intact, on a cardboard circle, with its bottom side down. With a cake spatula, spread a thin layer of Red Glaze on the cake. Next spread on a ⅛-inch-thick layer of frosting. Then place a closely touching layer of sliced strawberries on top of the frosting and cover them with another layer of frosting. Top with a second layer of cake and repeat the process, this time using the drained blueberries. Then top with the last layer of cake.

Spread Red Glaze thinly over the top and sides of the cake. Cover the cake closely with plastic wrap and refrigerate for at least a couple of hours to overnight.

After the cake has chilled, smoothly frost the top and sides of the cake with the rewhipped Whipped Cream/Cream Cheese Frosting, reserving 1 cup for piping the garnish. Place the reserved frosting in a pastry bag and decoratively pipe it around the top edge of the cake.

Cut the reserved 5 to 6 whole strawberries in half lengthwise through their leaves, leaving them intact. Heat the Red Glaze in a small pan. Holding the berries by their leaves, dip them one at a time into the hot glaze, and put them on a plate to dry for a moment. Place the drained blueberries in the center of the cake, forming a 3½-inch circle. Pipe a circle of frosting around the blueberry circle. Then pipe 10 to 12 rosettes of cream on the top of the cake in the space between the blueberries and the edge of the cake. Place a shining strawberry half on each rosette.

Refrigerate the cake for at least 1 hour before serving.

Baker's Tip

• Save the juice from draining the Blueberry Sauce. Use it as a topping for yogurt or ice cream, or use it to replace the water in any of the strawberry or raspberry sauces or in the Very-Berry Syrup (page 191).

German "Unchocolate" Cake

Yield:
10-inch cake
12 to 16 servings

German "Unchocolate" Cake is a variation of the similarly named cake from everyone's childhood. For many of my childhood friends other kinds of cake didn't exist.

This recipe is for a slightly more sophisticated version, teaming that delicious Coconut-Pecan Filling we all remember so fondly with a creamy and dark "unchocolate" frosting. I now have a few adult friends who continue to make German "Unchocolate" Cake their current birthday cake choice.

Including time for preparing and baking the cake, German "Unchocolate" Cake can be ready to serve in 2 to 3 hours.

2 ten-inch Carob Sponge Cake layers (page 147)
¾ cup Red Glaze (page 180)
1 recipe Coconut-Pecan Filling (page 179)
1 cup fruit-sweetened black cherry jam
½ recipe Creamy Carob Frosting (page 183)

Prepare and bake the Carob Sponge Cake layers according to the recipe directions, placing two-thirds of the batter in one pan and one-third of the batter in the other pan, so that you can slice the larger cake layer in half to make 2 layers.

Prepare the Red Glaze and let it come to room temperature.

Trim the cakes so that you have 3 level and equal-size layers of cake. Prepare the Coconut-Pecan Filling according to the recipe.

Place one layer of cake, preferably one with the bottom still intact, on a cardboard circle with its bottom-side down. With a cake spatula, spread a thin layer of black cherry jam on the cake. Next spread on 1½ cups of warm Coconut-Pecan Filling. Top with the next 2 layers of carob cake, repeating with the jam and the Coconut-Pecan Filling after each layer is in place, ending with the Coconut-Pecan Filling on top.

In a small pan, bring the Red Glaze to a boil and spread it onto the sides of the cake. Cover the sides closely with plastic wrap and refrigerate the cake while preparing the Creamy Carob Frosting according to the recipe directions.

Remove the cake from the refrigerator. Remove the plastic and smoothly frost the sides of the cake with the Creamy Carob Frosting. Decoratively pipe extra frosting through a pastry bag around both the top edge and foot of the cake.

Serve German "Unchocolate" Cake at room temperature for the best flavor and texture.

Mocha Almond Torte

Yield:
8-inch cake, 10 to 12 servings
10-inch cake, 12 to 16 servings

A rich, dark, delicious combination of flavors and textures. Mocha Almond Torte is a sophisticated multilayered torte with creamy Mocha Almond Frosting sandwiched between layers of rich Carob Sponge Cake. Mocha Almond Torte is worthy of your most elegant celebrations. An equally wonderful variation, Mocha Peach Praline Torte, evokes the ambience and grace of the South in its name as well as in its flavorful blending of tastes and textures—peach jam, Pecan Praline, creamy Mocha Frosting, and rich carob cake.

2 eight-inch or ten-inch Carob Sponge Cake layers (page 147)
1 recipe Mocha Almond Frosting (page 184)
1 to 1½ cups Yellow Glaze (page 181)
2 to 3 cups almonds

Prepare and bake the Carob Sponge Cake layers according to the recipe directions, placing two-thirds of the batter in one pan and one-third in the other pan. Then you can slice the larger cake layer into thirds and the smaller cake layer in half, making 5 level and equal-sized layers.

Prepare the Mocha Almond Frosting and the Yellow Glaze.

Toast the almonds in a preheated 350° F oven for 7 to 10 minutes, stirring occasionally. Allow the nuts to cool. Then process in a food processor, using the pulsing action, until finely ground. Do not overprocess, or you will end up with a paste.

Place one layer, preferably one with its bottom still intact, bottom-side down on a cardboard circle. Spread on a thin layer of room temperature Yellow Glaze. Spread on a ¼-inch-thick layer of Mocha Almond Frosting. Sandwich the remaining layers of cake in the same manner, ending with a layer of cake on top.

Cover the entire cake with a thin coat of Yellow Glaze. Smoothly frost the top and sides of the cake with Mocha Almond Frosting, reserving 1 cup for piping the garnish. Press the toasted ground almonds onto the sides of the cake. Place the reserved frosting into a pastry bag fitted with a large star tip, and pipe it decoratively around the top edge of the cake.

Chill the cake for at least 1 hour before serving.

Serve Mocha Almond Torte lightly chilled or at room temperature for the fullest flavor and best texture.

Variation

Mocha Peach Praline Torte. Replace the Yellow Glaze with unsweetened peach jam. Replace the Mocha Almond Frosting with Mocha Frosting (page 184). Press Pecan Praline (page 194) onto the sides and top of the frosted cake.

Black Forest Torte

Yield:
8-inch cake
10 to 12 servings

Black Forest Torte is one of the world's great desserts, with the richness and complexity of its tart and sweet flavors and the pleasurable texture of tender cake with sumptuous cream. I was shown this particular technique for assembling Black Forest Torte by a French pastry chef, Jacques Auber, under whom I worked in California. The method of assembly is unique and, because of the many steps and different layers, a bit of fun. I have combined what Jacques taught me with other techniques taught to me by a German pastry chef in Portland, Oregon, to come up with this "original" recipe.

One gentleman diner at The Ranch Kitchen said he had traveled through both Europe and America sampling Black Forest Tortes as he went. After he tried a bite, he said ours was the best he'd eaten! I must admit that even I was surprised—for this recipe is made without using refined sugar, the traditional Kirschwasser (cherry-flavored liqueur), or even chocolate!

It is best if you can assemble your Black Forest Torte up to 12 hours before frosting the cake. This allows the filling to firm up and the many flavors in the cake to marry.

Also, be sure to make the Tart Red Cherry Sauce at least 24 hours in advance, in order for the cherries to have the best flavor when you use them.

1 recipe Tart Red Cherry Sauce (page 187)
2 eight-inch Carob Sponge Cake layers (page 147)
½ recipe Creamy Carob Frosting (page 183)
1 recipe Whipped Cream/Cream Cheese Frosting (page 182)
1 cup Red Glaze (page 180)

Garnish

2 to 4 tablespoons carob powder
10 to 12 fresh cherries with their stems attached

Prepare the Tart Red Cherry Sauce the day before you plan to assemble the Black Forest Torte.

Prepare and bake the Carob Sponge Cake layers according to the recipe directions, placing two-thirds of the batter in one pan and one-third in the other pan. Then you can slice the larger cake layer into thirds and the smaller cake layer in half, making 5 level and equal-sized layers.

Prepare the Red Glaze and let it come to room temperature. Place the Cherry Sauce in a strainer to drain the cherries from the sauce, saving the juice for another use.

Cover the cakes lightly with plastic wrap while you prepare the Creamy Carob Frosting. Prepare the Whipped Cream/Cream Cheese Frosting, substituting almond extract for the peach extract.

Place one layer of cake, preferably one with its bottom still intact, bottom-side down on a cardboard circle. Spread a thin coat of Red Glaze on the cake. Then spread on a ¼-inch-thick layer of Creamy Carob Frosting. Distribute one-third of the well-drained cherries on top of the frosting. Top with a second layer of cake.

Spread a thin coat of glaze on the cake. Then spread on a ¼-inch-thick layer of Whipped Cream/Cream Cheese Frosting. Top with a third layer of cake.

Spread a thin coat of glaze on the cake. Place some of the carob frosting in a pastry bag fitted with a large #6 plain round tip, and pipe a ½-inch wide circle of carob frosting around the inside edge of the cake. Pipe a solid 1-inch diameter circle at the center of the cake. Fill in the space between the carob circles with well-drained cherries. Top with a fourth layer of cake.

Spread a thin coat of glaze on the cake. Spread on a ¼-inch-thick layer of carob frosting. Top with the last layer of cake.

Spread the glaze thinly over the top and sides of the cake. Cover the cake closely with plastic wrap and refrigerate it for at least a couple of hours to overnight. Remove the plastic and smoothly frost the cake with the rewhipped Whipped Cream Frosting, reserving a cup of frosting for piping the garnish. Use your decorating spatula to slightly mound the frosting on the top of the cake.

Place the carob powder in a fine strainer. Hold the cake at a 20° angle and *lightly* sprinkle carob powder over the cake. Pipe 10 to 12 rosettes of frosting around the inside edge of the top of the cake.

Bring the Red Glaze to a boil in a small pan. One at a time, dip each of the fresh cherries by its stem into the glaze, then place one cherry on each rosette, with its stem upright.

Refrigerate your Black Forest Torte for at least 1 hour before serving.

Baker's Tip

• Save the juice from the drained Tart Red Cherry Sauce. Use it to replace the water in other sauce recipes, such as in Very-Berry Syrup, Apple Currant Sauce, or in any of the strawberry or raspberry sauces.

Carob Raspberry Cream Roll

Yield:
14½-inch cake roll, 7 to 8 servings
16-inch cake roll, 8 to 10 servings

Carob Raspberry Cream Roll is an exquisite blend of carob and raspberry. When fresh raspberries abound, sprinkle some on the Raspberry Cream Filling before rolling the cake. Or you could serve this cake with Red Raspberry Sauce (page 175) to make any occasion even more sensational.

During the winter holidays, prepare a traditional Bûche de Noël (French Yule Log) using the Carob Raspberry Cream Roll as its base. Inspired by the French custom of keeping a log burning throughout the Christmas supper, this traditional Yule log is quite beautiful when decorated with "bark," "stumps," and vines. At The Ranch Kitchen, our Bûche de Noël is usually the most popular item on the holiday dessert buffets.

Many other variations are possible with the versatile Carob Cake Roll. Just alter the filling and the glaze, and perhaps add a sauce. For example, pair Peaches 'n' Cream or Apricot Cream filling (page 177) with Yellow Glaze (page 181) and a sauce of Carob Glaze (page 192). Or perhaps try Strawberry Cream Filling (page 177) and Red Glaze (page 180) with either fresh or frozen Strawberry Sauce (pages 188 and 189).

Bon appetit!

Quantities		Ingredients
14½-inch roll	16-inch roll	
1	1	Carob Cake Roll (page 150)
⅓ cup	½ cup	Red Glaze (page 180)
1½ cups	2 cups	Raspberry Cream Filling (page 176)

Garnish

Carob Powder (optional)

Prepare and bake the Carob Cake Roll. Within 10 to 15 minutes of removing the cake from the oven, use the point of a small knife to loosen the sides of the cake from the pan. Invert the cake onto a piece of baking paper and trim the edges. Gently peel off the baking paper from the bottom of the cake.

Cover the bottom of the cake with a thin layer of room-temperature Red Glaze.

Prepare the Raspberry Cream Filling and spread it evenly on the cake. Use the point of a small knife to score the cake along its length, ½ inch in from the edge closest to you. Beginning at this side closest to you, roll the cake up, jelly roll fashion, using the bottom piece of baking paper as support. Place the cake seam-side down directly on a flat serving platter. Serve the cake immediately or refrigerate it, well wrapped in plastic, for up to 2 days before serving.

Just before serving, sprinkle the Carob Raspberry Cream Roll with sifted carob powder. Cut the roll on the diagonal to serve oval slices.

Variations

Carob Apricot Cream Roll. Roll the Carob Cake Roll with Yellow Glaze (page 181) and Apricot Cream Filling (page 177).

Carob Strawberry Cream Roll. Roll the Carob Cake Roll with Red Glaze (page 180) and Strawberry Cream Filling (page 177) into which you have folded 1 cup of sliced strawberries.

Bûche de Noël (French Yule Log). Reserve ¼ cup of the Raspberry Cream Filling for coloring green for piping vines and leaves on the finished log. Trim a ¾-inch to 1-inch diagonal slice from each end of the Carob Raspberry Cream Roll. Reroll each slice tightly and place them on the roll to become "stumps." Prepare

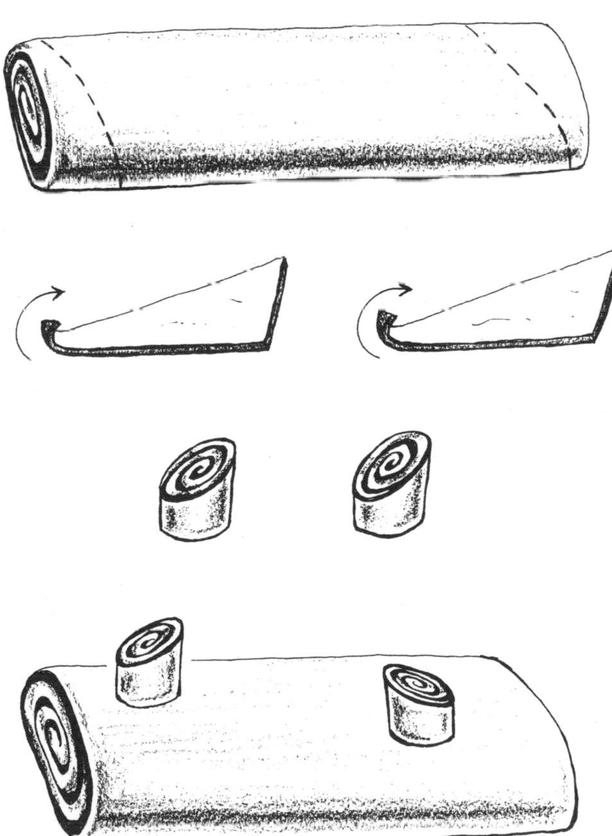

½ recipe of Carob Raspberry Cream Frosting. Pipe it through a pastry bag fitted with a #18 star tip over the cake roll and stumps to simulate bark. Be sure to include an occasional knot hole or two. (Alternatively, you could spread the frosting on the cake and use the tines of a fork to mark the cake to simulate the bark.) Decorate the log with the reserved green frosting making vines and runners (plain #3 tip), and leaves (#67 leaf). Place a few cranberries (drained from Cranberry Topping, page 187) as berries on the vine, for color. To set the frosting, refrigerate the Yule Log for 1 hour before serving.

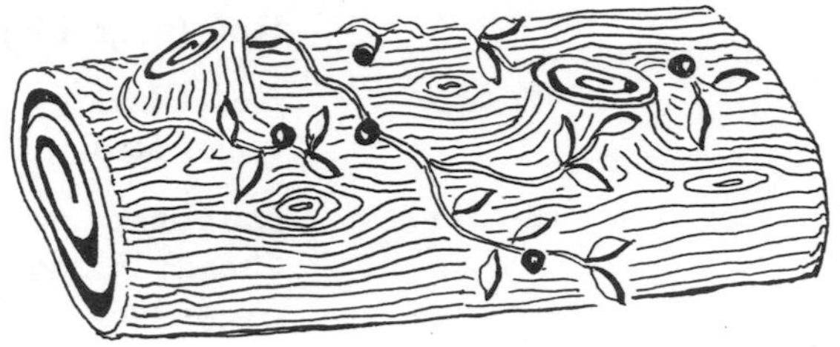

6

Fillings, Frostings, Sauces, Glazes, and Garnishes

The pâtissière's palette consists of the many colors, textures, and tastes of the frostings, fillings, sauces, glazes, and garnishes she uses to embellish her perfectly baked cakes, pies, and tarts. At the restaurant, we fill and decorate our favorite cakes according to the season, choosing between fresh fruits or frozen fruit fillings and a creamy custard or curd. Then we either frost our cakes and pastries with billowy whipped cream, glaze them with dark rich carob, paint them with a sparkling jam glaze, or perhaps top them with a fruited sauce. The choices are many, and the recipes can be combined in so many creative ways that your own palette will become almost limitless.

As you create your own masterpieces, here are a few guidelines to keep in mind:

Always think in terms of flavor, texture, color, and appearance, for it is the blending and contrasting of flavors, textures, and colors in a dessert that helps you create perfection. Some desserts need the unifying effect of a sauce to luxuriously blend their flavors and textures. Other simpler desserts are made complete and almost elegant when dressed with a flavorful sauce. In order to have enough sauce for each delicious mouthful, plan on 4 to 5 servings per cup of sauce, if you are dishing up each serving; plan on fewer servings per cup if your guests are to help themselves. At a large dinner party recently I noticed that the guests enjoyed the Apple Currant Sauce (page 191) so much, they were actually putting it in their bowls after they had eaten the dessert and then eating the sauce as if *it* were the dessert.

Jam glazes, with their natural sparkle, are a wonderful choice for beautifying cakes and tarts. Besides keeping fruits moist and heightening and brightening their natural color, these simple glazes can also be brushed on the bottom of fruit tarts to provide a bit of "waterproofing" for the crust. As jam glazes are really just jam, their special effects will last for a day at the most. So it is best to glaze fruit for the tops of pies, tarts, or cakes on the same day they are to be served.

With cakes, jam glazes are used as a "crumb-coat." They are spread thinly on a filled, unfrosted cake to keep the crumbs on the cake, so that they do not come off in the frosting. Sometimes, as an alternative to a rich, high-calorie frosting, I prefer to glaze the top and sides of the cake and then press on toasted chopped or sliced nuts.

Jam glazes are made from full-flavored jams like raspberry, strawberry, grape, and apricot. Even though the glazes are spread on thinly, they do provide a hint of a contrasting flavor which adds to the delicious complexity of the finished cake.

Traditionally, the glaze used depends upon the color of the fruit to be glazed. Red Glaze is suitable for red or dark-colored fruits, such as plums, purple grapes, strawberries, blackberries, raspberries, cherries, and blueberries; and Yellow Glaze is appropriate with light-colored fruits, such as pineapples, bananas, mangoes, oranges, kiwis, green grapes, apples, and pears.

The final detail in making pies and cakes is their garnish, just as with that very first pastry rose I baked on an apple pie. The first person to receive the pie opened her eyes wide and immediately reached for the object of her attention, plucking the rose from the pie. Garnishes can often be like that—a glaze-dipped dark-sweet cherry with its stem jauntily in the air is either eaten first or saved until the very last. At other times garnishes add to the texture of the dessert, becoming an integral part of it, such as chopped nuts on the edge of a tart or the sides of a cake, or crushed praline sprinkled on a topping of cream.

Garnishes should always enhance the finished appearance. Artfully place a few deep green mint leaves next to thin twists of lemon, and the image of springtime bursts forth in the mind of the beholder. Place glistening glazed strawberries with their pretty green leaves atop a cake, and you have uplifted that cake to a *gâteau*. Pipe rosettes of cream on a pumpkin pie, and it becomes the *pièce de résistance* of the meal.

Perfect your basic skills, and open your heart and your imagination and you will create satisfying works of beauty that will delight the eye as well as the palate.

Red Raspberry Filling

Yield:
2 cups

As a cake filling, this can't be beat for wonderful raspberry flavor. I'm inclined to think that I even prefer it to fresh raspberries (though I never thought it possible that anything would be preferable to fresh raspberries!).

Try Red Raspberry Filling with Raspberry Cream Filling and Frosting (page 176) for a truly unforgettable cake.

To make a superb Red Raspberry Sauce, just increase the water to ½ cup. As a sauce it is especially delicious served hot over a slice of Poppy Seed Cake (page 149), Toasted Almond Torte (page 142), or even just ice cream.

2¼ cups frozen unsweetened raspberries
2 cups frozen unsweetened strawberries
¼ cup fruit sweetener
2 tablespoons cornstarch
2½ tablespoons water

Bring the berries and sweetener to a boil in a heavy saucepan over medium-high heat. In a cup, mix the cornstarch and water and add to the berries. Use a whisk to thoroughly mix in the cornstarch. Continue stirring until the mixture returns to the boil. Reduce the heat and simmer for 5 minutes to stabilize the cornstarch. Remove from the heat.

Refrigerate until cold before using as a cake filling. Red Raspberry Filling can be stored in the refrigerator for 7 to 10 days.

Variation

Red Raspberry Sauce. Increase the amount of water to ½ cup. If there are too many seeds for your liking, pass the Red Raspberry Sauce through a fine sieve to remove them.

Spiced Peach Filling

Yield:
2 cups

Light and fresh-tasting, Spiced Peach Filling combines well with Vanilla Custard (page 178) or Peaches 'n' Cream Frosting (page 177) to sandwich between layers of Vanilla Sponge Cake (page 146) or Toasted Almond Torte (page 142). Spiced Peach Filling can also be a quick and easy topping for a Vanilla Custard parfait. For a lively Sunday brunch, pour hot Spiced Peach Filling over pancakes or waffles.

4 cups frozen sliced peaches
2 tablespoons fruit sweetener
1½ teaspoons cornstarch
Pinch salt
½ teaspoon cinnamon
⅛ teaspoon nutmeg
⅛ teaspoon ginger
½ teaspoon vanilla extract
¼ teaspoon peach extract

Defrost the frozen peaches and drain them, saving the juice. Place 2 tablespoons of the juice in a small bowl. Place the remaining juice in a sauté pan over high heat. Cook until the juice is reduced by one-half. Add the defrosted peaches, stirring until heated through.

Add the sweetener, cornstarch, salt, and spices to the reserved peach juice, stirring to blend well. When the peaches are hot, whisk in the cornstarch mixture, stirring continuously until the liquid is thickened and clear. Reduce the heat and simmer for 5 minutes, stirring occasionally. Turn off the heat and stir in the vanilla and peach extracts.

Place the Spiced Peach Filling in a container and refrigerate it thoroughly before using as a cake filling. As a sauce, it can be served hot or cold.

Raspberry Cream Filling and Frosting

Yield:
4 cups

Fruit-sweetened raspberry jam gives this cream exceptional taste and texture. You won't believe there is no other sweetener in it. Raspberry Cream Filling and Frosting is sensational enfolded in a Carob Cake Roll (page 150) or as the frosting and/or filling for the Vanilla or Carob Sponge Cakes (pages 146 and 147). This luscious recipe has been adapted from one from the creative and talented baker and author, Rose Levy Beranbaum.

½ cup seedless, fruit-sweetened raspberry jam
1½ teaspoons vanilla extract
2 cups heavy whipping cream
Few drops red food color (optional)

Use an electric mixer to whip the jam and vanilla smooth. Stir in the cream and, if desired, a drop or two of red food coloring. Increase the mixer speed to medium-high and whip until the cream is stiff. Use immediately.

Variations

Strawberry Cream Filling and Frosting. Substitute fruit-sweetened strawberry jam for the raspberry jam.

Apricot Cream Filling and Frosting. Substitute fruit-sweetened apricot jam for the raspberry jam and a drop or two of yellow food coloring for the red.

Peaches 'n' Cream Filling and Frosting. Substitute fruit-sweetened peach jam for the raspberry jam and use 1 teaspoon each vanilla and peach extracts. Add a drop of yellow food coloring in addition to a drop of red food coloring, if desired.

Baker's Tip

• If any of these jam and cream fillings sit for more than half an hour, they will need to be rewhipped to regain their original consistency. These fillings store well for at least a week, covered in the refrigerator; however, be sure to rewhip them before using.

Lemon Curd

 *

Yield:
1¾ cups

With very good reason, Lemon Curd is an English favorite and mine, too. Lemon Curd has just the right amount of delicious tartness to make you pucker a bit. Enjoy it as it is on toast, or use it as the base of Blueberry Lemon Tartlets (page 112) or Lemon Cream Pie (page 101), or spread it between the layers of a Kiwi Lemon Cake (page 159).

½ cup (¼ pound) butter* ***(substitute margarine for dairy-free)***
5 egg yolks
Grated zest of 1½ lemons
Juice of 2 lemons
½ cup fruit sweetener

Cut the butter or margarine into ½-inch pieces.

Combine the egg yolks, lemon zest and juice, and sweetener in a medium-size stainless steel bowl. Place the bowl directly in a pan of boiling water. Whisk the mixture continuously until it becomes very thick and light. Remove the bowl from the boiling water and whisk in the butter or margarine.

Store Lemon Curd in the refrigerator, where it will keep for 2 to 3 months.

Baker's Tip

• If you don't think you can stir fast enough to keep the Lemon Curd from getting too hot and curdling, you can make it in the top of a double boiler, instead of in a bowl placed directly in the boiling water as suggested in the recipe.

Vanilla Custard

Yield:
1, 2, 3 or 4 cups

Almond Milk makes this traditional crème pâtissière not only rich and creamy, but also dairy-free. Very versatile and delicious, Vanilla Custard can be used as a base in fruit tarts, as a filling for cakes, or as a quick dessert parfait.

Here are the ingredients for making Vanilla Custard in 4 different quantities, depending upon how much you need. Once made, Vanilla Custard will keep for at least a week under refrigeration.

Blend the almonds and water in the blender for 5 minutes. Strain the milk through a dampened piece of cheesecloth. Measure the remaining liquid and add additional water, if necessary, to make the required quantity of almond milk.

Place the almond milk in a heavy bottom saucepan over medium-high heat.

In a small bowl, whip together the yolks, sweetener, and cornstarch with an electric mixer on medium-high speed until light and fluffy. When the almond milk comes to the boil, reduce the heat so that the milk is simmering. Reduce the mixer speed to low and pour in ¼ of the hot milk. (This will accustom the yolks to the heat and prevent them from curdling when they are added to the boiling milk.) Pour the yolk mixture into the milk on the stove, whisking constantly. Raise the heat to medium-high again, and use both a whisk and a rubber spatula to keep the custard free of lumps as it returns to a boil.

Once the custard begins to boil, reduce the heat and simmer for 5 minutes, whisking constantly. Remove the custard from the heat and stir in the vanilla. Pour the custard into a bowl and cover its surface directly with plastic wrap to prevent a skin from forming. Refrigerate the

Quantities				Ingredients
1 cup	**2 cups**	**3 cups**	**4 cups**	
1 cup	**1⅞ cups**	**2½ cups**	**3¾ cups**	**almond milk (4:1)**
2	**4**	**6**	**9**	**egg yolks**
2½ tablespoons	**5⅓ tablespoons**	**7 tablespoons**	**10 tablespoons**	**fruit sweetener (see Baker's Tips)**
⅛ cup	**¼ cup**	**⅓ cup**	**½ cup**	**cornstarch**
½ teaspoon	**¾ teaspoon**	**1 teaspoon**	**1½ teaspoons**	**vanilla extract**

Prepare the almond milk using the following quantities of almonds and water for each of the yields:

1 cup almond milk: ¼ cup almonds, 1 cup water

1⅞ cups almond milk: ½ cup almonds, 1⅞ cups water

2½ cups almond milk: ⅔ cup almonds, 2½ cups water

3¾ cups almond milk: 1 cup almonds, 3¾ cups water

custard until it is thoroughly cold. Then purée it in a food processor or blender to return it to a smooth creamy consistency. (The custard will thicken again as it sits.)

Variations

Dairy Vanilla Custard. Substitute regular homogenized milk for the almond milk.

Vanilla Custard Parfaits. Spoon blended Vanilla Custard into parfait glasses and top with any fruit-filled sauce for an always welcome dessert.

Baker's Tips

• For the best flavor, use 3P, the peach, pear, and pineapple mixed fruit sweetener, when making Vanilla Custard. Apple or grape juice concentrate is not recommended for this recipe as either one gives an unusual flavor to the finished custard.

• When the custard is coming to a boil, it is helpful to stir with both a whisk and a rubber spatula. Use the rubber spatula around the inside edges of the pot to bring the thickening custard to the center, where it can be whisked smooth.

Coconut-Pecan Filling

Yield:
3½ cups
Filling for one 10-inch cake

This is the Coconut-Pecan Filling that makes German "Un-Chocolate" Cake (page 167) so memorable. Admittedly rather rich, sweet, and gooey for an everyday dessert, it is best reserved for special celebrations.

1 cup (3½ ounces) shredded, unsweetened coconut
½ cup pecans
6-ounce can evaporated milk
¼ cup fruit sweetener
¼ cup butter
2 eggs, slightly beaten
Pinch salt
1 teaspoon vanilla extract

Preheat the oven to 350° F.

To lightly toast the coconut, place it on a cookie sheet in the preheated oven for approximately 7 minutes. Stir the coconut 2 or 3 times during baking so that it browns evenly. Toast the pecans in the preheated oven for 7 to 10 minutes, stirring occasionally. Allow the nuts to cool. Then coarsely chop them with a knife or with a pulsing action in a food processor.

Combine the evaporated milk, sweetener, butter, and salt in a medium-size saucepan over medium heat. When the mixture is warm and the butter is melted, whisk in the eggs. Stir constantly over medium heat until just before the boiling point, when the filling slightly thickens. *Do not let this mixture come to a boil or the filling will curdle.* Remove the pan from the heat and stir in the vanilla. Stir the mixture for 1 minute to cool it slightly. Stir in the toasted coconut and the pecans. Use Coconut-Pecan Filling while it is still warm and spreadable.

Baker's Tips

• As the temperature of this sauce is very important for its proper consistency, you may prefer to prepare Coconut-Pecan Filling in the top of a double boiler.

• Egg yolks are often used to thicken sauces and custards. As eggs can easily curdle from overheating (above 180° F), they must be heated carefully. It is preferable to add them near the end of the cooking process, and then to cook them only until the mixture has slightly thickened. The restaurant test is to dip a metal spoon in the custard. If you can make a track on the back of the spoon with your finger, the mixture is done and should immediately be removed from the heat.

Red Glaze

Yield:
2 cups

Making Red Glaze from fruit-sweetened raspberry, strawberry, and concord grape jams give a very rich and full flavor that seems to complement every fruit, pie, tart, or cake with which it is used. Of course, Red Glaze can be made with a single red jam instead, as in the recipe for Yellow Glaze. Red Glaze is used over red, purple, or other dark-colored fruits to make them sparkle. The sparkle will last for about 1 day.

Glaze can be made in a large quantity and used over and over again but be careful to strain out any crumbs that get into it. The glaze will keep for 2 to 3 months stored in the refrigerator.

1 cup fruit-sweetened raspberry jam
½ cup fruit-sweetened strawberry jam
½ cup fruit-sweetened concord grape jelly
½ cup water

Combine the jams and the water in a small pot. Bring the mixture to a boil over medium heat. Continue to cook at a low boil for 5 minutes. Pour the hot glaze through a strainer to remove all seeds and chunks of fruit.

Check your recipe to see whether the glaze is to be used hot, warm, or cold. Store leftover glaze in the refrigerator.

Yellow Glaze

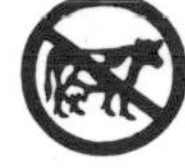  

Yield:
1 cup

Use fruit-sweetened apricot or peach jam for making this glaze. Yellow Glaze is used over yellow, green, or other light-colored fruits to make them sparkle. The sparkle will last for about 1 day.

Glaze can be made in a large quantity and used over and over again but be careful to strain out any crumbs that get into it. The glaze will keep for 2 to 3 months stored in the refrigerator.

1 cup fruit-sweetened apricot or peach jam
¼ cup water

Combine the jam and water together in a small pot. Bring the mixture to a boil over medium heat. Continue to cook at a low boil for 5 minutes. Pour the hot glaze through a strainer to remove all chunks of fruit.

Check your recipe to see whether the glaze is to be used hot, warm, or cold. Store leftover glaze in the refrigerator.

Whipped Cream

Yield:
4 cups

There is nothing like the exquisite flavor and texture of whipped cream. So soft and billowy white, it is unsurpassed in Strawberry Shortcake (page 156), with a bowl of fresh-picked raspberries, or as an accompaniment to pumpkin and pecan pies. Have the cream and all the utensils well chilled before you begin so that the cream doesn't overwhip and lose its glorious texture.

2 cups heavy whipping cream
¼ cup fruit sweetener
2 teaspoons vanilla extract

Place all of the ingredients in a cold mixing bowl. Begin whipping the cream with an electric mixer on medium speed. Once the cream begins to thicken, increase the speed to high and continue to whip until the cream forms stiff peaks. Whipping Cream has the best texture when it is used immediately after whipping.

Baker's Tip

- Here is another hint I learned from Jacques Auber: If cream is whipped exclusively on high speed there will be a lot of air and volume but not much strength. Therefore, whip cream most of the way on medium speed, building strength into the cream. Then raise the speed to high to give it volume as it stiffens.

Whipped Cream/Cream Cheese Frosting

Yield:
5 cups
Frosting and filling for an 8-inch cake

This is our sensational basic frosting. Because of the strengthening quality of the cream cheese, this becomes an even more delicious, all-purpose frosting. By using the larger amount of cream cheese, the frosting holds its shape well enough to fancifully decorate wedding cakes. The smaller amount of cream cheese is sufficient for almost every other kind of cake, from a Strawberry Cream Cake (page 163) to a Banana Walnut Cake (page 145) to a red, white, and blue July Fourth Cake (page 166).

For the smoothest texture, have the cream cheese at room temperature when you begin.

¼ to ½ pound cream cheese, at room temperature
⅓ cup fruit sweetener
1 teaspoon vanilla extract
1 teaspoon peach extract
2 cups heavy whipping cream

Use an electric mixer on medium-high speed to whip the cream cheese until smooth. Reduce the speed and stir in the sweetener and the extracts until the mixture is smooth and well blended. With the mixer on low speed, add half of the cream. Use a rubber spatula to remove any unmixed cream cheese from the bottom of the bowl. When the mixture is smooth, gradually add the rest of the whipping cream. Increase the speed to high and whip until stiff. Use immediately for the best decorating texture.

Variation

Coconut Cream Frosting. Lightly toast 1¼ cups thinly shredded, unsweetened coconut in a 350°F oven for 7 to 10 minutes. When the coconut has completely cooled, prepare the Whipped Cream/Cream Cheese Frosting and fold in the toasted coconut.

Baker's Tip

- If frostings with whipped cream sit for more than half an hour, they will need to be re-whipped to regain their firm consistency. These frostings store very well for at least a week, covered, in the refrigerator. Be sure to whip them stiff again before using.

Creamy Carob Frosting

Yield:
4½ cups
Frosting and filling for one 8-inch cake

A sumptuous, creamy texture with rich, deep flavor makes Creamy Carob Frosting the perfect "unchocolate" frosting with German "Unchocolate" Cake (page 167) or as the filling with Black Forest Torte (page 169). For the richest flavor and deepest color, use the greater amount of Carob Fudge Sauce. For more of a milk-carob flavor, use the lesser amount of sauce. And for the smoothest texture, have the cream cheese at room temperature when you begin.

1 to 1¾ cups Carob Fudge Sauce (page 192)
3 ounces cream cheese, at room temperature
1½ teaspoons vanilla extract
1½ cups heavy whipping cream

Prepare the Carob Fudge Sauce. Use an electric mixer on medium-high speed to whip the cream cheese until smooth. Reduce the speed to low and add the warm Carob Fudge Sauce (according to your taste) and the vanilla. Increase the speed to medium-high and beat until light and creamy. Reduce to low speed again and stir in ½ cup of the whipping cream. Use a rubber spatula to remove any unmixed cream cheese from the bottom of the bowl. When the mixture is smooth, gradually add the rest of the whipping cream. Increase the speed to high and whip until stiff. Use immediately for the best decorating texture.

Baker's Tip

• Cream cheese is used in these whipped cream frosting recipes to give extra body to the frosting so that it can hold its form when piped through a pastry bag.

Carob Raspberry Cream Frosting

Yield:
4½ cups
Frosting and filling for one 8-inch cake

Elegant Carob Raspberry Cream Frosting was developed a couple of years ago for decorating our holiday Yule Logs. Its rich color and lovely texture make for realistic "bark" and "stumps."

When preparing Carob Raspberry Cream Frosting, the Carob Glaze should be at room temperature or (only) slightly warmer. If it is too warm, the frosting will not whip up well and will be too soft to use for decorating.

½ cup Carob Glaze (page 192)
½ cup seedless fruit-sweetened raspberry jam
1½ teaspoons vanilla extract
2 cups heavy whipping cream

Prepare the Carob Glaze and let it cool to room temperature before proceeding. Use an electric mixer on medium speed to whip the jam and vanilla and Carob Glaze smooth. Stir in the cream. Increase the mixer speed to medium-high and whip until the cream is stiff. Use immediately for the best decorating texture.

Mocha Frosting

Yield:
6 cups
Frosting and filling for one 8-inch or 10-inch cake

Mocha has always been one of my favorite flavors. I once traveled through Europe testing and comparing mocha ice cream in each city—the winner of my very informal survey was from a restaurant somewhere in London. Mocha Frosting is especially wonderful with carob cakes, such as the elegant Mocha Almond Torte (page 168), or rolled in the middle of a Carob Cake Roll (page 150).

For the smoothest texture, have the cream cheese at room temperature when you begin.

5 ounces cream cheese, at room temperature
¼ cup instant coffee powder
5 teaspoons carob powder
⅔ cup fruit sweetener
1¼ teaspoons vanilla extract
2½ cups heavy whipping cream

Use an electric mixer on medium-high speed to whip the cream cheese until smooth. In a small bowl, stir the instant coffee and carob powders into the fruit sweetener. Stir the coffee mixture and the vanilla into the cream cheese until the mixture is smooth and well blended. With the mixer on low speed, add half of the cream. Use a rubber spatula to remove any unmixed cream cheese from the bottom of the bowl. When the mixture is smooth, gradually add the rest of the whipping cream. Increase the speed to high and whip until stiff. Use immediately for the best decorating texture.

Variation

Mocha Almond Frosting. Add ½ teaspoon almond extract in addition to the 1¼ teaspoons vanilla extract.

Cream Cheese Frosting with Raisins and Nuts

Yield:
5 cups
Frosting and filling for one 8-inch cake

Carrot cake and cream cheese frosting just seem to go together, as in the fifties song "you can't have one without the other."

This cream cheese frosting is at its creamiest when both the cream cheese and the butter are at room temperature when you begin. It is best to prepare the frosting just before you are ready to fill and ice your cake, so that the frosting's creamy texture makes finishing the cake almost effortless.

⅓ cup walnuts
¼ cup raisins
1 pound cream cheese, at room temperature
10 tablespoons butter, softened
½ cup fruit sweetener, at room temperature
2 teaspoons vanilla extract
2 teaspoons peach extract (optional)

Preheat the oven to 350° F.

Toast the walnuts in the preheated oven for 7 to 10 minutes, stirring occasionally.

Bring ½ cup of water to a boil and add the raisins. When the water returns to the boil, turn off the heat. Let the raisins plump in the water for at least 10 minutes. Drain the raisins, saving any raisin water for another use.

Whip the cream cheese with an electric mixer on medium speed until the cream cheese is very smooth and lump-free. Add the softened butter and continue to cream them both on high speed until they are light and fluffy. Use a rubber spatula to scrape the bottom of the bowl to keep the frosting free from lumps. Reduce the speed to medium and whip in the sweetener and the extracts.

Meanwhile, use a chef's knife to finely chop the plumped raisins and toasted walnuts. With the mixer on low speed, stir the raisins and walnuts into the frosting.

Use the frosting as soon as it is made, when it has the lightest and creamiest texture.

Baker's Tip

• Peach extract is optional but it gives a delicious flavor. If you do not use it, substitute 1 teaspoon almond extract for the peach extract, or use all vanilla extract.

Royal Icing

Yield:
2 cups

To fancifully decorate cookies such as Gingerbread Girls and Boys (page 73), classic Royal Icing is almost the perfect choice—its only drawback is that it is made from powdered sugar. Royal Icing is very easy to prepare and to work with, it quickly dries hard, and it is easily tinted from the lightest pastels to the deepest, holiday colors.

2 egg whites
2 cups plus 2 tablespoons powdered sugar
A few drops lemon juice
Assorted food colors

Sift the powdered sugar three times.

Using an electric mixer, whip the egg whites and the powdered sugar on low speed until the sugar is incorporated. Raise the speed to high and whip the mixture 7 to 10 minutes until the icing is light and can stand in peaks. Return the mixer to low speed and stir in a few drops of lemon juice to bring the icing to decorating consistency.

Divide the icing into small bowls and color as desired.

Keep Royal Icing covered with a damp cloth as it dries quickly.

Blueberry Sauce

Yield:
2 cups

This very quickly made, delicious, and sparkling Blueberry Sauce is made with frozen blueberries. They have excellent flavor and give a rich, deep-blue color. Blueberry Sauce is exceptional over Cheesecake (page 152) and delightful with Lemon Curd (page 177) in tartlets. When the fruit is drained a bit from the sauce, the blueberries make a mouth-watering filling and topping for cakes, such as the July Fourth Cake (page 166).

Blueberry Sauce will keep for 3 or more weeks in the refrigerator.

4½ cups frozen blueberries
⅓ cup fruit sweetener
½ cup water
2 tablespoons cornstarch

Bring the blueberries and sweetener to a boil in a heavy saucepan. Mix the cornstarch and water in a small bowl. Whisk the dissolved cornstarch into the boiling berry mixture, stirring continuously. When the mixture returns to a boil, reduce the heat and simmer for 5 minutes. Remove from the heat.

Refrigerate the Blueberry Sauce until needed.

Baker's Tip

• In order to keep dissolved cornstarch from lumping when it is added to a boiling mixture, use a wire whisk to quickly and thoroughly incorporate the cornstarch. Continue to whisk until the mixture returns to a boil.

Tart Red Cherry Sauce

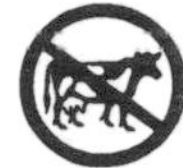

Yield:
1¾ Cups

Frozen tart red cherries need to be infused in this sauce for at least 24 hours to develop their incomparably delicious and unique tartness.

The acid in the cherries tends to thin this sauce if it sits for more than a couple of days. You may have to thicken it again with arrowroot the next time you use it.

¼ orange, peel and juice
2½ tablespoons fruit sweetener
½ teaspoon cinnamon
2 cups frozen tart red cherries
1½ teaspoons arrowroot
1 tablespoon cold water
¼ teaspoon vanilla extract

Use a vegetable peeler to remove long strips of peel from a quarter of an orange. Measure the juice squeezed from one quarter of an orange, and add enough water to make 3 tablespoons liquid altogether. Place the juice and water, sweetener, cinnamon, and orange peel in a medium saucepan, and bring to a boil.

Stir in the cherries and return the mixture to a boil. In a cup, dissolve the arrowroot in the cold water and stir it into the pot. As soon as the sauce thickens remove the pan from the heat and stir in the vanilla.

Refrigerate the sauce for 24 hours to develop its rich cherry flavor.

Cranberry Topping

Yield:
3 cups

When wonderful red cranberries first come into the markets, they bring an immediate spot of bright color and assertive flavor to the mellower fall and winter amber, green, and gold fruits.

I love to use this full-flavored Cranberry Topping as a sauce on Cheesecake (page 152) or as the fruit topping on tarts or tartlets, or over a base of Vanilla Custard (page 178). The tartness of the cranberries can add a delicious and unexpected contrast when used as the filling in a Carob Sponge Cake (page 147) frosted with Creamy Carob Frosting (page 183).

If you have thought ahead in November and frozen extra cranberries, you can prepare Cranberry Topping in the middle of the summer to everyone's surprise and delight.

Juice and peel of ½ orange
¼ cup fruit sweetener
½ teaspoon cinnamon
3 cups fresh or frozen cranberries
1 teaspoon arrowroot
1 tablespoon cold water
½ teaspoon vanilla extract

Use a vegetable peeler to remove long strips of peel from half an orange. Measure the juice squeezed from half an orange, and add enough water to make ¼ cup liquid altogether. Place the juice and water, sweetener, cinnamon, and orange peel in a medium-size saucepan, and bring to a boil.

Stir in the cranberries and return the mixture to a boil. Reduce the heat and simmer for about 5 minutes, until the skins of the cranberries begin to pop.

Dissolve the arrowroot in 1 tablespoon cold water. Stir the dissolved arrowroot into the simmering cranberry mixture. As soon as the sauce thickens remove the pan from the heat and stir in the vanilla.

Store Cranberry Topping refrigerated for 3 to 4 weeks.

Variation

Cranberry Raspberry Topping. Stir ⅓ cup fruit-sweetened raspberry jam into the hot topping, along with the vanilla extract.

Baker's Tips

- Drain a few of the whole cranberries from this topping and use them as decorative berries on your Bûche de Noël (page 171).
- Cranberries and raspberries are very complementary flavors. The addition of raspberry jam fills out and enhances the flavor of the cranberries.

Fresh Strawberry Sauce

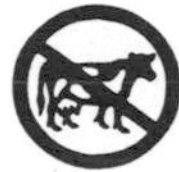

Yield:
3 cups

When you want to extend the life of your strawberries just a little bit longer, make them into a beautiful Fresh Strawberry Sauce. Bright red in color, Fresh Strawberry Sauce provides a refreshing contrast of flavors and textures. Try it as an accompaniment to Cheesecake (page 152), Poppy Seed Cake (page 149), or Vanilla Custard (page 178).

3 cups strawberries
1½ teaspoons cornstarch
1½ teaspoons arrowroot
2 tablespoons cold water
3 tablespoons fruit sweetener
2 tablespoons fruit-sweetened raspberry jam
Few drops red food color (optional)

Quickly wash the strawberries by dipping them in cool water and removing them immediately. Dry the berries in a single layer on a clean kitchen towel. Use the tip of a vegetable peeler to remove the hulls from the berries. Leave small berries whole, and cut large and medium-size berries in half.

Dissolve the cornstarch and arrowroot in the cold water. In a medium-size saucepan, whisk the cornstarch mixture together with the sweetener and the jam over medium-high heat until they come to a boil. Stir in the fresh strawberries and cook, stirring carefully to avoid mashing the berries.

At this point the mixture will become very thick and sticky. Then, as the berries begin to release their juices, the sauce will thin down and become more manageable. Continue to cook until the berries are heated through.

Remove the pan from the heat and stir in a few drops of food color, if necessary, to enhance the color of the sauce.

Store Fresh Strawberry Sauce under refrigeration for about 7 days.

Frozen Strawberry Sauce

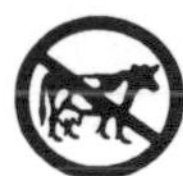  

Yield:
2 cups

When fresh strawberries are out of season, use unsweetened frozen strawberries to make a delightful Frozen Strawberry Sauce. The flavor is pure strawberry and the color is often more naturally red than the color of fresh berries. Use Frozen Strawberry Sauce in all the same delicious ways you would use Fresh Strawberry Sauce.

2½ cups frozen unsweetened strawberries
1 tablespoon cornstarch
⅓ cup cold water
¼ cup fruit sweetener

Place the strawberries in a bowl to thaw, saving their juice. In a small bowl, dissolve the cornstarch in the cold water, and stir in the sweetener. Place everything in a medium-size saucepan over medium heat. Bring the sauce to a boil, stirring gently and frequently with a wooden spoon. Reduce the heat and simmer for 5 minutes.

Store Frozen Strawberry Sauce under refrigeration for 7 to 10 days.

Lemon Sauce

  *

Yield:
2 cups

This is an irresistibly wonderful Lemon Sauce. It is the kind of Lemon Sauce that is lemon at its best—tart yet slightly sweet—perfect with Poppy Seed Cake (page 149) or warm Gingerbread (page 141). It stores well, for about three weeks under refrigeration.

¼ cup butter* ***(substitute margarine for dairy-free)***
½ cup fruit sweetener
1¾ tablespoons cornstarch
1½ cups cold water
Pinch salt
Grated zest of ½ lemon
2 tablespoons fresh lemon juice
A drop or two of yellow food color (optional)

Cut the butter or margarine into walnut-size pieces.

Mix the sweetener, cornstarch, water, salt, and lemon zest together in a saucepan. Whisk the mixture continuously over high heat until it comes to a boil. Reduce the heat and simmer for 5 minutes.

Remove the pan from the heat and whisk in the pieces of butter or margarine and the lemon juice. Add a drop or two of yellow food color, if necessary, to enhance the color of the finished sauce.

Store Lemon Sauce refrigerated. However, Lemon Sauce tastes best and has the best consistency when served hot or at room temperature.

Raspberry Purée

Yield:
1 cup

This recipe couldn't be simpler, and the flavor is pure raspberry. Raspberry Purée seems to go with just about everything, over or under cakes or tarts where it completes the balancing, blending, and contrasting of flavors and textures.

2 cups unsweetened frozen raspberries
1 to 3 tablespoons fruit sweetener

Thaw the raspberries in a bowl, saving their juice. Purée the berries with their juice in a blender until smooth. Strain the purée through a sieve to remove all of the seeds. Add sweetener to taste. Store under refrigeration for 1 week or for 2 months in the freezer.

Strawberry-Raspberry Sauce

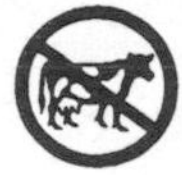

Yield:
3 cups

Raspberry Purée adds an extra dimension of flavor to sliced fresh strawberries, making them extra special in both color and taste. Place Strawberry-Raspberry Sauce on a plate under a wedge of Toasted Almond Torte (page 142) or Banana Walnut Cake (page 145), or use it as a topping for Vanilla Custard (page 178).

1 pint basket fresh strawberries
1 cup Raspberry Purée (this page)

Quickly wash the strawberries by dipping them in cool water and removing them immediately. Dry the berries in a single layer on a clean kitchen towel. Use the tip of a vegetable peeler to remove the hulls from the berries. Slice the strawberries and toss them into the Raspberry Purée.

Store Strawberry-Raspberry Sauce refrigerated for 1 week.

Very-Berry Syrup

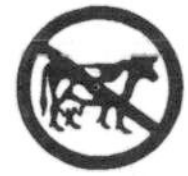  

Yield:
4 cups

This is the exceptionally delicious syrup that has been offered with pancakes and waffles at The Ranch Kitchen since 1982. Delectable and beautiful at breakfast, by itself or combined with other fruit sauces, it becomes a well-balanced dessert sauce to be spooned over Vanilla Custard (page 178).

In making Very-Berry Syrup, once you have added the berries, stir very gently to keep them from breaking down.

3 cups (¾ pound) frozen strawberries
2 cups (½ pound) frozen blueberries
2⅓ cups (½ pound) frozen boysenberries or blackberries
2 cups water
¾ cup fruit sweetener
¾ cup water
⅜ cup cornstarch

Place all of the berries in a bowl to thaw, saving their juices. Bring the 2 cups water and sweetener to a boil in a large, heavy saucepan. Mix the ¾ cup water and the cornstarch together in a small bowl, and whisk into the boiling mixture. Continue to whisk until the mixture thickens, becomes clear, and returns to a boil. Reduce the heat and simmer for 5 minutes. Add the thawed berries with their juices and cook just until the berries are hot all the way through. To avoid breaking down the berries, stir carefully once they are added.

Very-Berry Syrup can be stored for 7 to 10 days in the refrigerator. It can be used either hot or cold.

Variation

Parfait Topping. Combine 1 cup Very-Berry Sauce with ½ cup Blueberry Sauce (page 186) and ½ cup of the cherries drained from Tart Red Cherry Sauce (page 187).

Apple Currant Sauce

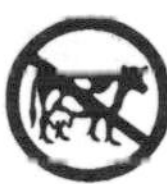  

Yield:
2 cups

A light and spicy sauce. Serve it hot over warm Gingerbread (page 111). Refrigerated, Apple Currant Sauce will keep for a month. If you have no currants, chopped raisins can be substituted.

2 tablespoons dried currants
2 cups unsweetened apple juice
1½ tablespoons cornstarch
½ teaspoon cinnamon
¼ teaspoon nutmeg

In a small saucepan, bring the currants and 1½ cups of the apple juice to a boil over medium heat. Combine the cornstarch, cinnamon, and nutmeg in a small bowl. Stir in the remaining ½ cup of cold apple juice. Whisk the diluted cornstarch mixture into the boiling apple juice, stirring constantly. When the sauce returns to a boil, reduce the heat and simmer for 5 minutes.

Apple Currant Sauce has the best flavor when served hot.

Carob Glaze

Yield:
1 cup

Elegant Carob Glaze with its rich, dark color and flawless, shiny finish is perfect for coating the tops of Eclairs (page 130), flavoring Carob Raspberry Cream Frosting (page 183), dipping stemmed strawberries, and pouring hot over homemade ice cream or poached pears.

Carob Glaze is made from sifted carob powder. It will keep for 2 to 3 weeks in the refrigerator, or for 2 months in the freezer.

⅔ cup heavy whipping cream
½ cup fruit sweetener
5 tablespoons butter
1 cup carob powder
1½ teaspoons vanilla extract

Combine the cream, sweetener, and butter in a medium-size saucepan. Whisk together over medium heat until the butter is melted. Sift in the carob powder in 3 parts, whisking smooth after each addition. Continue cooking for about 5 more minutes, just until the glaze comes to a boil, whisking continuously until the glaze is completely smooth and thickened. Remove it from the heat and stir in the vanilla. Store under refrigeration.

To reuse Carob Glaze, heat it in the top pan of a double boiler. Add about a tablespoon of cream if necessary to return the glaze to its proper consistency.

Carob Fudge Sauce

Yield:
2 cups

Unsweetened carob chips are the reason Carob Fudge Sauce is so richly flavored. When you use it as a base for Mocha Mud Pie (page 102) or Creamy Carob Frosting (page 183), stir in the smaller amount of water. For use as a rich carob sauce, stir in the larger amount of water.

Store Carob Fudge Sauce in the refrigerator for 2 weeks, or for a couple of months in the freezer.

9 ounce can evaporated milk
⅓ cup fruit sweetener
1¼ cups unsweetened carob chips
¼ to ¾ cup water

Combine the milk and sweetener in a medium-size saucepan over medium heat. As the milk becomes hot, gradually whisk in half of the carob chips. As the chips melt, add the remaining chips, continuing to whisk until the chips have melted and the sauce is totally smooth. Stir in the water.

Store Carob Fudge Sauce under refrigeration.

Our Famous Apple Butter

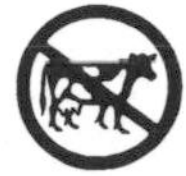  

Yield:
6 cups (made with applesauce)
7½ cups (made with fresh apples)

This is the recipe for the incomparable Apple Butter that is and has been served with every breakfast at The Ranch Kitchen since our first morning 10 years ago. In the early years we used to purchase Winesap apples to make our apple butter. Then we discovered we could save a great deal of time and energy if we used unsweetened applesauce instead of the whole apples. The well-balanced taste is still spicy and delicious, the color is still rich and deep, the texture is still thick and spreadable, and the kitchen still smells marvelous as the apple butter cooks. You can see why we have switched to this more efficient method. However, here are ingredients for both methods, as the choice is yours.

When you have the time, make a large quantity of Apple Butter, as it can be easily frozen or canned for long-term storage, or stored in the refrigerator for daily use.

7 pounds red apples or 12 cups unsweetened applesauce
1½ cups apple juice concentrate
1 tablespoon cinnamon
½ teaspoon nutmeg

If you are using fresh apples, cook the apples with the apple juice concentrate and enough water to just cover the apples. Cook until the apples are tender. Purée the mixture in a blender and strain out all the seeds and skin. Stir in the spices.

If you are using unsweetened applesauce, stir the apple concentrate and spices into the unsweetened applesauce.

Preheat the oven to 375° F. Pour the apple mixture into a heavy baking pan and place it in the preheated oven. After the first hour of baking, stir the apple butter every 30 minutes, continuing for 5 to 6 hours, until the Apple Butter is done. It should be a rich, dark brown, and when a drop is placed on a cold plate, no water should separate out.

To can the Apple Butter for long-term storage, spoon it into hot, sterilized half-pint jars. Seal the jars and process them in a boiling water bath for 10 minutes.

Tofu Cream

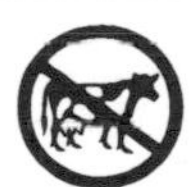  

Yield:
½ cup

Tofu Cream is a nondairy garnish for pies such as the Boysenberry or Apple Custard. Tofu Cream has the best flavor when made with very fresh tofu. After it is made, it must be stored in the refrigerator, where it will keep for 2 to 3 days.

4 ounces firm tofu
1 tablespoon fruit sweetener
¾ teaspoon vanilla extract
½ teaspoon peach or almond extract

Remove the tofu from its carton and wash it in fresh water. Dry the tofu with paper towels, then press it with a weight for about 30 minutes to remove any excess water.

Place all of the ingredients in a blender and process until smooth and creamy.

Pecan Praline

Yield:
3 cups

Pecan Praline is finely ground pecans enveloped in caramelized sweetener. It is delicious sprinkled on the top of Mocha Mud Pie (page 102) or pressed onto the sides and top of a Mocha Peach Praline Torte (page 168).

Once made, Pecan Praline can be stored for many months in an airtight container in the freezer. As praline made with a liquid sweetener is stickier than praline made with white sugar, it is usually necessary to reprocess it in the food processor before each use.

2 cups pecans
1½ cups fruit sweetener
1 tablespoon butter

Preheat the oven to 350° F.

Toast the pecans in the preheated oven for 7 to 10 minutes, stirring occasionally.

Cook the fruit sweetener in a medium-size heavy saucepan until the mixture reaches 310° F on a candy thermometer. Remove the pot from the heat and carefully stir in the butter and the toasted pecans. Pour the mixture onto a lightly oiled baking pan, spreading it evenly.

As the praline cools, it hardens. When it is cold, break it into large chunks and finely chop them in a food processor. Praline can be stored almost indefinitely in a covered container in the freezer.

Coconut Powder

Yield:
2¼ cups

Substitute Coconut Powder for powdered sugar, and dust it on freshly baked puff pastry strudel, on a classic Linzertorte (page 110), or on a Cream Puff Swan (page 131) to give each a more finished appearance.

It is always possible to have Coconut Powder on hand, as it can be quickly prepared and easily stored in the refrigerator for many months in a tightly closed container.

2 cups dried unsweetened coconut
¼ cup nonfat, non instant milk powder

Use an herb and spice grinder to grind the coconut into as fine a powder as possible. Place the Coconut Powder in a small bowl and use a fork to stir in the milk powder. Store in a tightly closed container.

To use Coconut Powder, sift it through a fine strainer.

Baker's Tip

• Nonfat, non-instant milk powder can be purchased in many natural food stores.

INDEX

Adrenal glands
and blood sugar level, 6
Almond(s)
RECIPES USING:
Almond Blossoms, 127
Almond Cookies, 68
Almond Macaroons, 75
Almond Oatmeal Cookies, 65
Almond Paste, 75
Almond Straws, 127–28
Applesauce Almond Cake, 145
Carob Almond Cookies, 65
Maple Almond Cookies, 68
Mocha Almond Frosting, 184
Mocha Almond Torte, 168
Raspberry Toasted Almond Torte, 158
Toasted Almond Torte, 142
Almond milk, 12
in Vanilla Custard, 178–79
Almond Paste, 75
Aluminum compounds
in baking powder, 12
Aluminum pie tins, 23
Amazake, 12
American Beauty Apple Pie, 85–87
American Fruit Processors, 16
Angel Biscuits, 60
Apple(s), 12
peeling and coring, 94
RECIPES USING:
American Beauty Apple Pie, 85–87
Apple Butter, 193
Apple Currant Sauce, 191
Apple Custard Parfait, 98
Apple Custard Pie, 98
Apple Nut Strudel, 125
Apple Strudel, 126
Apple Turnovers, 123
Cranberry Apple Pie, 87–88
Crustless French Apple Tart, 110
French Apple Tart, 110
Molded Apple Custard, 98
Tarte Tatin, 118–19
Apple butter, 10, 193
Apple juice
concentrate, 16
Apple peeler-corer-slicer, 24
Applesauce
in Our Famous Apple Butter, 193
Applesauce Almond Cake, 145
Applesauce Spice Cake, 148–49
in Gâteau Normandy, 160–61
Apricot(s), 18–19
RECIPES USING:
Apricot Cream Filling and Frosting, 177
Carob Apricot Cream Roll, 171
Fresh Apricot Tart, 106–7
Arrowroot, 13, 17

Baker's knife, 23, 27
Baker's Tip(s)
about activating yeast, 32
about aluminum pie tins, 23
for Angel Biscuit dough, 61
for avoiding lavender blueberry muffins, 55
for baking pies, 90
for blueberry pies, 90
for Carob Cake Roll, 151
for cheesecake, 153
for Coconut-Pecan Filling, 180
for coloring cookies, 69
about cranberries, 52, 188
for Cranberry Apple Pie, 88
for cream cheese frosting, 185
about cream cheese in whipped cream frosting, 183
for custard, 179
for custard cake, 162
for dissolving gelatin, 100–101
for egg-free pies, 84
for freezing sponge cakes, 147
for freezing strudel, 125
for frostings with whipped cream, 182
for fruit tarts, 106
for fruitcake, 156
for granola crust, 84
about hazelnuts, 68
for jam and cream fillings, 177
for juice from Blueberry Sauce, 167
for juice from Tart Red Cherry Sauce, 170
for keeping dissolved cornstarch from lumping, 186

for Kiwi Lemon Cake, 159–60
lacing explained, 156
for macaroons, 75
macerate explained, 157
for making a Linzertorte, 111
for making Lemon Curd, 177
for making smaller cinnamon rolls, 38
for mixed fruit tarts, 119–20
about Monarch rolls, 36
about non-fat, non-instant milk powder, 194
for Nutty-Oat Crusts, 83
for Peach 'n' Berry Crisp, 104
for peach pies, 93
for peeling and coring pears and apples, 94
for pie crusts, 81
for pie dough, 81
for quick breads, 50
for Raspberry Thumbprint Cookies, 70
for ripe pears, 94
for rolling pins, 81
for scalding milk, 36
about shelf life of spices, 95
for slowing down rising dough, 32
about spelt, 65
"sponge" explained, 100–101
for stabilizing fresh fruit in cake, 165
about substituting for canned pumpkin, 95
for thickening sauces and custards, 180
"torte" defined, 142
for whipped cream, 181
Baking
blind baking of crusts, 80
essential elements of, 9–11
organization tips for, 11
recommended equipment for, 21–24
Baking pans, 22–23
Baking paper
and cookies, 63
and pie crusts, 79, 80, 81
Baking powder, 12, 13
Baking soda, 13, 160
Banana(s)
in mixed fruit tarts, 120
RECIPES USING:
Banana Cream Pie, 100
Banana Nut Bread, 50
Banana Walnut Cake, 145
Cranberry Banana Walnut Bread, 51
Fresh Banana Tart, 122–23
Very Banana Nut Muffins, 59
Basic Carrot Cake, 144
Basic Pie Crust, 82
Basic Shortbread Cookies, 69
Bickford Laboratories, 19
Biscuit cutters, 23
Biscuits, 10
and flour, 14–15
RECIPES:
Angel Biscuits, 61
Southern-Style Buttermilk Biscuits, 60
Black Forest Torte, 169–70
Blackberry(ies)
cleaning, 19–20
in custard cake, 162
in mixed fruit tarts, 120
substitute for boysenberries, 99
RECIPES USING:
Blackberry Cream Tartlets, 114
Very-Berry Syrup, 191
Blind baking
of crusts, 80
Blood sugar level, 5–6
Blueberry(ies)
in mixed fruit tarts, 120
RECIPES USING:
Blueberry Lattice Pie, 89–90
Blueberry Lemon Tartlets, 112
Blueberry Muffins, 54–55
Blueberry Sauce, 186
Cheesecake with Blueberry Sauce, 152–53
Crimson Pie, 88–89
July Fourth Cake, 166–67
Peach 'n' Berry Crisp, 104
Very-Berry Syrup, 191
Blueberry Sauce, 186
juice from, 167
RECIPES USING:
Cheesecake with Blueberry Sauce, 152–53
July Fourth Cake, 166–67
Bowl(s)
mixing, 22
for rising dough, 28
Boysenberry(ies)
Boysenberry Custard, 99
Boysenberry Custard Pie, 99
in Very-Berry Syrup, 191
Bread
baking, 31–32
cooling, 32
Egg Wash for, 45
freezing, 32
slicing, 32
yield given in recipes, 25
see also Quick breads; Yeasted breads
Bread dough, 10
mixing and kneading, 26–28
punching the dough down, 29
raising, 28–29, 32
in the refrigerator, 26, 32
second rising, 25, 29
shaping, 29–31
see also Dough
Bread pans, 22
Brown rice
cultured, 12
flour, 15
Bûche de Noël (French Yule Log), 170, 171–72, 188
Butter, 13
alternative to, 17
and cream puff pastry, 128
creaming with fruit sweetener, 10, 16
oil substituted for, 18
unsalted, 13
Buttermilk Biscuits, 60–61
in Strawberry Shortcake, 156–57

Cake(s)
cutting and trimming, 135
decorating equipment, 23
decorating with a pastry bag, 138–40
decorating with fruit, 137–38
decorating with nuts, 137
filling and frosting, 135–37
and flour, 15
importance of technique, 10
jam glazes as a "crumb coat" on, 136, 174
measuring and folding, 133–34
removing from pans, 134–35

rolling, 151
sweetener and egg yolks in, 14
and unrefined oils, 18
RECIPES FOR BASIC CAKES:
Applesauce Almond Cake, 145
Applesauce Spice Cake, 148–49
Banana Walnut Cake, 145
Basic Carrot Cake, 144
Carob Cake Roll, 150–51
Carob Sponge Cake, 147
Cheesecake with Blueberry Sauce, 152–53
Coffee Cake, 143
Dairy-Free Coffee Cake, 143
Gingerbread, 141
Holiday Cake, 153–54
Poppy Seed Cake, 149–50
The Ranch Kitchen Fruitcake, 154–56
Toasted Almond Torte, 142
Toasted Hazelnut Torte, 142
Vanilla Sponge Cake, 146–47
RECIPES FOR SPECIALTY CAKES:
Black Forest Torte, 169–70
Bûche de Noël (French Yule Log), 170, 171–72
Carob Apricot Cream Roll, 171
Carob Raspberry Cream Roll, 170–72
Carob Strawberry Cream Roll, 171
"Carobou" Cake, 145
Celebration Carrot Cake, 158–59
Gâteau Normandy, 160–61
German "Unchocolate" Cake, 167
July Fourth Cake, 166–67
Kiwi Lemon Cake, 159–60
Mocha Almond Torte, 168
Mocha Peach Praline Torte, 168
Peach Hazelnut Torte, 157–58
Peaches 'n' Cream Cake, 164–65
Raspberry Cream Cake, 164
Raspberry Custard Torte, 158
Raspberry Toasted Almond Torte, 158
Strawberry Cream Cake, 163–64
Strawberry Custard Cake, 161–62
Strawberry Shortcake, 156–57
Strawberry Toasted Almond Torte, 158
Cake pans, 22
and lecithin spray, 17
Calcium
in carob, 13
in fruit sweetener and white sugar, 7
and sugar in the bloodstream, 5
in tahini, 20
Calcium oxalate, 13
Calories
in fruit sweetener and white sugar, 7
and sugar, 5, 6
Cancer, 6
Canola oil, 18
Carbohydrates
in amazake, 12
in fruit sweetener and white sugar, 7
Cardboard cake rounds (circles), 24, 134–35
Carob, 13
carob cake, 146
RECIPES USING:
Black Forest Torte, 169–70
Bûche de Noël (French Yule Log), 170, 171–72
Carob Almond Cookies, 65
Carob-Almond Pinwheel Cookies, 72
Carob Apricot Cream Roll, 171
Carob Cake Roll, 150–51
Carob Chip Cookies, 74–75
Carob Cream Eclairs, 130
Carob Fudge Sauce, 192
Carob Glaze, 192
Carob Raspberry Cream Frosting, 183–84
Carob Raspberry Cream Roll, 170–72
Carob Sponge Cake, 147
Carob Strawberry Cream Roll, 171
Carob Strawberry Eclairs, 130
"Carobou" Cake, 145
Creamy Carob Frosting, 183
Crunchy Carob Almond Cookies, 65
German "Unchocolate" Cake, 167
Mocha Almond Frosting, 184
Mocha Almond Torte, 168
Mocha Frosting, 184
Mocha Mud Pie, 102–3
Carob Glaze, 192
RECIPES USING:
Carob Cream Eclairs, 130
Carob Strawberry Eclairs, 130
Fresh Banana Tart, 122–23
Carob Sponge Cake, 147
RECIPES USING:
Black Forest Torte, 169–70
German "Unchocolate" Cake, 167
Mocha Almond Torte, 168
Strawberry Custard Cake, 161–62
"Carobou" Cake, 145
Carrot bread, 39–40
Carrot cake, 144, 158–59
Cast iron skillet
and Tarte Tatin, 118–19
Center for Science in the Public Interest
on sugar, 5
Cheesecake
Baker's Tips for, 153
Cheesecake with Blueberry Sauce, 152–53
Cherry(ies)
in Black Forest Torte, 169–70
Fresh Cherry Pie, 90–91
Tart Red Cherry Sauce, 187
Chocolate
substitute for, 13
Cholesterol, 2
in baked goods, 18
Banana Nut Muffins low in, 59
Dairy-free Blueberry Muffins lower in, 54–55
Cholesterol-free recipes
Apple Custard Pie, 98
Boysenberry Custard Pie, 99
Cholesterol-Free Oatmeal Cookies, 66
Raisin Oat Bran Muffins, 57–58
Sesame Raisin Cookies, 66–67
see also Dairy-free recipes; Egg-free recipes
Chromium
and sugar in the bloodstream, 5
Cinnamon rolls, 37–38
Cinnamon swirl raisin bread, 42–43
Citrus fruits
zest of, 21
Cocoa powder
substitute for, 13

Coconut
RECIPES USING:
Coconut Cream Frosting, 182
Coconut-Pecan Filling, 179–80
Coconut Powder, 194
Coconut Powder, 194
to replace powdered sugar, 3
RECIPES USING:
Cream Puff Swans, 131
Peach Strudel, 126
Coffee Cake, 143
Coloring
cookies, 69
Cookie crumbs
and Linzertorte, 111
Cookie cutters, 23, 63
Cookie sheets, 22, 63
Cookies, 62–75
pointers for success, 62–63
RECIPES:
Almond Cookies, 68
Almond Macaroons, 75
Basic Shortbread Cookies, 69
Carob-Almond Pinwheel Cookies, 72
Carob Chip Cookies, 74–75
Cholesterol-Free Oatmeal Cookies, 66
Crunchy Almond Oatmeal Cookies, 65
Crunchy Carob Almond Cookies, 65
Gingerbread Girls and Boys, 73
Hazelnut Cookies, 68
Jan Hagels, 71
Maple Almond Cookies, 68
Maple Hazelnut Cookies, 68
Maple Pecan Cookies, 68
Maple Walnut Cookies, 67–68
Old-Fashioned Oatmeal Raisin Cookies, 64
Pecan Butter Cookies, 71
Raspberry Thumbprint Cookies, 70
Sesame Raisin Cookies, 66–67
Spice Cookies, 74
Wheat-less Shortbread Cookies, 69
Corn
in cornbread, 48
Cornbread, 48
Cornstarch, 13, 186
Couplers, 23, 138
Cranberry(ies), 52
and raspberries, 188
RECIPES USING:
Cranapple Walnut Muffins, 52
Cranberry Apple Pie, 87–88
Cranberry Banana Walnut Bread, 51
Cranberry Raspberry Topping, 188
Cranberry Topping, 187–88
Crimson Pie, 88–89
Cream cheese
in Cream Cheese Frosting with Raisins and Nuts, 185
in Creamy Carob Frosting, 183
in Whipped Cream/Cream Cheese Frosting, 182
Cream puff pastries, 128–31
RECIPES USING:
Carob Cream Eclairs, 130
Carob Strawberry Eclairs, 130
Cream Puff Swans, 131
Cream Puff Pastry, 129
Crimson Pie, 88–89
Crisp
Crisp Topping, 104
Peach 'n' Berry Crisp, 104
Croutons, 45
Crunchy Almond Oatmeal Cookies, 65
Crunchy Carob Almond Cookies, 65
Crust(s)
fluted, 78
fork-edged, 78
partially baking, 79–80
pie, 10, 76–84
prebaking, 80
rolling out, 77–78, 81
tart pan, 78
for tartlet pans, 78–79
for tartlets in muffin tins, 79, 80
RECIPES:
Basic Pie Crust, 82
Granola Crust, 83–84
Nutty-Oat Crust, 83
Cups
measuring, 22
Currants
in Apple Currant Sauce, 191
Custard
Baker's Tips for, 179
custard fillings, 79
Dairy Vanilla Custard, 179
Vanilla Custard, 178–79
RECIPES USING:
Apple Custard Parfait, 98
Apple Custard Pie, 98
Boysenberry Custard, 99
Boysenberry Custard Pie, 99
Molded Apple Custard, 98
see also Vanilla Custard
Cutting board, 22

Dairy-free recipes
American Beauty Apple Pie, 85–87
Apple Butter, 193
Apple Currant Sauce, 191
Apple Custard Parfait, 98
Apple Custard Pie, 98
Applesauce Almond Cake, 145
Applesauce Spice Cake, 148–49
Banana Nut Bread, 50
Banana Walnut Cake, 145
Basic Carrot Cake, 144
Basic Pie Crust, 82
Basic Shortbread Cookies, 69
Blueberry Lattice Pie, 89–90
Blueberry Sauce, 186
Boysenberry Custard, 99
Boysenberry Custard Pie, 99
Carob-Almond Pinwheel Cookies, 72
Carob Chip Cookies, 74–75
Carob Sponge Cake, 147
Cholesterol-Free Oatmeal Cookies, 66
Cranapple Walnut Muffins, 52
Cranberry Apple Pie, 87–88
Cranberry Banana Walnut Bread, 51
Cranberry Raspberry Topping, 188
Cranberry Topping, 187–88
Crimson Pie, 88–89
Crunchy Almond Oatmeal Cookies, 65
Crunchy Carob Almond Cookies, 65
Crusty French Bread, 33–34
Dairy-free Blueberry Muffins, 54–55
Dairy-Free Coffee Cake, 143
Date Nut Bread, 49–50
Egg Wash for Bread, 45
Fresh Cherry Pie, 90–91
Fresh Peach Ginger Pie, 94

Fresh Peach Pie, 91–92
Fresh Pear Ginger Pie, 93–94
Fresh Strawberry Sauce, 188–89
Frozen Peach Pie, 92–93
Frozen Strawberry Sauce, 189
Gâteau Normandy, 160–61
Gingerbread, 141
Gingerbread Girls and Boys, 73
Golden Carrot Bread, 39–40
Granola Crust, 83–84
Hazelnut Cookies, 68
Jan Hagels, 71
Kiwi Lemon Cake, 159–60
Lemon Curd, 177
Lemon Sauce, 189–90
Maple Pecan Pie, 97
Maple Walnut Cookies, 67–68
Mock Mincemeat, 96
Molded Apple Custard, 98
Nutty-Oat Crust, 83
Old-Fashioned Oatmeal Raisin Cookies, 64
Parfait Topping, 191
Peach 'n' Berry Crisp, 104
Peach Hazelnut Torte, 157–58
Peach Oat Bran Muffins, 56–57
Peach Roses, 112–13
Pecan Butter Cookies, 71
Pineapple Pecan Muffins, 53
Poppy Seed Cake, 149–50
Pumpkin Mincemeat Pie, 96–97
Pumpkin Pie, 95
Raisin Oat Bran Muffins, 57–58
Raspberry Custard Torte, 158
Raspberry Purée, 190
Raspberry Thumbprint Cookies, 70
Raspberry Toasted Almond Torte, 158
Red Glaze, 180
Red Raspberry Filling, 175
Red Raspberry Sauce, 175
Royal Icing, 185
Sesame Raisin Cookies, 66–67
Spice Cookies, 74
Spiced Peach Filling, 176
Spicy Pumpkin Muffins, 58
Squaw Bread, 43–44
Strawberry Cream Tartlets, 113–14
Strawberry Custard Cake, 161–62
Strawberry-Raspberry Sauce, 190
Strawberry Toasted Almond Torte, 158
Tart Red Cherry Sauce, 187
The Ranch Kitchen Whole Wheat Bread, 40–41
Toasted Almond Torte, 142
Toasted Hazelnut Torte, 142
Tofu Cream, 193
Vanilla Custard, 178–79
Vanilla Custard Parfaits, 179
Vanilla Sponge Cake, 146–47
Very Banana Nut Muffins, 59
Very-Berry Syrup, 191
Whole Wheat Cinnamon Swirl Raisin Bread, 42–43
Yellow Glaze, 181
Zucchini Bread, 48–49
Dairy-free symbol
explained, vi
Dairy Vanilla Custard, 179
Date Nut Bread, 49–50
Decorating equipment, 23
Dessert
guidelines, 173–74
Diabetes, 5, 6
Diet
and sugar intake, 7
and sweets, 5
Dietary Guidelines
Department of Agriculture's, 5
Double pan
for baking cookies, 63
Dough
absorbs flour easily, 15
pie, 77–81, 82
see also Bread dough
Dough hook, 28
Dough scraper, 23, 27, 29

Eclairs
Carob Cream Eclairs, 130
Carob Strawberry Eclairs, 130
Egg bread, 34–35
Egg-free recipes
Almond Macaroons, 75
Almond Straws, 127–28
American Beauty Apple Pie, 85–87
Angel Biscuits, 61
Apple Butter, 193
Apple Currant Sauce, 191
Apple Custard Parfait, 98
Apple Custard Pie, 98
Apple Strudel, 126
Apple Turnovers, 123
Apricot Cream Filling and Frosting, 177
Basic Pie Crust, 82
Basic Shortbread Cookies, 69
Blueberry Lattice Pie, 89–90
Blueberry Sauce, 186
Boysenberry Custard, 99
Boysenberry Custard Pie, 99
Carob Fudge Sauce, 192
Carob Glaze, 192
Carob Raspberry Cream Frosting, 183–84
Cholesterol-Free Oatmeal Cookies, 66
Coconut Cream Frosting, 182
Coconut Powder, 194
Cranberry Apple Pie, 87–88
Cranberry Raspberry Topping, 188
Cranberry Topping, 187–88
Cream Cheese Frosting with Raisins and Nuts, 185
Creamy Carob Frosting, 183
Crimson Pie, 88–89
Crunchy Almond Oatmeal Cookies, 65
Crunchy Carob Almond Cookies, 65
Crustless French Pear or Apple Tarts, 110
Crusty French Bread, 33–34
French Apple Tart, 110
French Pear Tart, 109–10
Fresh Apricot Tart, 106–7
Fresh Cherry Pie, 90–91
Fresh Peach Pie, 91–92
Fresh Peach Tart, 107
Fresh Plum Tart, 105–6
Fresh Strawberry Sauce, 188–89
Frozen Peach Pie, 92–93
Frozen Strawberry Sauce, 189
Golden Carrot Bread, 39–40
Granola Crust, 83–84
Hazelnut Cookies, 68
Lemon Sauce, 189–90
Mocha Almond Frosting, 184
Mocha Frosting, 184
Mock Mincemeat, 96
Molded Apple Custard, 98
Nutty-Oat Crust, 83
Parfait Topping, 191
Peach 'n' Berry Crisp, 104
Peach Hazelnut Torte, 157–58

Peach Strudel, 126
Peaches 'n' Cream Filling and Frosting, 177
Pecan Butter Cookies, 71
Pecan Praline, 194
Raisin Oat Bran Muffins, 57–58
Raspberry Cream Filling and Frosting, 176–77
Raspberry Purée, 190
Raspberry Toasted Almond Torte, 158
Red Glaze, 180
Red Raspberry Filling, 175
Red Raspberry Sauce, 175
Royal Icing, 185
Sesame Raisin Cookies, 66–67
Southern-Style Buttermilk Biscuits, 60
Spiced Peach Filling, 176
Spicy Pumpkin Muffins, 58
Squaw Bread, 43–44
Strawberry Cream Filling and Frosting, 177
Strawberry-Raspberry Sauce, 190
Strawberry Shortcake, 156–57
Strawberry Toasted Almond Torte, 158
Tart Red Cherry Sauce, 187
Tarte Tatin, 118–19
Toasted Almond Torte, 142
Toasted Hazelnut Torte, 142
Tofu Cream, 193
Very Banana Nut Muffins, 59
Very-Berry Syrup, 191
Whipped Cream, 181
Whipped Cream/Cream Cheese Frosting, 182
Yellow Glaze, 181
Egg-free symbol
explained, vi
Egg wash
for bread, 31, 35, 45
on double-crusted pie, 79
for pies and tarts, 84
Egg whites
folding into cake batter, 134
whipping, 14
Egg yolks
in cakes, 14
Eggs
and cream puff pastry, 128
in quick breads, 46
separating, 14
to thicken sauces and custards, 180
Equipment
recommended, 21–24

Fats
in fruit sweetener and white sugar, 7
Filberts, 68
Fillings
Apricot Cream Filling and Frosting, 177
Coconut-Pecan Filling, 179–80
Lemon Curd, 177
Peaches 'n' Cream Filling and Frosting, 177
Raspberry Cream Filling and Frosting, 176–77
Red Raspberry Filling, 175
Spiced Peach Filling, 176
Strawberry Cream Filling and Frosting, 177
Whipped Cream, 181
Flour, 14–15
in a bread recipe, 26
brown rice, 15
and cream puff pastry, 128
and kneading dough, 27, 28, 29
measuring, 15
oat, 15
and rolling out a rope of dough, 30
unbleached white, 14
white cake, 15
whole wheat bread, 15
whole wheat pastry, 15
on the work surface, 15
and yeasted dough, 28
Folding
for making cakes, 133–34
Food and Drug Administration, 7
Food processor, 23
French Apple Tart, 110
French bread, 33–34
French Pear Tart, 109–10
Fresh Apricot Tart, 106–7
Fresh Banana Tart, 122–23
Fresh Cherry Pie, 90–91
Fresh Peach Ginger Pie, 94
Fresh Peach Pie, 91–92
Fresh Peach Tart, 107
Fresh Pear Ginger Pie, 93–94
Fresh Plum Tart, 105–6
Fresh Strawberry Sauce, 188–89
Fresh Strawberry Tart, 108
Frosting
cakes, 135–37
RECIPES:
Apricot Cream Filling and Frosting, 177
Carob Raspberry Cream Frosting, 183–84
Coconut Cream Frosting, 182
Cream Cheese Frosting with Raisins and Nuts, 185
Creamy Carob Frosting, 183
Mocha Almond Frosting, 184
Mocha Frosting, 184
Peaches 'n' Cream Filling and Frosting, 177
Raspberry Cream Filling and Frosting, 176–77
Royal Icing, 185
Strawberry Cream Filling and Frosting, 177
Whipped Cream, 181
Whipped Cream/Cream Cheese Frosting, 182
Frozen Peach Pie, 92–93
Frozen Strawberry Sauce, 189
Fructose, 6
Fruit(s)
and arrowroot, 13
between cake layers, 135–36, 165
decorating cakes with, 137–38
dried, 14
frozen, 15
Mixed Fruit Tarts, 119–20
in Peach 'n' Berry Crisp, 104
Fruit juice
concentrates, 3, 4–5, 6
frozen, 3
Fruit sweetener(s), 16
in combination with baking soda, 13
comparison of nutrients in sugar and, 6, 7
composed of monosaccharides, 6
replace molasses with, 18
where to purchase, 16
Fruitcake, 153–56
Fudge sauce
carob, 192

Garnishes, 174–75
RECIPES:
Coconut Powder, 194

Pecan Praline, 194
Tofu Cream, 193
Gâteau Normandy, 160–61
Gelatin
dissolving, 100–101
German "Unchocolate" Cake, 167
Ginger
in Fresh Peach Ginger Pie, 94
in Fresh Pear Ginger Pie, 93–94
Gingerbread, 141
Gingerbread cookies, 73
Gingerbread Girls and Boys, 73
Glaze(s), 174
as a "crumb coat" on cakes, 136, 174
RECIPES:
Carob Glaze, 192
Red Glaze, 180
Yellow Glaze, 181
Glucose
in amazake, 12
in the blood, 5–6
Gluten, 15
in pie dough, 78
and shaping of bread dough, 29, 30
Graham cracker crust
alternative to, 83–84
Granola
and Linzertorte, 111
Granola Crust, 83–84
in Cheesecake with Blueberry Sauce, 152–53

Hazelnut(s), 68
RECIPES USING:
Hazelnut Cookies, 68
Maple Hazelnut Cookies, 68
Peach Hazelnut Torte, 157–58
Toasted Hazelnut Torte, 142
Heart disease, 5, 6
Hokaido pumpkin, 95
Holiday Cake, 153–54
Hyperactivity, 5
Hypoglycemia, 4, 5

Ice cream scoop(s), 23
for cookies, 62
to form muffins, 46
Ingredients
measuring, 24
at room temperature for cookies, 62
and temperature, 10
Irish Soda Bread, 47
Irish Soda Bread Muffins, 55–56
Iron
in amazake, 12
in fruit sweetener and white sugar, 7
in tahini, 20

Jams
fruit-sweetened, 16
Jan Hagels, 71
Jelly roll pan, 22
July Fourth Cake, 166–67
Junk food eaters, 6

Kabocha squash, 95
Kitchen scale, 24
Kiwi fruits, 17
in custard cake, 162
in Kiwi Lemon Cake, 159–60
in mixed fruit tarts, 120
Kneading
bread dough, 26–28
Knife
for slicing bread, 32
Knives, 22, 23
Koji, 12
Kudzu, 17
Kuzu, 17

Lacing
explained, 156
Lattice-crusted pie, 79
Lattice strips
on Blueberry Lattice Pie, 89–90
defrosted, 81
refrigerated, 78
Leaves
for American Beauty Apple Pie, 85–86
Lecithin
in tahini, 20
Lecithin spray, 17, 29, 30
on muffin pans, 46
Lemon(s)
to keep pears from browning, 19
on peeled, sliced or cut apples, 12
and whipping egg whites, 14
RECIPES USING:
Blueberry Lemon Tartlets, 112
Kiwi Lemon Cake, 159–60
Lemon Cream Pie, 101–2
Lemon Curd, 177
Lemon Sauce, 189–90
Lemon Curd, 10, 177
RECIPES USING:
Blueberry Lemon Tartlets, 112
Kiwi Lemon Cake, 159–60
Lemon Cream Pie, 101–2
Linzertorte, 110–11
Loaves
baking, 32
of carrot bread, 39–40
of cinnamon swirl raisin bread, 43
of egg bread, 35
egg wash to glaze, 31, 45
forming, 29–30
of French bread, 33–34
slash the tops of, 31
of squaw bread, 44
of whole wheat bread, 41
yield given in recipes, 25
Love, 9–10

Macaroons
almond, 75
Macerate
explained, 157
Magnesium
and sugar in the bloodstream, 5
Maltose
in amazake, 12
Mango, 120
Maple Almond Cookies, 68
Maple Hazelnut Cookies, 68
Maple Pecan Cookies, 68
Maple Pecan Pie, 97
Maple Walnut Cookies, 67–68
Maranatha Foods, 20
Marble surface, 24
Margarine, 17
Measuring cups, 22, 133
Measuring spoons, 22
Milk
alternative to, 12, 20
nonfat, non-instant powder, 194
scalding, 36
Mincemeat
Pumpkin Mincemeat Pie, 96–97
Minerals
in fruit sweeteners, 6

to metabolize sugar, 5
needed for metabolism of calories, 6
in sea salt, 20
Mixed Fruit Tarts, 119–20
Mixer
heavy-duty, 23
and kneading dough, 28
for making sponge cakes, 146–47
Mixing bowls, 22
Mocha Almond Frosting, 184
Mocha Almond Torte, 168
Mocha Frosting, 184
Mocha Mud Pie, 102–3
Mocha Peach Praline Torte, 168
Mock Mincemeat, 96–97
Molasses, 18
Molded Apple Custard, 98
Montana
The Ranch Kitchen in, 1–2
wheat from, 14
Muffin tins
crusts for tartlets in, 79, 80
tartlets made in, 77, 79
Muffins, 46
RECIPES:
Blueberry Muffins, 54–55
Cranapple Walnut Muffins, 52
Dairy-free Blueberry Muffins, 54–55
Irish Soda Bread Muffins, 55–56
Peach Oat Bran Muffins, 56–57
Pineapple Pecan Muffins, 53
Raisin Oat Bran Muffins, 57–58
Spicy Pumpkin Muffins, 58
Very Banana Nut Muffins, 59
Mystic Lake Dairy, 16

Nectarines, 18–19
in custard cake, 162
Niacin
in fruit sweetener and white sugar, 7
Nut Crumb Filling, 105, 106–7
in Fresh Apricot Tart, 106–7
in Fresh Peach Tart, 107
in Fresh Plum Tart, 105–6
Nut Strudel, 124–25
Nutritional deficiencies
and sugar, 5, 6
Nuts
decorating with, 137
toasting, 18
Nutty-Oat Crust, 83
in Apple Custard Pie, 98
in Boysenberry Custard Pie, 99

Oat bran
in Peach Oat Bran Muffins, 56–57
in Raisin Oat Bran Muffins, 57–58
Oat flour, 15
Oatmeal cookies, 66
Oatmeal raisin cookies, 64
Oats, rolled, 18
RECIPES USING:
Blueberry Muffins, 54–55
Cholesterol-Free Oatmeal Cookies, 66
Crunchy Almond Oatmeal Cookies, 65
Crunchy Carob Almond Cookies, 65
Dairy-free Blueberry Muffins, 54–55
Nutty-Oat Crust, 83
Old-Fashioned Oatmeal Raisin Cookies, 64
Peach Oat Bran Muffins, 56–57
Sesame Raisin Cookies, 66–67
Obesity, 5, 6
Oil, 18
Orange juice
concentrate, 16
Organization
in baking, 10, 11
Oven
and baking bread, 32
and baking pies, 76, 80
knowing your, 10
opening the door of, 11
preheating, 11, 31
for puff pastry, 115
raising dough in, 28, 30
steaming the, 34

Pam, 17
Pan(s)
baking, 22–23
to cut a circle of dough, 77
double, 63
for Tarte Tatin, 118–19
Pancreas
and blood glucose level, 6
and fructose, 6
Papaya, 120
Parfait(s)
Apple Custard Parfait, 98
Vanilla Custard Parfaits, 179
Pastries
and flour, 14–15
Pastry bag(s), 23
and cream puff pastry, 129
decorating with, 138–40
Pastry brush, 23
Pastry wheel, 24
Peach(es), 18–19
in custard cake, 162
extract, 19
fruit concentrate from, 16
peeling, 18–19
RECIPES USING:
Fresh Peach Ginger Pie, 94
Fresh Peach Pie, 91–92
Fresh Peach Tart, 107
Frozen Peach Pie, 92–93
Mocha Peach Praline Torte, 168
Peach 'n' Berry Crisp, 104
Peach Hazelnut Torte, 157–58
Peach Oat Bran Muffins, 56–57
Peach-Raspberry Rectangle, 121–22
Peach Roses, 112–13
Peach Strudel, 126
Peaches 'n' Cream Cake, 164–65
Peaches 'n' Cream Filling and Frosting, 177
Spiced Peach Filling, 176
Pear(s), 19
Baker's Tips about, 94
fruit concentrate from, 16
RECIPES USING:
Crustless French Pear Tart, 110
French Pear Tart, 109–10
Fresh Pear Ginger Pie, 93–94
Pecan(s)
RECIPES USING:
Coconut-Pecan Filling, 179–80
Maple Pecan Cookies, 68
Maple Pecan Pie, 97
Pecan Butter Cookies, 71
Pecan Praline, 194
Pineapple Pecan Muffins, 53
Spicy Pumpkin Muffins, 58
Phosphorous
in fruit sweetener and white sugar, 7
in tahini, 20
Pie(s), 85–103
baking, 80, 90
on baking sheets, 80

bubbling to within 3 inches of the center test, 90
double-crusted, 79
egg wash for, 84
lattice-crust, 79
partially baking single-crusted, 79–80
RECIPES:
American Beauty Apple Pie, 85–87
Apple Custard Pie, 98
Banana Cream Pie, 100
Blueberry Lattice Pie, 89–90
Boysenberry Custard Pie, 99
Cranberry Apple Pie, 87–88
Crimson Pie, 88–89
Fresh Cherry Pie, 90–91
Fresh Peach Ginger Pie, 94
Fresh Peach Pie, 91–92
Fresh Pear Ginger Pie, 93–94
Frozen Peach Pie, 92–93
Lemon Cream Pie, 101–2
Maple Pecan Pie, 97
Mocha Mud Pie, 102–3
Pumpkin Mincemeat Pie, 96–97
Pumpkin Pie, 95
Pie crust(s), 10, 76–84
Pie pan(s), 22, 77, 78, 79
Pie weights, 79–80, 81
Pineapple(s)
fruit concentrate from, 16
Pineapple Pecan Muffins, 53
Plum
Fresh Plum Tart, 105–6
Poppy seed(s), 31
Poppy Seed Cake, 149–50
Potassium
in fruit sweetener and white sugar, 7
and sugar in the bloodstream, 5
Praline
Mocha Peach Praline Torte, 168
Pecan Praline, 194
Protein
in fruit sweetener and white sugar, 7
in fruit sweeteners, 6
spelt as a complete, 65
in tahini, 20
Puff pastry, 115
purchased, 76
tart shells from, 115–17
RECIPES:
Almond Blossoms, 127
Almond Straws, 127–28
Apple Nut Strudel, 125
Apple Strudel, 126
Apple Turnovers, 123
Fresh Banana Tart, 122–23
Mixed Fruit Tarts, 119–20
Nut Strudel, 124–25
Peach-Raspberry Rectangle, 121–22
Peach Strudel, 126
Raspberry Treasure Chests, 120–21
Tarte Tatin, 118–19
Puff pastry tart shells
baking, 116, 117
rectangular, 115–16
round, 116–17
small, 117
Pumpkin
substituting for canned, 95
RECIPES USING:
Pumpkin Mincemeat Pie, 96–97
Pumpkin Pie, 95
Spicy Pumpkin Muffins, 58

Quick breads, 46–51
RECIPES:
Banana Nut Bread, 50
Cornbread, 48
Cranberry Banana Walnut Bread, 51
Date Nut Bread, 49–50
Irish Soda Bread, 47
Zucchini Bread, 48–49

Raisin(s)
in granola, 84
plumped, 19
RECIPES USING:
Cream Cheese Frosting with Raisins and Nuts, 185
Holiday Cake, 153–54
Old-Fashioned Oatmeal Raisin Cookies, 64
Our Famous Cinnamon Rolls, 37–38
Raisin Oat Bran Muffins, 57–58
The Ranch Kitchen Fruitcake, 154–56
Sesame Raisin Cookies, 66–67
Spicy Pumpkin Muffins, 58
Whole Wheat Cinnamon Swirl Raisin Bread, 42–43
Raisin water, 19
Ranch Kitchen, The Restaurant and Bakery, 1–2
Rancidity
and brown rice flour, 15
and oat flour, 15
and tahini, 20
and unrefined oils, 18
and unsalted butter, 13
Raspberry(ies)
cleaning, 19–20
in custard cake, 162
enhance the flavor of cranberries, 188
frozen, 15
in mixed fruit tarts, 120
RECIPES USING:
Bûche de Noël (French Yule Log), 170, 171–72
Carob Raspberry Cream Frosting, 183–84
Carob Raspberry Cream Roll, 170–72
Cranberry Raspberry Topping, 188
Cream Puff Swans, 131
Peach-Raspberry Rectangle, 121–22
Raspberry Cream Cake, 164
Raspberry Cream Filling and Frosting, 176–77
Raspberry Cream Tartlets, 114
Raspberry Custard Torte, 158
Raspberry Purée, 190
Raspberry Thumbprint Cookies, 70
Raspberry Toasted Almond Torte, 158
Raspberry Treasure Chests, 120–21
Red Raspberry Filling, 175
Red Raspberry Sauce, 175
Strawberry-Raspberry Sauce, 190
Recipes
how to get the most out of, 11
Red Glaze, 120, 180
Red Raspberry Filling, 175
Red Raspberry Sauce, 175
Refrigerator
bread dough in, 26, 32
Riboflavin
in fruit sweetener and white sugar, 7
Rice
rice milk, 12
see also Brown rice
Rolled oats
see Oats, rolled

Rolling pin, 23, 77, 81
Rolls
  baking, 32
  of carrot bread, 39–40
  of egg bread, 35
  egg wash to glaze, 31, 45
  forming, 30–31
  Monarch, 36
  Our Famous Cinnamon Rolls, 37–38
  of whole wheat bread, 41
  yield given in recipes, 25
Rosebuds
  for American Beauty Apple Pie, 85–86
Rosette design
  for cake decorating, 139–40
Royal Icing, 185

Saint John's Bread, 13
Salt
  sea, 20
  table, 20
  and whipping egg whites, 14
  and yeasted dough, 28
Sauce(s)
  servings per cup, 174
  RECIPES:
  Apple Currant Sauce, 191
  Blueberry Sauce, 186
  Carob Fudge Sauce, 192
  Carob Glaze, 192
  Cranberry Raspberry Topping, 188
  Cranberry Topping, 187–88
  Fresh Strawberry Sauce, 188–89
  Frozen Strawberry Sauce, 189
  Lemon Sauce, 189–90
  Parfait Topping, 191
  Raspberry Purée, 190
  Red Raspberry Sauce, 175
  Strawberry-Raspberry Sauce, 190
  Tart Red Cherry Sauce, 187
  Very-Berry Syrup, 191
Saucepan(s), 22
  lid to cut a circle of dough, 77
Sea salt, 20
Sesame Raisin Cookies, 66–67
Sesame seeds, 31
  in Sesame Raisin Cookies, 66–67
  tahini from, 20
Shell design(s)
  for cake decorating, 139, 140
Shortbread cookies, 69
Sifter
  drum, 23
Soda bread
  Irish Soda Bread, 47
  Irish Soda Bread Muffins, 55–56
Sodium
  in fruit sweetener and white sugar, 7
  and sugar in the bloodstream, 5
Southern-Style Buttermilk Biscuits, 60
Soy milk, 20
Spelt, 65
Spice
  Applesauce Spice Cake, 148–49
Spice Cookies, 74
"Sponge"
  explained, 100–101
Sponge cake(s)
  freezing, 147
  Vanilla Sponge Cake, 146–47
Spoons
  measuring, 22
Squaw Bread, 43–44
Stems
  for American Beauty Apple Pie, 85–86
Strainer, 22
Strawberry(ies)
  frozen, 15
  in mixed fruit tarts, 120
  removing the hulls, 20
  washing, 20
  RECIPES USING:
  Carob Strawberry Cream Roll, 171
  Carob Strawberry Eclairs, 130
  Fresh Strawberry Sauce, 188–89
  Fresh Strawberry Tart, 108
  Frozen Strawberry Sauce, 189
  July Fourth Cake, 166–67
  Peach 'n' Berry Crisp, 104
  Red Raspberry Filling, 175
  Strawberry Cream Cake, 163–64
  Strawberry Cream Filling and Frosting, 177
  Strawberry Cream Tartlets, 113–14
  Strawberry Custard Cake, 161–62
  Strawberry-Raspberry Sauce, 190
  Strawberry Shortcake, 156–57
  Strawberry Toasted Almond Torte, 158
  Very-Berry Syrup, 191
Stress, 6
Streusel Topping
  in Fresh Peach Ginger Pie, 94
  in Fresh Pear Ginger Pie, 94
Strudel
  Apple Nut Strudel, 125
  Apple Strudel, 126
  Nut Strudel, 124–25
  Peach Strudel, 126
Sucrose, 5, 18
Sugar, 5–8
  alternative to, 4–5
  in amazake, 12
  comparison of nutrients in fruit sweetener and, 6, 7
  consumption by Americans, 6
  effects of, 3, 4, 5, 7
  replacements for, 3
  replacing with fruit sweetener in a recipe, 3, 16
Sugar Association, 6
Sulfur dioxide, 18
  fruit dried with, 14
Swans
  Cream Puff Swans, 131
Sweet and Dangerous, 7
Sweetener(s)
  fruit, 3, 16
  fruit juice concentrates as, 3
  and whipping egg whites, 14
Syrup
  Very-Berry Syrup, 191

Tahini, 20–21
Tart(s), 105–11, 118–23
  Baker's Tip for, 106
  egg wash for, 84
  glazes brushed on the bottom of, 174
  partially baking, 79–80
  RECIPES:
  Crustless French Pear or Apple Tarts, 110
  French Apple Tart, 110
  French Pear Tart, 109–10
  Fresh Apricot Tart, 106–7
  Fresh Banana Tart, 122–23
  Fresh Peach Tart, 107
  Fresh Plum Tart, 105–6
  Fresh Strawberry Tart, 108
  Mixed Fruit Tarts, 119–20
  Linzertorte, 110–11
  Peach-Raspberry Rectangle, 121–22